Diagnosis and Management Guide for Anorectal Disease

A Clinical Reference

Diagnosis and Management Guide for Anorectal Disease

A Clinical Reference

Waqar Qureshi, MD, FRCP, FACP, FACG, FASGE

Professor of Medicine, Baylor College of Medicine
Faculty Physician, Baylor St. Luke's Medical Center
Staff Physician, VA Medical Center
Faculty, Texas Children's Hospital Pavilion for Women
Houston, Texas

CRC Press
Taylor & Francis Group
Boca Raton London New York

CRC Press is an imprint of the
Taylor & Francis Group, an **informa** business

First published 2020 by SLACK Incorporated

Published 2024 by CRC Press
2385 NW Executive Center Drive, Suite 320, Boca Raton FL 33431

and by CRC Press
4 Park Square, Milton Park, Abingdon, Oxon, OX14 4RN

CRC Press is an imprint of Taylor & Francis Group, LLC

Cover Artist: Lori Shields

Library of Congress Cataloging-in-Publication Data

Names: Qureshi, Waqar (Waqar Ahmed), 1957- editor.
Title: Diagnosis and management guide for anorectal disease : a clinical reference / [edited by] Waqar Qureshi.
Description: Thorofare, NJ : SLACK Incorporated, [2020] | Includes bibliographical references and index.
Identifiers: LCCN 2019028121 (print) | ISBN 9781630914929 (paperback) |
Subjects: MESH: Rectal Diseases--diagnosis | Rectal Diseases--therapy
Classification: LCC RC864 (print) | NLM WI 603 | DDC 616.3/5--dc23
LC record available at https://lccn.loc.gov/2019028121

ISBN: 9781630914929 (pbk)
ISBN: 9781003523826 (ebk)

DOI: 10.1201/9781003523826

Dedication

To my Mother for her unconditional love and support and my Father for instilling the importance of education and focus.

To my wife, Linda, and sons, Liam, Shan, and Dean, who let me sit at the computer for endless hours.

Contents

Acknowledgments

This book would not have been possible without the contributing authors who took time off their busy schedules to write for us. I selected them because they are outstanding in their fields, and I cannot thank them enough for their time and effort. Dr. Marcus Aquino provided excellent images that have added immensely to the quality of this publication.

About the Editor

Waqar Qureshi, MD, FRCP, FACP, FACG, FASGE spent his early years in the United Kingdom, where he earned his medical degree at the Royal Free Hospital School of Medicine, University of London. Following residency training in Rochester, NY and fellowship training in Gastroenterology at the University of Arkansas for Medical Sciences in Little Rock, he was recruited to Baylor College of Medicine, Houston, TX, in 1997 to be Chief of Endoscopy. He is now Professor in the Section of Gastroenterology and Hepatology at Baylor. He recognized that, despite the widespread popularity of gastroenterology, few programs provided comprehensive training in anorectal disorders. Dr. Qureshi started an anorectal clinic, which is now included as an essential rotation by the fellows in training so as to learn the details regarding managing anorectal disease in the outpatient setting. The national gastroenterology societies have since recognized this deficiency in training and have begun to offer workshops on anorectal disease, some of which Dr. Qureshi has directed. In addition, he obtained a grant from the American Society of Gastrointestinal Endoscopy to produce a DVD on anorectal examination (https://learn.asge.org/Public/Catalog/Home.aspx).

This book covers most aspects of nonsurgical anorectal disease management as well as topics that need surgical intervention but provide the underlying disease processes for the nonsurgeon. Dr Qureshi hopes that this book, being the first of its kind, will assist fellows in training and for practicing gastroenterologists to provide state-of-the-art comprehensive care for their patients.

Contributing Authors

Ihsan Al-Bayati, MD (Chapter 5)
Department of Internal Medicine
Texas Tech University Health Sciences Center
Paul L. Foster School of Medicine
El Paso, Texas

Sarah Al-Obaidi, MD (Chapter 5)
Department of Internal Medicine
Texas Tech University Health Sciences Center
Paul L. Foster School of Medicine
El Paso, Texas

Avo Artinyan, MD, MS (Chapter 12)
Director Surgical Oncology, Colorectal Surgery
Verity Medical Foundation
Los Angeles, California

Noemi Baffy, MD (Chapter 1)
Tufts University School of Medicine
Maine Medical Center
Portland, Maine

J. Michael Berry-Lawhorn, MD (Chapter 17)
Clinical Professor of Medicine
Division of Hematology Oncology
Associate Director, HPV-Related Clinical Studies
Anal Neoplasia Clinic, Research, and Education Center
University of California San Francisco
San Francisco, California

Lisa S. Brubaker, MD (Chapter 4)
Micheal E. DeBakey Department of Surgery
Baylor College of Medicine
Houston, Texas

Bidhan Das, MD, FACS (Chapter 8)
Assistant Professor
University of Texas—Houston
McGovern Medical School
Colon and Rectal Clinic of Houston
Houston, Texas

Samer Doughan, MD, FRCSEd (Gen Surg) (Chapter 15)
American University of Beirut Medical Center
Beirut, Lebanon

Gulchin A. Ergun, MD, AGAF, FACG (Chapter 9)
Professor of Clinical Medicine, Weill Medical College
David M. Underwood Distinguished Professor of Medicine in Digestive Disorders
Medical Director, Digestive Disease Endoscopy & Reflux Center
Houston Methodist Gastroenterology Associates
Lynda K. and David M. Underwood Center for Digestive Disorders
Houston, Texas

Yezaz A. Ghouri, MD (Chapter 7)
Department of Internal Medicine
Division of Gastroenterology and Hepatology
University of Missouri School of Medicine
Columbia, Missouri

Vineet S. Gudsoorkar, MD (Chapter 9)
Lynda K. and David M. Underwood Center for Digestive Disorders
Houston Methodist Hospital and Weill Cornell Medical College
Houston, Texas

Mitchel Guttenplan, MD, FACS (Chapter 3)
Medical Director
CRH Medical
Bellevue, Washington

Lisa M. Haubert, MD, MS, FASCRS (Chapter 4)
Division of General Surgery
Baylor College of Medicine
Houston, Texas

Stephen Landreneau, MD (Chapter 16)
Section of Gastroenterology
Department of Medicine
Louisiana State University School of Medicine
New Orleans, Louisiana

Richard McCallum, MD, FACP, FRACP (AUST), FACG, AGAF (Chapter 5)
Department of Internal Medicine
Texas Tech University Health Sciences Center
Paul L. Foster School of Medicine
El Paso, Texas

Tejal Mistry, MD (Chapter 14)
Internal Medicine Department
University of Texas Health Science Center at Houston
Houston, Texas

Van Morris, MD (Chapter 14)
Department of Gastrointestinal Medical Oncology
University of Texas
MD Anderson Cancer Center
Houston, Texas

Rishi D. Naik, MD, MSCI (Chapter 13)
Assistant Professor of Medicine
Division of Gastroenterology, Hepatology, and Nutrition
Vanderbilt University Medical Center
Nashville, Tennessee

Leila Neshatian, MD, MSc (Chapter 6)
Clinical Assistant Professor
GI Director, Pelvic Health Center
Department of Gastroenterology and Hepatology
Stanford University
Redwood City, California

Keith L. Obstein, MD, MPH, FASGE, FACG, AGAF (Chapter 13)
Associate Professor of Medicine
Division of Gastroenterology, Hepatology, and Nutrition
Vanderbilt University Medical Center
Nashville, Tennessee

Roman Sargsyan, MD, PhD (Chapter 12)
Faculty Colorectal Surgeon
Department of Surgery
Central Clinical Military Hospital
Yerevan, Armenia

Mehnaz A. Shafi, MD (Chapter 10)
Professor of Medicine
Deputy Department Chair
Director, GI Motility
Department of Gastroenterology, Hepatology and Nutrition
University of Texas MD Anderson Cancer Center
Houston, Texas

Yasser Shaib, MD, MPH, FASGE (Chapter 15)
Associate Professor of Medicine
American University of Beirut Medical Center
Beirut, Lebanon

Bo Shen, MD (Chapter 7)
Professor of Medicine
Ed and Joey Story Endowed Chair
Department of Gastroenterology/Hepatology
Cleveland Clinic
Cleveland, Ohio

Andy Tau, MD (Chapter 11)
Austin Gastroenterology
Austin, Texas

Sarah B. Umar, MD (Chapter 1)
Mayo Clinic
Phoenix, Arizona

Sai Sruthi Veerisetty, MD (Chapter 16)
Section of Gastroenterology
Department of Medicine
Louisiana State University School of Medicine
New Orleans, Louisiana

Zachary Yeung, MD (Chapter 14)
Hematology and Oncology
Department of Medicine
Baylor College of Medicine
Houston, Texas

Preface

As practicing gastroenterologists, we frequently are presented with patients complaining of one or more of a number of anorectal symptoms. For whatever reason, the evaluation and treatment of these common ailments is not included within the core curriculum of most gastrointestinal (GI) fellowship training programs, and so has not, until fairly recently, been incorporated into a typical GI practice. In addition, I was unable to find a text that reviewed the care of these issues in a manner directed to nonsurgeons (particularly gastroenterologists), which was the impetus behind the development of this text.

In the patient's mind, any symptoms experienced in the perianal or anorectal region are due to "hemorrhoids." Symptomatic hemorrhoids are an incredibly common ailment, but as the chapters that follow will make clear, there are many other processes that must also be taken into consideration.

The vast majority of these perianal and anorectal problems can be successfully treated nonsurgically; the following chapters review a number of diseases that gastroenterologists should be able to effectively manage in their office. Common problems such as symptomatic hemorrhoids, anal fissures, and anorectal dyssynergia are among the many diagnoses that should be managed within the realm of the gastroenterologist. Currently, all too often, these patients are referred to our surgical colleagues when surgery is not necessary, adding to the cost, inconvenience, and frustration of our patients.

A thorough history and physical examination with a properly performed digital rectal examination and anoscopy will provide the correct diagnosis in the majority of patients. However, a role for anorectal manometry, pelvic magnetic resonance imaging, and behavior therapy is increasingly recognized.

Hemorrhoidal problems have been recorded as a plague of mankind since biblical times. Sclerotherapy, one of the oldest forms of nonoperative treatment, was first described in 1869 by Morgan in Dublin, Ireland. Gastroenterologists are now able to offer office-based, effective treatment of symptomatic hemorrhoids in most cases, and this often obviates the need for a surgical hemorrhoidectomy. Office-based hemorrhoid treatment is both quick and generally painless. Acutely thrombosed hemorrhoids can be drained in the office quickly. Anal fissures are easy to diagnose and to effectively treat with topical vasodilators. There are a number of functional disorders of the GI tract and the pelvic floor that present with anorectal symptoms, and these are discussed as well. While the majority of these issues can be treated nonsurgically, an understanding of the circumstances that call for a surgical consultation is key, along with a good working relationship with your surgical colleagues for those patients in whom conservative management is not sufficient. I have also included a chapter on the care of patients at an increased risk of anal cancer (eg, those with human papillomavirus infection), including an understanding of the need for screening these patients. This area presents a liability risk for gastroenterologists who may not think of sending high-risk patients for high-resolution anoscopy or anal Papanicolau (Pap) smears.

The gastroenterologist occupies a unique position between conservative treatment offered by primary care physicians and the more invasive procedures offered by the surgeon. This book, probably the first of many, is designed to provide gastroenterologists with a comprehensive understanding of anorectal diseases that they can manage and, therefore, improve the care of their patients.

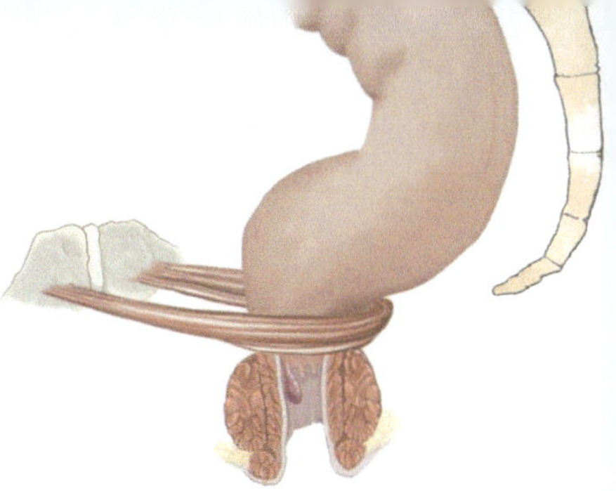

Section 1

Anatomy and Examination

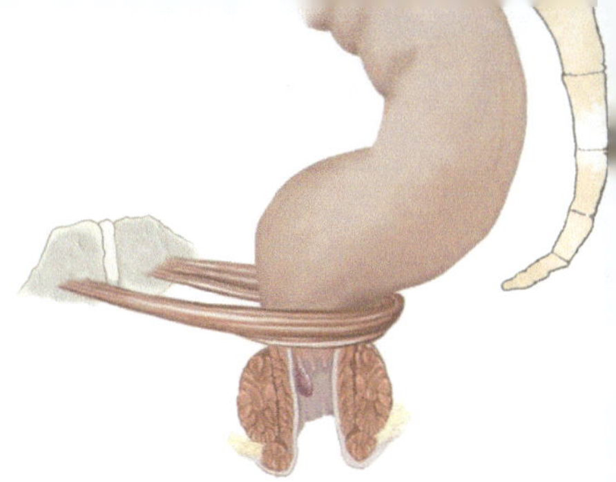

1

Anatomy and Physiology of the Pelvic Floor

Noemi Baffy, MD and Sarah B. Umar, MD

Key Points

- The 4 phases of defecation include the basal phase, preparatory phase, expulsive phase, and termination phase.
- The sigmoid colon and rectum are the intraperitoneal and extraperitoneal gastrointestinal (GI) structures, respectively, occupying the pelvis.
- Innervation to the internal anal sphincter (IAS) is both sympathetic and parasympathetic. Sympathetic nerves mediate IAS contraction, and parasympathetic nerves mediate IAS relaxation.
- The IAS is composed of slow twitch, smooth muscle, and the external anal sphincter (EAS) is composed of striated muscle.
- An acceptable frequency of defecation ranges from 3 times per day to 3 times per week.
- High-amplitude propagating phasic contractions propel colonic content distally and occur approximately 5 to 6 times daily.
- Together, the pubococcygeus, iliococcygeus, and puborectalis muscles comprise the levator ani.
- The arterial blood supply to the sigmoid colon and rectum is derived from the inferior mesenteric artery (IMA).

The pelvic floor represents the convergence of 3 separate but closely related organ systems: the digestive, urinary, and reproductive systems. There are many pathologic processes that can affect any one of these systems and, in turn, may secondarily affect the others. This chapter focuses on the anatomy and physiology of the posterior pelvic GI structures, more specifically the anorectum. A

Qureshi W, ed. *Diagnosis and Management Guide for Anorectal Disease: A Clinical Reference* (pp 3-10).

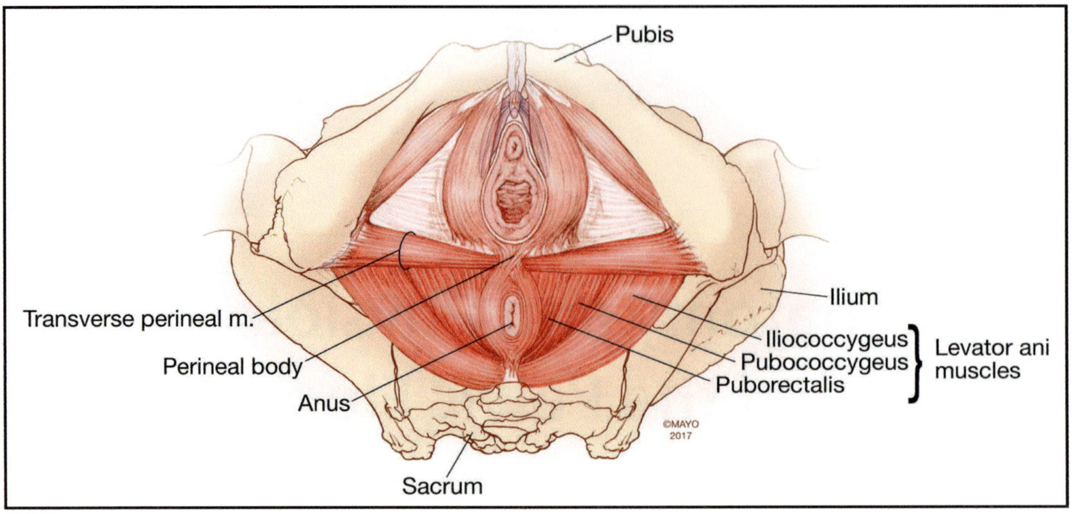

Figure 1-1. Pelvic floor bony anatomy. (Used with permission of Mayo Foundation for Medical Education and Research, all rights reserved.)

thorough understanding of anatomy and physiology is a critical starting point for understanding the complexities of anorectal disorders.

Anatomy of the Pelvic Floor

The pelvic floor is a finite space enclosed by the pelvic bones and numerous muscles, which serve varying functions (Figure 1-1). The bony structures include the anterior pubis and pubic symphysis, the ischium and ilium, and, to the posterior, the sacrum and coccyx. Ligaments connect these structures and form foramina, which contain the blood vessels and nerves supplying the pelvic floor.

The portions of the GI tract that occupy the pelvis are the sigmoid colon and the rectum. The sigmoid colon is an intraperitoneal structure and represents the most distal portion of the colon. It is the narrowest, most tortuous segment of the colon and is highly mobile, all of which predispose the sigmoid to problems, such as volvulus and obstructive symptoms. Within the sigmoid mesentery reside the nerves and blood vessels that supply it, and coursing deep and retroperitoneal to the sigmoid mesocolon is the left ureter.

The rectum, while a continuation of the sigmoid colon, is largely extraperitoneal with a small portion of the upper rectum being intraperitoneal. It lacks haustra, epiploic appendages, and a true mesentery. In contrast to the sigmoid colon, it is wide and very compliant. The length of the rectum is between 12 and 15 cm, with the anorectal junction being located 2 to 3 cm anterior to the tip of the coccyx. When performing digital rectal examination, anteriorly, one can palpate the uterine cervix and posterior wall of the vagina in women and the prostate in men. Posteriorly, the sacrum and coccyx are palpable, and the ischial tuberosities and ischiorectal fossae are palpable laterally.

The termination of the GI tract is at the anus. The anus is a 4- to 5-cm–long structure that is separated from the rectum by the dentate line. There are 6 to 14 columns of Morgagni, longitudinal folds of rectal mucosa that terminate in the anal papillae at the level of the dentate. These columns are joined together by the anal valves, and between these anal valves are the anal crypts. About half of the anal crypts drain anal glands, which are most often located in the anterior anal canal. The majority of the anal glands terminate within the intersphincteric space.

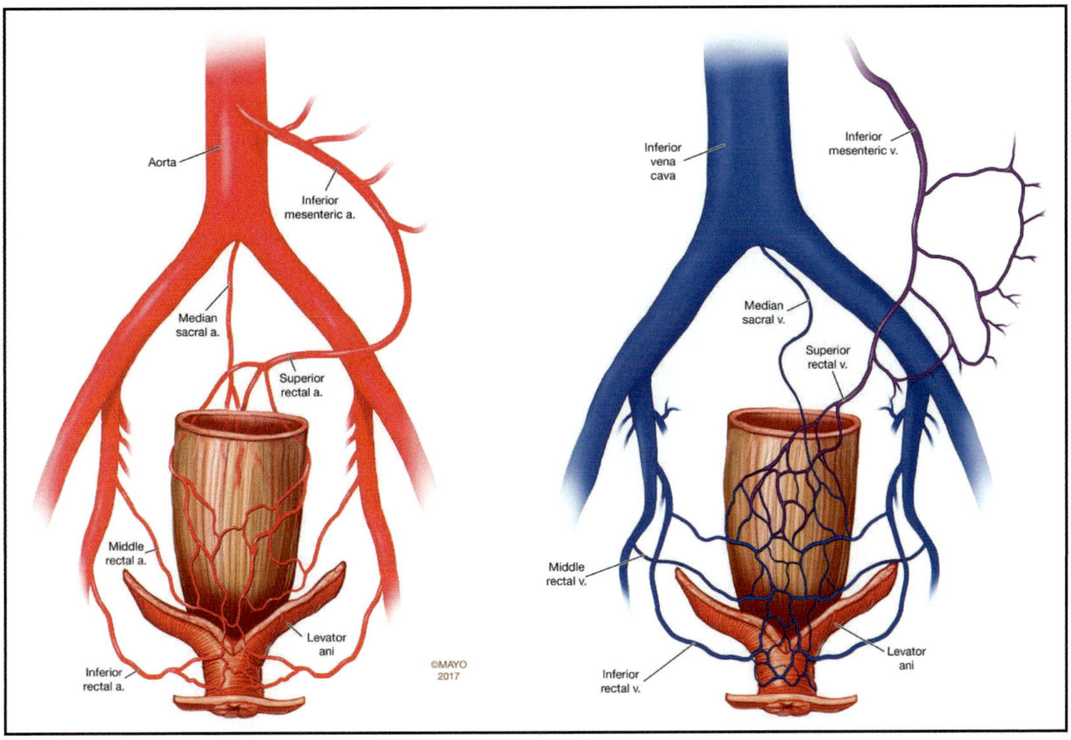

Figure 1-2. Vasculature of the pelvic floor. (Used with permission of Mayo Foundation for Medical Education and Research, all rights reserved.)

PELVIC FLOOR MUSCULATURE (SEE FIGURE 1-1)

The anal sphincters encircle the anal canal and play a critical role in the maintenance of continence, which is discussed in further detail later. The IAS represents a continuation and thickening of the circular smooth muscle layer of the rectal wall. It ends approximately 1 cm distal to the dentate line and superior to the EAS. It has a high spontaneous tone and is critical to maintaining continence. The EAS is a larger skeletal muscle that encircles the entire anal canal, in contrast to the IAS, which only surrounds the superior two-thirds of the anal canal. The deepest component of the EAS extends into the puborectalis; however, these 2 muscles are separate and do not share the same innervation. The EAS has a high resting tone as well, but this tone is able to be modified by voluntary efforts.

The levator ani is another important muscular structure of the pelvic floor and acts to support the pelvic organs; both the levator ani and the coccygeus muscles constitute the pelvic diaphragm, which is shaped like a bowl and attached superiorly to the walls of the pelvis. The levator ani muscles are divided into 3 groups of muscle fibers: the iliococcygeus, pubococcygeus, and puborectalis muscles. These groups of muscles join together at the midline. It is the central puborectalis portion of the levator ani that forms a U-shaped sling posterior to the anorectal junction and maintains the perineal flexure, also known as the *anorectal angle*.

PELVIC FLOOR VASCULATURE (FIGURE 1-2)

The arterial blood supply to the sigmoid colon and the upper rectum is derived from branches of the IMA, which originates from the aorta approximately 3 to 4 cm from the aortic bifurcation. The IMA gives rise to the left colic artery and the sigmoid arteries and then continues as the superior rectal (superior hemorrhoidal) artery. The superior rectal artery provides the majority of the blood supply to the upper and middle portions of the rectum, with the lower rectum and anal canal being supplied primarily by branches of the internal iliac artery. The median sacral artery may serve as a minor contributor to the rectal blood supply and arises directly from the posterior aspect of the aorta. The middle rectal (hemorrhoidal) artery provides blood flow to the inferior rectum and the proximal anus, whereas the inferior rectal (hemorrhoidal) artery supplies the distal anal canal. The inferior rectal artery arises from the internal pudendal artery, which is a branch of the internal iliac artery.

The veins of the pelvis closely track the arterial supply, with the inferior mesenteric vein positioned to the left of the IMA and aorta. Venous drainage of the pelvic floor occurs via both the systemic and portal systems. The inferior mesenteric vein drains the superior rectal (hemorrhoidal) veins and then empties into the splenic vein just posterior to the pancreas. The splenic vein then unites with the superior mesenteric vein to form the portal vein. The middle and inferior rectal veins drain to systemic venous circulation through the internal iliac vein, with the inferior rectal veins first draining to the internal pudendal veins.

PELVIC FLOOR INNERVATION (FIGURE 1-3)

The autonomic nervous system innervates the GI tract and includes the sympathetic, parasympathetic, and enteric nerves. The sympathetic and parasympathetic nerves constitute the extrinsic supply, and these connect with the intrinsic enteric nerve supply. The enteric nervous system is the largest component of the autonomic nervous system, containing more neurons than the parasympathetic and sympathetic divisions combined.

The sources of innervation for the IAS and EAS are different. The IAS is supplied by both the sympathetic and parasympathetic nerves, with the sympathetic fibers originating from the superior hypogastric plexus and the parasympathetic from the inferior hypogastric plexus. It is the sympathetic nerves that mediate IAS contraction. Stimulation of the parasympathetic nerves causes IAS relaxation. The EAS is innervated through the pudendal nerve by motor and sensory neurons as well as the perineal nerve. The levator ani is innervated by the direct sacral nerves and the perineal branch of the pudendal nerve, all of which are branches from the sacral nerve roots of S2, S3, and S4.

Physiology of the Pelvic Floor

Anorectal physiology is complex, with an interplay of sensory and motor inputs to the pelvic floor muscles coordinated to result in timely and controlled defecation. For defecation to occur in a predicted manner, fecal continence needs to be maintained by a set of factors that are closely related. Stool volume and consistency, rectal sensation, and mechanical factors are mutually involved to ensure continence and defecation transpire as anticipated. Dysfunction of anorectal physiology will be reviewed in the corresponding chapters; however, an understanding of normal physiology is essential to developing direct and effective diagnostic and treatment options.

CONTINENCE

Fecal continence is ultimately dependent on the tension present in the IAS and EAS, which at rest exerts approximately 30 to 80 mm Hg resting pressure, with many factors such as age and sex influencing it.[1] The IAS, which is made up of slow twitch, smooth muscles, is primarily responsible for maintaining continence at rest. The EAS, also in a state of constant tonic activity at rest, consists of a layer of striated muscle that is under voluntary control. The anal vascular cushion, which is composed of the superior hemorrhoidal plexus, adds to the basal anal tone but, more importantly, provides an airtight seal to help preserve continence.

The distal part of the colon functions as a reservoir of its contents, aided in part by the lateral angulation of the sigmoid and the valves of Houston, which provide a physical barrier. Once stool

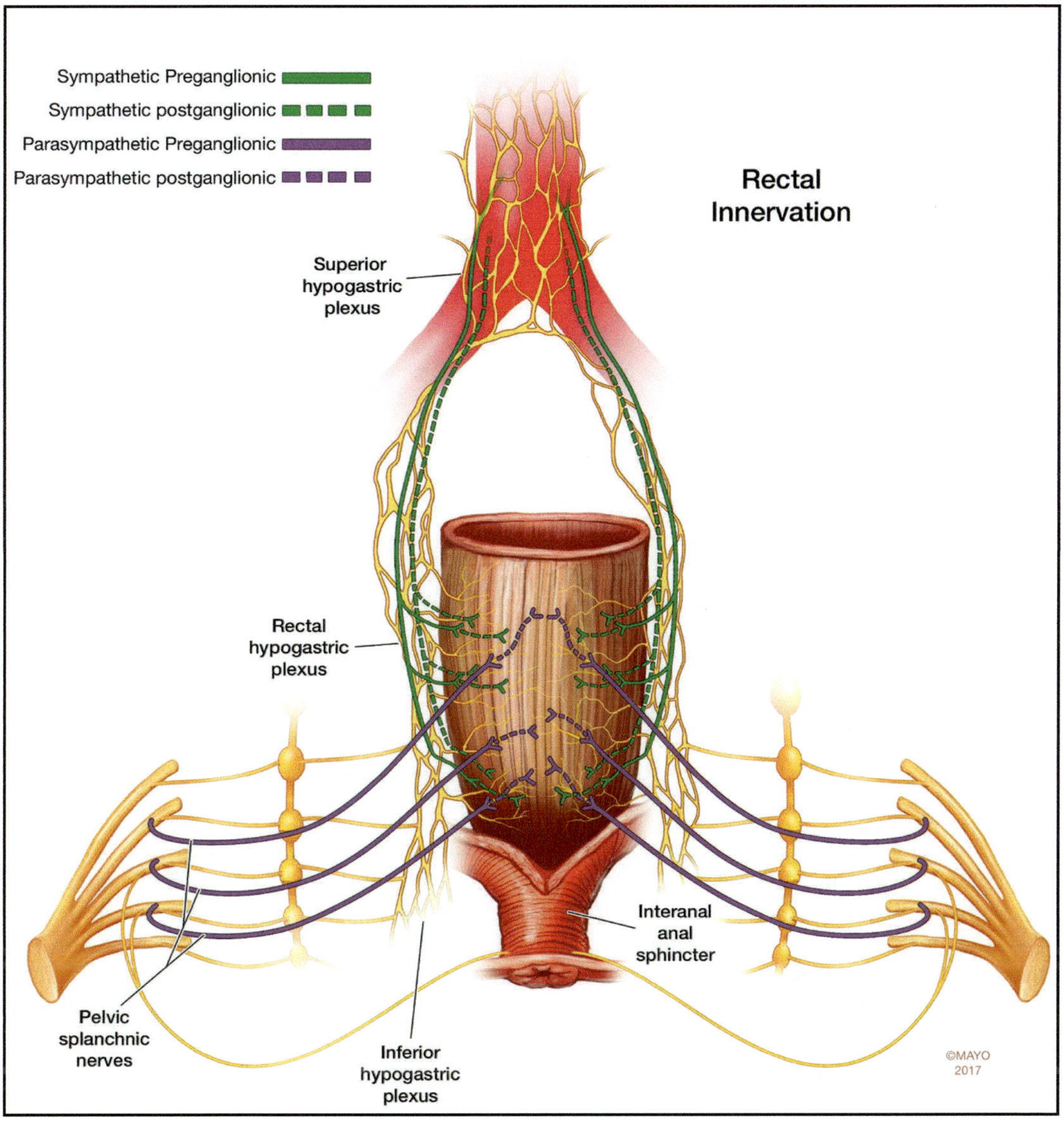

Figure 1-3. Innervation of the pelvic floor. (Used with permission of Mayo Foundation for Medical Education and Research, all rights reserved.)

or gas reaches the rectum, it distends the lumen, allowing it to stretch and accommodate its content. When rectal distension reaches a threshold of compliance, sensory reflexes via the myenteric plexus involving the anal canal result in relaxation of the IAS via the rectoanal inhibitory reflex, allowing "sampling" of intraluminal contents by the more sensitive anal mucosa.[2] This enables an individual to discriminate between solid, liquid, and gas and may lead to defecation when socially acceptable. When defecation is deferred, voluntary contraction of the EAS is often needed to maintain continence. Suppression of the urge to defecate leads to increased compliance of the rectum and gradual retrograde propulsion of its content back to the sigmoid colon.

Liquid stool, especially in large volumes, may overpower the continence mechanisms and can become difficult to retain, even in those with normal anal sphincter tone. Furthermore, if rectal sensation is impaired, it has the potential to compromise defecatory function or continence, resulting in definable symptoms and the clinical syndromes reviewed in the chapters that follow.

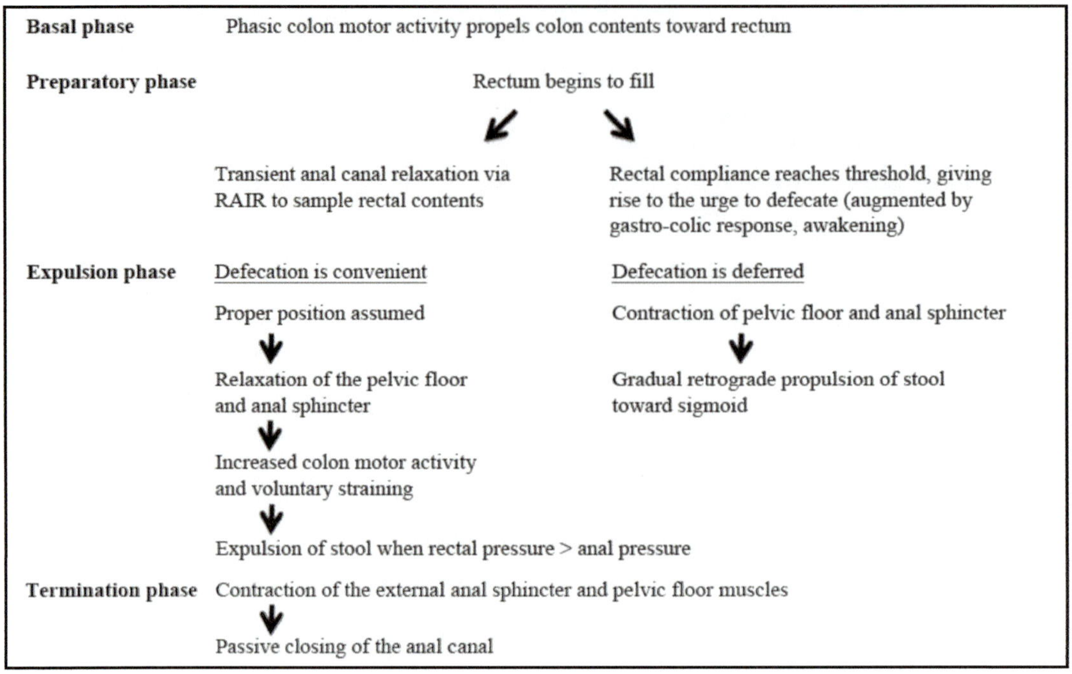

Figure 1-4. Four phases of defecation. (Used with permission of Mayo Foundation for Medical Education and Research, all rights reserved.)

DEFECATION

The frequency of defecation varies between individuals and is a measure often used to define constipation. Anywhere from 3 bowel movements daily to 3 times weekly is generally considered acceptable.[3] Frequently, there is discordance between what is "normal" and patients' perception of disordered function. Stool volume and consistency influence GI transit time and, as a general rule, loose stools are associated with a more rapid colonic transit.[4] The assessment of colon transit time with radiopaque markers or scintigraphy can be performed to assist in the planning of therapeutic interventions.

Defecation was believed to be exclusively a function of the anorectum; however, it is now clear that the entire colon is integrated in the defecatory sequence. Colonic motor activity is characterized by phasic and sustained contractions. Phasic contractions are further classified as propagating or nonpropagating based on whether they move along the colon. Manometric studies have provided useful insight into this complex process. High-amplitude propagating pressure waves have amplitudes > 100 mm Hg and occur in a sequence starting in the proximal colon, successively propelling colonic content distally and resulting in intermittent filling of the rectum.[5] These occur on average 5 to 6 times per day. Low-amplitude propagating sequences typically have amplitudes < 50 mm Hg and propagate for short distances either antegrade or retrograde. Nonpropagating contractions are less well understood and are believed to aid in mixing of the intraluminal contents.[6] Motor activity in the rectum is characterized by recurrent motor complexes, with amplitudes 15 to 60 mm Hg in range shown to propagate in a retrograde direction to retard the flow of colonic contents. Although incompletely understood, rectal motor complexes appear to be triggered by propagating pressure waves and are inhibited during defecation, providing a "break" to keep the rectum empty between bowel movements and control challenges to continence.[7]

Four distinct phases of defecation have been described[2] (Figure 1-4). In the basal phase, normal colorectal motor activity occurs as described previously without the desire to defecate. The preparatory phase can start 1 hour before the expulsion of stool, intensifying in the 15 minutes preceding

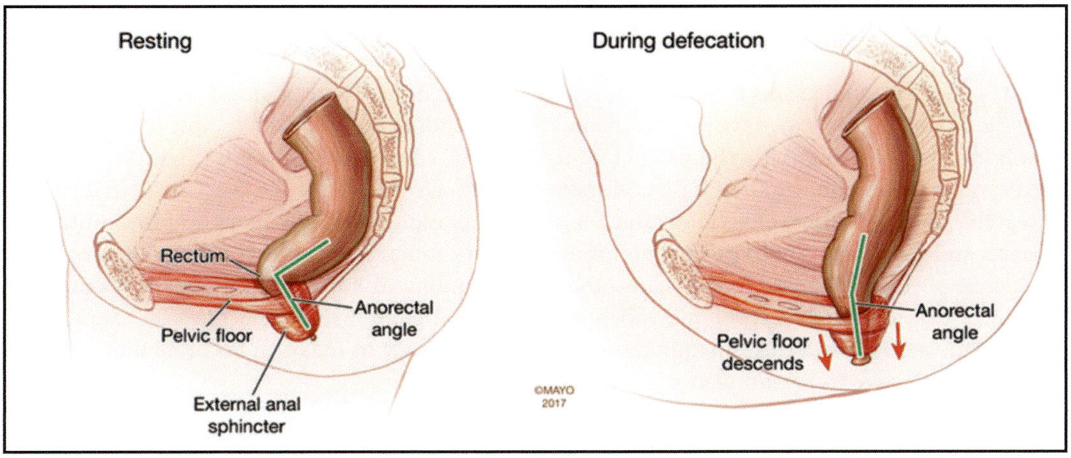

Figure 1-5. Demonstration of the anorectal angle at rest and with defecation. (Used with permission of Mayo Foundation for Medical Education and Research, all rights reserved.)

evacuation, and result in the "urge" to have a bowel movement. Ingestion of a meal is one of the most potent stimuli that increase colonic activity, which is most pronounced in the transverse and descending colon, and is often referred to as the *gastrocolic response*.[8] The meal response is dependent on a minimal caloric load of 300 kcal as well as the fat content.[9] Morning awakening also stimulates an increase in propagating pressure waves, undoubtedly explaining the common habit of defecation shortly after awakening.

Distension of the distal sigmoid and rectum leads to the activation of sacral spinal afferent mechanoreceptors that give rise to the defecatory urge. As long as this occurs at a convenient time, a conscious decision to evacuate is made, initiating the expulsive phase of defecation. Sacral parasympathetic innervation of the distal bowel increases peristalsis and inhibits the IAS; this relaxes the pelvic floor muscles, allowing for defecation to occur. When the rectal pressure becomes greater than the anal canal pressure, the expulsion of stool occurs. Even under normal circumstances, voluntary suppression of defecation may be overcome by the volume and consistency of stool.

The efficacy of evacuation is helped in part by proper positioning and voluntary straining. Adequate pelvic floor relaxation coupled with elevated intra-abdominal pressure leads to pelvic floor descent, which is essential for effective evacuation. The anorectal angle at rest is approximately 90 degrees (normal range, 70 to 140 degrees; Figure 1-5). As the pelvic floor relaxes, this angle becomes more obtuse, the levator ani muscles contract, and the perineum descends, funneling stool into the anal canal. Further straightening of the angle occurs with hip flexion, allowing for easier evacuation.[10] Thus, it is not surprising that complete rectal evacuation is easiest in the squatting posture and most difficult lying down.[11] Inadequate pelvic floor relaxation coupled with paradoxical contraction of the anal sphincter uncovered via high-resolution anorectal manometry is a hallmark of dyssynergic defecation, which is discussed elsewhere.

The final termination phase of defecation commences with a sense of complete rectal emptying. This begins with involuntary contraction of the EAS and pelvic floor, which closes the anal canal and reverses the pressure gradient in the rectum. Once straining ceases, the intra-abdominal pressure decreases, and the pelvic floor muscles constrict, increasing traction on the anorectal junction and elongating the anal canal to allow it to passively close.[6]

There is increasing recognition that many previously under-recognized factors also influence evacuation. Psychological and behavioral events experienced in childhood may lead to long-term effects on voluntary and involuntary suppression of defecation.[12] Stress, physical activity, and emotional factors may modulate colonic activity by activating the autonomic nervous system. Autonomic dysfunction has been implicated in a number of colonic disorders; however, research in this area is sparse.[3]

Conclusion

The pelvic floor represents a complex interaction between the GI, urologic, and reproductive systems, and it is important to have a fundamental understanding of both the anatomy and physiology of this area because multiple systems are frequently involved with the pathology. The physiology of the pelvic floor functions to maintain continence and to allow for effective evacuation in a socially acceptable time and place. Defecation and continence are under both voluntary and involuntary influence, and the disruption of normal motor and sensory function or reflexes can result in complex problems, posing challenges to clinicians. The understanding of normal physiology is necessary to recognize disordered defecation and incontinence. A complete history and physical examination along with radiographic and functional tests may be necessary to make an accurate diagnosis and develop an effective treatment plan.

References

1. Noelting J, Ratuapli SK, Bharucha AE, Harvey DM, Ravi K, Zinsmeister AR. Normal values for high-resolution anorectal manometry in healthy women: effects of age and significance of rectoanal gradient. *Am J Gastroenterol.* 2012;107(10):1530-1536.
2. Palit S, Lunniss PJ, Scott SM. The physiology of human defecation. *Dig Dis Sci.* 2012;57(6):1445-1464.
3. American Gastroenterological Association, Bharucha AE, Dorn SD, Lembo A, Pressman A. American Gastroenterological Association medical position statement on constipation. *Gastroenterology.* 2013;144(1):211-217.
4. Degen LP, Phillips SF. How well does stool form reflect colonic transit? *Gut.* 1996;39(1):109-113.
5. Bampton PA, Dinning PG, Kennedy ML, Lubowski DZ, deCarle D, Cook IJ. Spatial and temporal organization of pressure patterns throughout the unprepared colon during spontaneous defecation. *Am J Gastroenterol.* 2000;95(4):1027-1035.
6. Brookes SJ, Dinning PG, Gladman MA. Neuroanatomy and physiology of colorectal function and defaecation: from basic science to human clinical studies. *Neurogastroenterol Motil.* 2009;21(suppl 2):9-19.
7. Feldman M, Friedman LS, Brandt LJ. *Sleisenger and Fordtran's Gastrointestinal and Liver Disease: Pathophysiology, Diagnosis, Management.* 10th ed. Philadelphia, PA: Saunders/Elsevier; 2016.
8. Rao SS, Sadeghi P, Beaty J, Kavlock R. Ambulatory 24-hour colonic manometry in slow-transit constipation. *Am J Gastroenterol.* 2004;99(12):2405-2416.
9. Di Stefano M, Miceli E, Missanelli A, Mazzocchi S, Corazza GR. Meal induced rectosigmoid tone modification: a low caloric meal accurately separates functional and organic gastrointestinal disease patients. *Gut.* 2006;55(10):1409-1414.
10. Bell AM, Pemberton JH, Hanson RB, Zinsmeister AR. Variations in muscle tone of the human rectum: recordings with an electromechanical barostat. *Am J Physiol.* 1991;260(1, pt 1):G17-G25.
11. Rao SS, Kavlock R, Rao S. Influence of body position and stool characteristics on defecation in humans. *Am J Gastroenterol.* 2006;101(12):2790-2796.
12. Drossman DA. Abuse, trauma, and GI illness: is there a link? *Am J Gastroenterol.* 2011;106(1):14-25.

Bibliography

Bass LM, Wershil BK. Anatomy, histology, embryology, and developmental anomalies of the small and large intestine. In: Feldman M, Friedman LS, Brandt LJ, eds. *Sleisenger and Fordtran's Gastrointestinal and Liver Disease.* 10th ed. Philadelphia, PA: Saunders/Elsevier; 2016:1649-1678.

Drake RL, Vogl AW, Mitchell AWM. *Gray's Anatomy for Students.* 3rd ed. Philadelphia, PA: Churchill Livingstone; 2015:421-532.

Szmulowicz U. Anatomy and physiology of the pelvic digestive organs. In: Hull TL, ed. *Posterior Pelvic Floor Abnormalities.* Philadelphia, PA: Saunders/Elsevier; 2011:1-40.

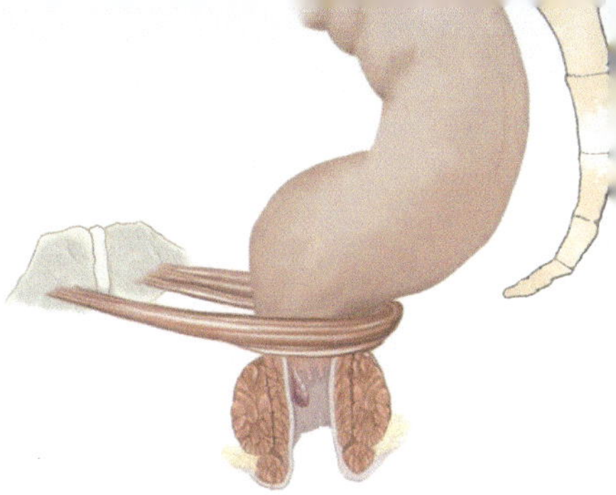

Section 2

Benign Anorectal Conditions

2

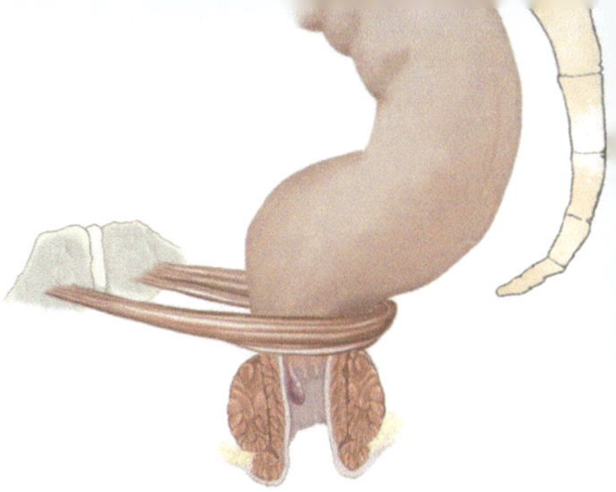

Hemorrhoids

Waqar Qureshi, MD, FRCP, FACP, FACG, FASGE

Key Points

- There is no cure for hemorrhoids. Even after surgery, they may recur, so it is critical that patients learn to eat fiber to keep their stools soft and bulky to avoid straining, sit on the toilet no longer than 5 minutes, and treat constipation aggressively.
- Hemorrhoids do not hurt unless acutely thrombosed. Look for another cause.
- Whenever possible, examine the anorectum, and treat hemorrhoids unsedated. This way, you can tell if the patient has a fissure you are just not seeing. Ask the patient if it hurts when you apply suction before you deploy the band.
- Anal sphincter spasm is sometimes associated with anal fissures or acutely thrombosed hemorrhoids. Nitroglycerin or nifedipine ointment can help relax the sphincter and reduce pain.
- Provide the patient with a 24/7 callback phone number for symptoms such as excessive pain, bleeding, fever, chills, or rigors, particularly after hemorrhoid banding.

Although hemorrhoids are a normal feature of anorectal anatomy, symptomatic hemorrhoids are relatively common, with an estimated prevalence in the United States of 4.4% and a peak prevalence between 45 and 65 years of age.[1] It is thought that only one-third of patients with symptomatic hemorrhoids seek help, making the true prevalence difficult to define.[1] It is estimated that over 23 million Americans suffer from hemorrhoid symptoms, resulting in about 3.5 million visits to the doctor and over $500 million in health care costs.[2,3] Many patients and even some physicians attribute symptoms in the anorectal area to hemorrhoid disease, although this is not always the case. Traditionally, a surgeon has managed hemorrhoid disease. Increasingly, gastroenterologists are beginning to manage many aspects of anorectal disease, including symptomatic hemorrhoids, in the office setting.

Qureshi W, ed. *Diagnosis and Management Guide for Anorectal Disease: A Clinical Reference* (pp 13-26).

Pathophysiology

Hemorrhoids are cushions of arteriovenous vascular plexuses with supporting connective tissues that surround the distal rectum and anal canal. There are usually 3 major anal cushions found in the right anterior, right posterior, and left lateral positions. Various changes occur with the development of symptomatic hemorrhoids. These include abnormal venous dilation, vascular thrombosis, and a degenerative process in the collagen and fibroelastic tissues that form the supportive scaffolding for the vessels and overlying mucosa.[4] An associated inflammatory response involving the blood vessels and surrounding connective tissues is seen on microscopy of hemorrhoidal tissue, leading to ulceration, ischemia, and thrombosis.[5]

Hemorrhoid symptoms arise as the anal cushions enlarge along with the blood vessels within them, leading to easily traumatized mucosa. This causes bleeding, which is typically bright red, from the arteriovenous communications. The enlarged cushions eventually prolapse through the anal canal. Constipation and prolonged straining are thought to lead to symptomatic hemorrhoids through increased abdominal pressure, causing engorgement of the hemorrhoidal plexus and hard stool, impacting a traumatizing force of the anal cushions. However, in some circles, this remains controversial because not all patients with hemorrhoidal symptoms are constipated. Pregnancy predisposes to symptomatic hemorrhoids that settle soon after delivery. Other factors such as a low-fiber diet, spicy foods, prolonged lavatory sitting, and a family history have been implicated, but the data are inconsistent. It is possible that an imbalance between endothelium-derived relaxing factors (nitric oxide and prostacyclin) and constricting factors (endothelin and reactive oxygen radicals) predisposes to the development of hemorrhoids.[6] The resting anal pressure in patients with hemorrhoids (prolapsing or not) is significantly higher than in those without hemorrhoids. It is not clear whether the increase in anal pressure contributes to or is the result of the symptomatic hemorrhoids, but this relationship may also explain why a significant number of hemorrhoid sufferers also have anal fissures.

Classification and Grading

Hemorrhoids are classified into internal hemorrhoids if they arise above the dentate line and external hemorrhoids when they arise below the dentate line. External hemorrhoids may be described as mild, moderate, or severe, which is rather subjective. Internal hemorrhoids are graded as follows according to the degree of prolapse:

- Grade I: do not prolapse below the dentate line, may cause painless bleeding
- Grade II: prolapse below the dentate line during defecation but spontaneously reduce
- Grade III: prolapse below the dentate line but require manual reduction
- Grade IV: prolapse and stay below the dentate line, not reducible; incarcerated internal hemorrhoids

Signs and Symptoms

Most hemorrhoid symptoms result from internal hemorrhoids becoming enlarged over time. Common symptoms include painless, bright red bleeding, which may range from streaks of blood on the toilet paper to less commonly significant bleeding with or without a bowel movement. Hemorrhoids may present with itching in the anal area caused by stool seepage due to interference in the continence mechanism by enlarged internal hemorrhoids or relative ischemia on the surface of hemorrhoids from their distention. Prolapsed internal hemorrhoids can also cause mucus

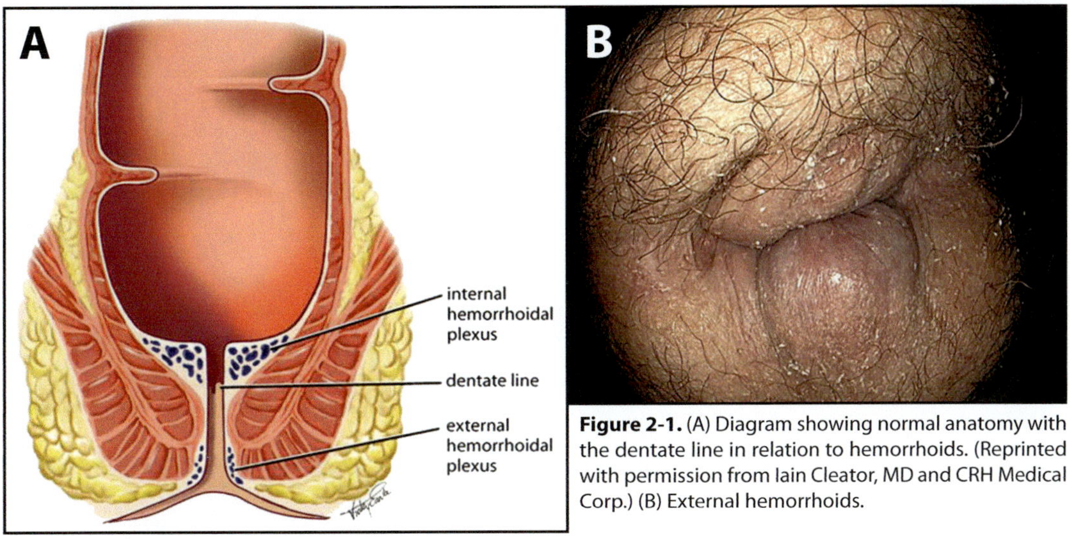

Figure 2-1. (A) Diagram showing normal anatomy with the dentate line in relation to hemorrhoids. (Reprinted with permission from Iain Cleator, MD and CRH Medical Corp.) (B) External hemorrhoids.

deposition in the perianal skin, leading to itchiness. Patients may report a bulge felt while wiping after a bowel movement that may reduce spontaneously or may need to be manually reduced. Pain is not a prominent feature of hemorrhoid disease, except when an external hemorrhoid becomes thrombosed or there is an anal fissure present. Up to 20% of patients with symptomatic hemorrhoids have a concomitant anal fissure.[7] Stool seepage or staining of underwear may be a result of hemorrhoidal prolapse.

Diagnosis

Accurate diagnosis requires a careful directed history and examination. Ask about the color of blood, its relationship to a bowel movement and whether it is covering or mixed in with stool, and the relationship between any bleeding and bowel movements. Ask about pain and what factors exacerbate or alleviate the symptoms. These elements will help greatly because the diagnosis is almost always a clinical one.

Visual Examination

Examinations performed in the office setting are usually done in the left lateral decubitus position with both the hips and knees bent. A good light source is required to inspect the perianal area. Findings may include external hemorrhoids (Figure 2-1), external and prolapsed internal hemorrhoids (Figure 2-2), prolapsed internal hemorrhoids (Figure 2-3), hemorrhoids with rectal prolapse (Figure 2-4), rectal prolapse (Figure 2-5), skin tags, sentinel tags, pilonidal disease, dermatitis, an anal fissure, a fistula-in-ano, warts, or malignancy. Malignancies are usually hard and ulcerated (Figure 2-6), whereas premalignant conditions such as Bowen's or Paget's disease appear erythematous.[8] A thrombosed external hemorrhoid has a bluish color from the clot underlying the anoderm (Figure 2-7). Prolapsed internal hemorrhoids are covered with pink mucosa, whereas external hemorrhoids are covered with the anoderm. If the patient complains of painful defecation, an anal fissure may be present, in which case gentle separation of the buttocks at the anal verge may cause pain or reveal a tear, usually in the posterior aspect of the anal verge. A perianal abscess (Figure 2-8) will likely require surgical drainage.

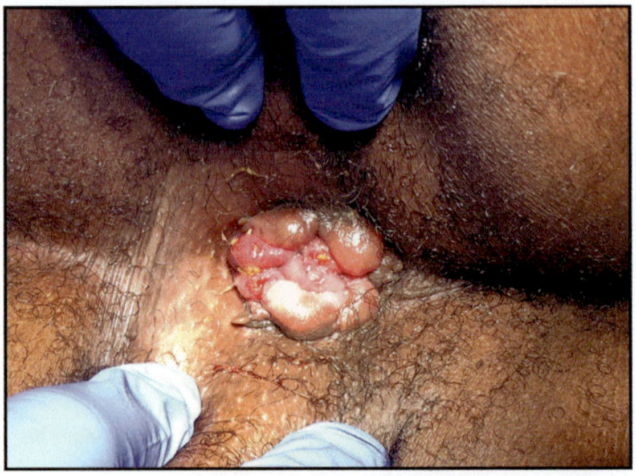

Figure 2-2. External hemorrhoids with prolapsed internal hemorrhoids at the center.

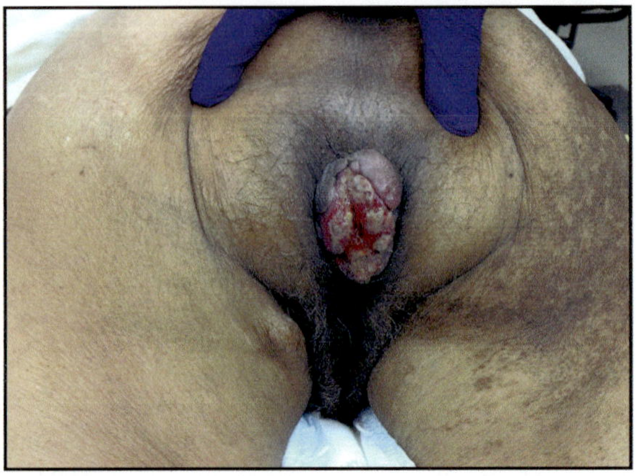

Figure 2-3. Prolapsed hemorrhoids. They could not be reduced and are therefore grade 4.

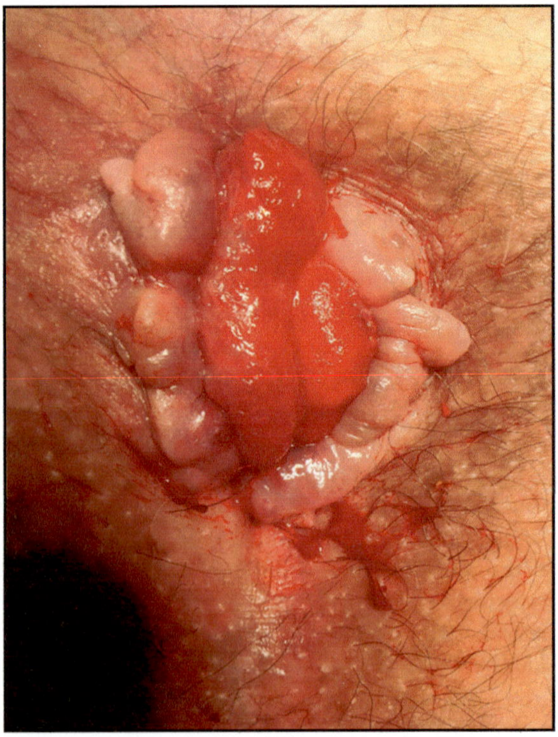

Figure 2-4. External hemorrhoids with rectal prolapse.

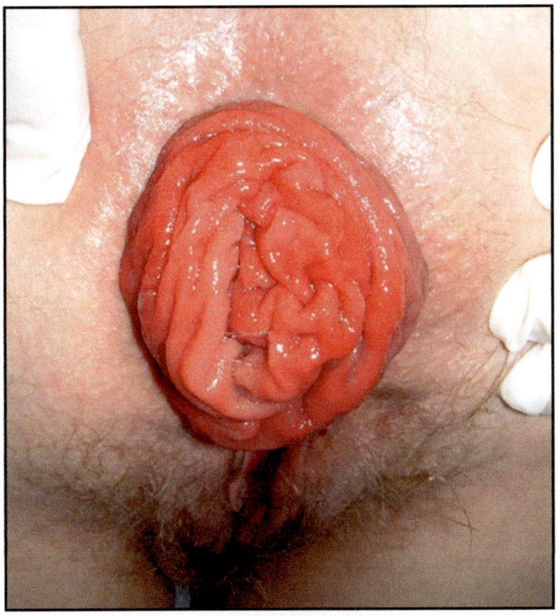

Figure 2-5. Rectal prolapse.

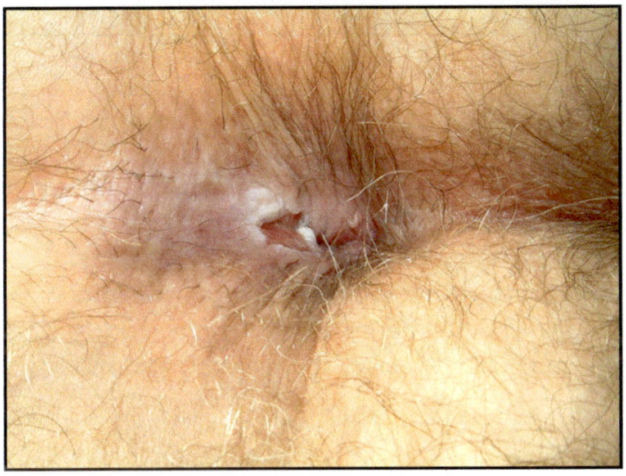

Figure 2-6. Squamous cell carcinoma of the anus.

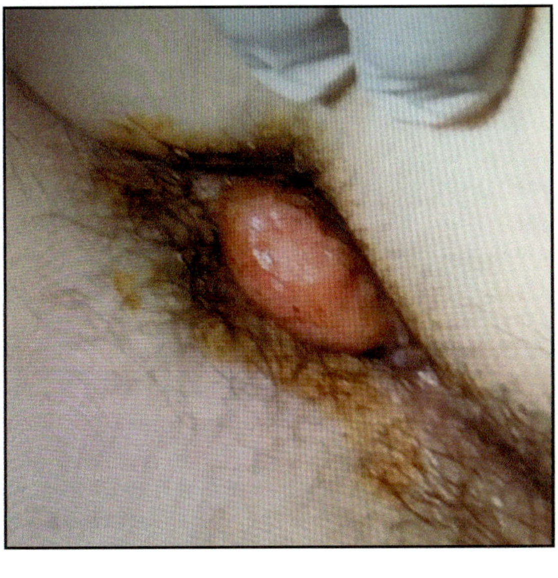

Figure 2-7. A thrombosed external hemorrhoid.

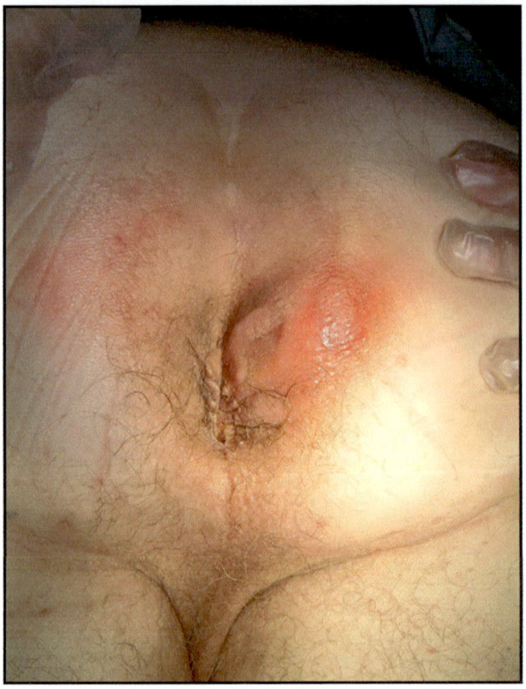

Figure 2-8. A perianal abscess.

DIGITAL RECTAL EXAMINATION

Digital examination is an anal as well as a rectal examination. Pathology is frequently missed in the anal canal. In addition to looking for a fissure, tenderness, or mass, the tone of the anal sphincter is evaluated. A partially healed anal fissure may be felt as a roughness in the otherwise smooth anal canal and may not be visualized. The resting sphincter tone is assessed, and a widened intersphincteric groove may indicate internal sphincter spasm. The puborectalis is felt posteriorly at the anorectal junction. The patient is asked to squeeze and strain to assess the symmetry and function of the sphincter.

ANOSCOPY

This is the only tool that allows thorough examination of the anal canal and distal rectum without any special preparation. There are several different types of anoscopes. I prefer a beveled anoscopy as opposed to a slotted one because it allows rotation without causing trauma. Disposable, clear plastic anoscopes with built-in lighting are cheap and convenient. A lubricated anoscope is inserted while the patient bears down to relax the anal canal. The anus is examined circumferentially, noting hemorrhoid bundles in the right anterior, right posterior, or left lateral positions (Figure 2-9). This is an extremely easy procedure to learn and is performed quickly; yet, it is essential for complete examination of the anal canal and to assess the size of the internal hemorrhoids (Figure 2-10).

Treatment and Follow-up

MEDICAL TREATMENT

Dietary and lifestyle modification is the first step in hemorrhoid treatment. Hard stool can cause damage to the anal cushions, leading to bleeding and eventually prolapse. The use of psyllium showed

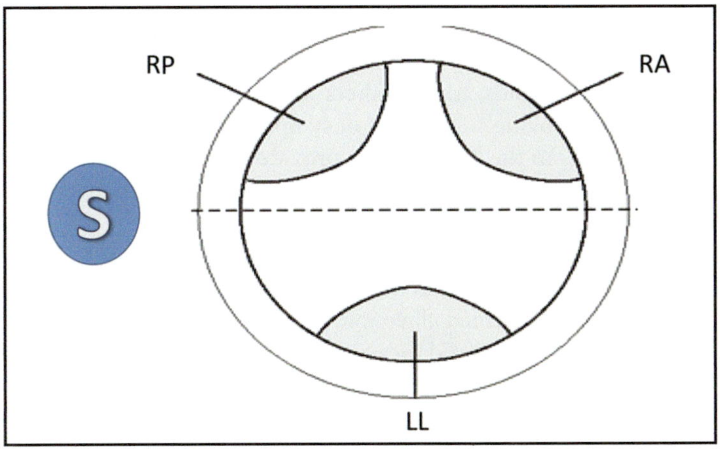

Figure 2-9. Schematic diagram showing the internal hemorrhoids through an anoscope. The patient is in the left lateral position with the sacrum to the left (S), the internal hemorrhoids are shown, right posterior (RP), right anterior (RA) and left lateral (LL).

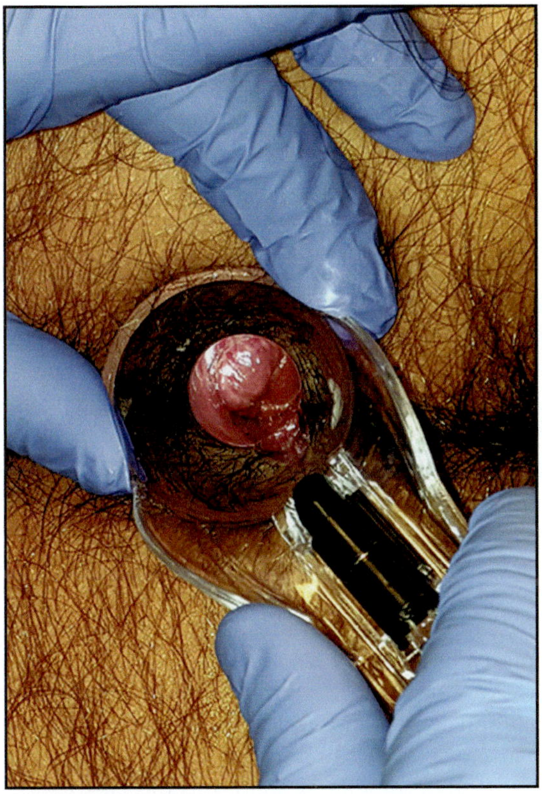

Figure 2-10. A view of the right posterior hemorrhoid during anoscopy.

a reduction in hemorrhoidal bleeding and painful defecation in a double-blind, placebo-controlled trial.[9] In another study, a fiber supplement reduced the risk of persisting symptoms and bleeding by 50%.[10] Dietary fiber is cheap and safe and is advised with all degrees of hemorrhoids, along with increased fluid intake. Most authorities advise 25 g/day soluble fiber. Both constipation and diarrhea can cause or worsen hemorrhoids and need to be treated. Patients should be instructed not to neglect the first urge to defecate and avoid straining.[11] They are encouraged to avoid reading, getting on social media, and answering emails while sitting on the toilet because it could make hemorrhoids worse.[12] In addition, regular exercise, a reduction in fat intake, and improving anal hygiene are advised. Sitz baths or warm water soaks can help ameliorate the symptoms, and ice packs may reduce the swelling of hemorrhoids.

Over-the-Counter Topicals

A variety of topical agents, such as Anusol (Johnson & Johnson), Preparation H (phenylephrine), Tucks (Blistex Inc), Balneol (Meda), and steroids, among others, are available over the counter. Although these creams or suppositories may provide some relief of symptoms, they are unlikely to significantly ameliorate hemorrhoid symptoms in the long term or provide a cure.[13] Steroid creams should not be used repeatedly because this might result in thinning of the perianal skin, making it more sensitive.

Flavonoids are oral drugs commonly used in Europe and Asia to treat hemorrhoids. These drugs increase the vascular tone and lymphatic drainage and normalize capillary permeability. Two placebo-controlled trials using oral micronized purified flavonoid fraction (MPFF) showed improvement with the use of MPFF.[14,15] MPFF is not approved for use in the United States by the Food and Drug Administration.

NONOPERATIVE TREATMENT

Nonoperative treatment modalities start with diet and lifestyle modifications followed by in-office treatment. In-office procedures attempt to reduce redundancy and vascularity and increase fixation of the anal cushion to its underlying muscle through scarring. This decreases the risk of bleeding and prolapse. These procedures are relatively well tolerated, all display variable recurrence rates, and all may require repeated application.[16]

RUBBER BAND LIGATION

Hemorrhoid ligation was initially described using suture material by Blaisdell in 1954, and Barron first described ligation using a rubber band in 1963; it has undergone various modifications over time to become a popular office-based procedure. Today, band ligation is a simple, relatively inexpensive, office-based procedure that is ideal for grades I, II, and III internal hemorrhoids. Several banding devices are available on the market (Figure 2-11A-C). Regardless of which one you use, the correct technique is essential for a satisfactory outcome. Although there are variations in the techniques of band placement (ie, some are performed "blind," whereas others require direct vision of the hemorrhoid to be banded), the end result is the same. The band causes necrosis and sloughing of the mucosa and hemorrhoid feeding vessels, resulting in an ulcer, which heals by fibrosis (Figure 2-11E-F). This has 2 results: it lessens the blood flow into the hemorrhoid and tacks the mucosa to the side of the rectal wall, helping to control prolapse.

The bands are placed about 2 cm above the dentate line so that discomfort is minimal postprocedure (Figure 2-11D). It is recommended that you place one band per session and certainly not more than 2 to avoid excessive postprocedure discomfort. After band placement, it is important to palpate the banded mucosa, which should feel like a mobile soft "polyp." If it feels fixed, you probably have the muscle layer caught in the band, which will cause immediate discomfort. When this happens, the "polyp" is simply rolled in a circular fashion and will become more mobile as the muscle layer is freed. Complications are uncommon if good technique and avoidance of placing multiple bands per session are observed. Rubber band ligation (RBL) as recommended here is associated with a low complication rate (<2%). The complications include anal pain, a vasovagal response, and in about 2% to 11%, thrombosis of the external hemorrhoid.[17] Pelvic sepsis is a rare but serious complication of hemorrhoid banding and should be managed emergently when diagnosed. RBL is well tolerated and effective in over 80% of patients.[18-21] RBL is the procedure of choice for first- through third-degree hemorrhoids.[21] There is controversy regarding how many hemorrhoidal columns can be safely banded at one time. Banding one hemorrhoid column per visit minimizes patient discomfort and might reduce the risk of complications, including pelvic sepsis.[22,23]

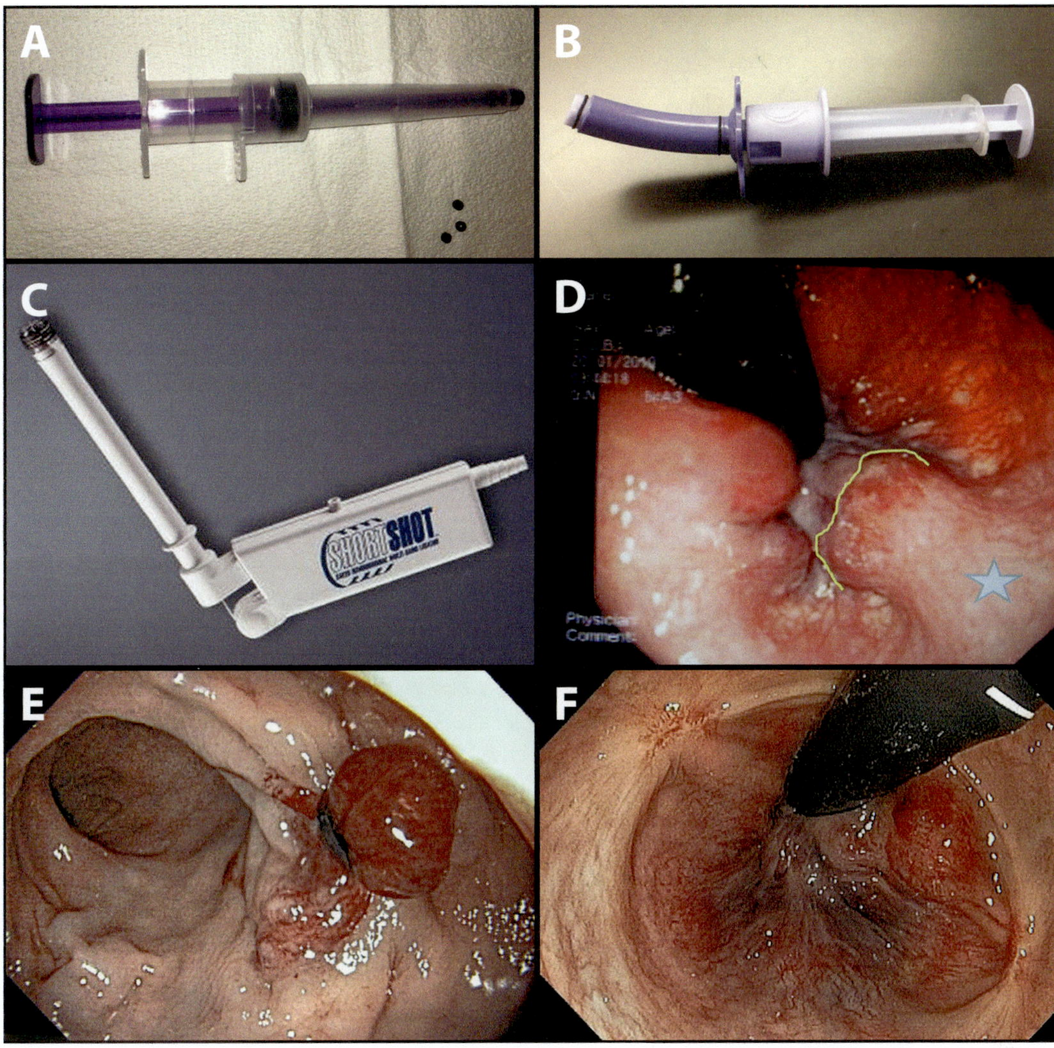

Figure 2-11. (A) The CRH O'Regan banding device by CRH Medical Corp. (B) The SpaceBander by ConMed. (C) The ShortShot Saeed multiband device by Cook Medical. (Permission for use granted by Cook Medical Incorporated, Bloomington, Indiana.) (D) This photograph shows the ideal position for a band application well away from the dentate line. (E) Shortly after banding, the tissue becomes necrotic and sloughs off. (F) The site of banding ulcerated and healed with fibrosis.

INFRARED COAGULATION

Infrared coagulation (IRC) of internal hemorrhoids uses infrared light to create heat for the thrombosis and scarring of hemorrhoid tissue. This technique requires direct vision of the hemorrhoid and contact of the probe with the mucosa. One device developed for office use by Redfield Corporation consists of a light generator and a handheld gun (Figure 2-12), which has a light bulb, trigger, and probe that are passed through an anoscope. The amount of energy delivered is selected on a dial on the generator and ranges from a fraction of a second to several seconds. A duration of 0.8 to 1.2 seconds per site with 4 to 6 sites per hemorrhoid seems to work well. Figures 2-13A and B show the best position to apply the IRC energy. With each treatment, a blanching of the mucosa is seen. Over the next few days, the treated tissue gets thrombosed and scars. All 3 internal hemorrhoids may be treated in one session and repeated in a few weeks if the symptoms are better but still present. The reported success rates are 67% to 96% from 2 prospective studies for the treatment of first- and second-degree hemorrhoids.[24]

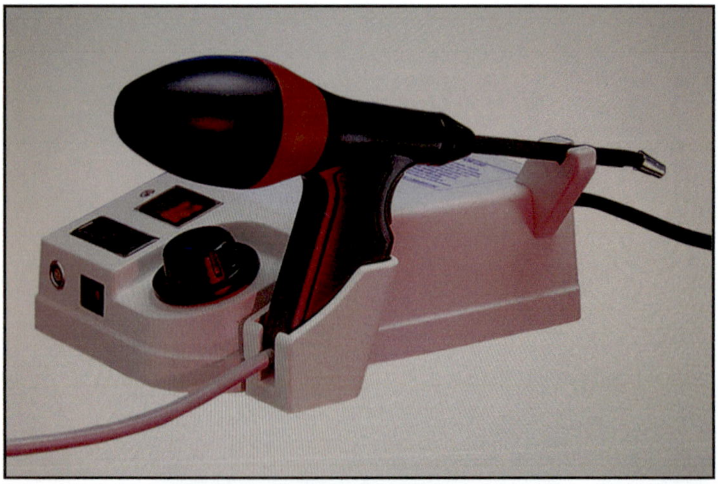

Figure 2-12. The IRC for internal hemorrhoid treatment. (Reprinted with permission from Redfield Corporation.)

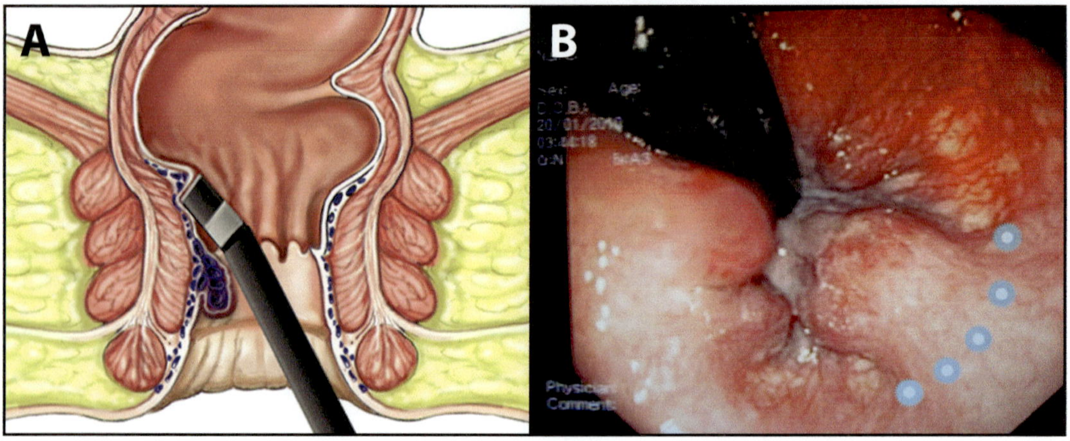

Figure 2-13. (A) An IFR probe makes contact with the base of the internal hemorrhoid well above the dentate line. (Reprinted with permission from Redfield Corporation.) (B) The blue circles demonstrate the area for infrared energy delivery.

BIPOLAR DIATHERMY AND DIRECT CURRENT ELECTROTHERAPY

Hemorrhoid energy therapy (HET, Medtronic/Covidien) is a newer device (Figure 2-14) that uses bipolar energy approved for grades I and II internal hemorrhoids. This device is a modified anoscope with a treatment window through which the hemorrhoid tissue just proximal to the internal hemorrhoid base is caught, and energy is applied until the temperature reaches about 50°F in order to cause low-energy coagulation of the hemorrhoid. All 3 hemorrhoids are treated at one visit. In a retrospective study of 23 patients, it was shown to be safe and effective, with sedation being optional.[25] A more recent prospective case series of 20 patients showed it to be comparable with hemorrhoid banding for grades I and II internal hemorrhoids.[26]

Direct current electrotherapy requires a prolonged application of 110-V direct current (up to 15 mA) for periods up to 15 minutes or more to the base of each hemorrhoidal complex. Both the current and time requirements increase for larger hemorrhoids. It has lost its appeal because of the lengthy treatment times.[27]

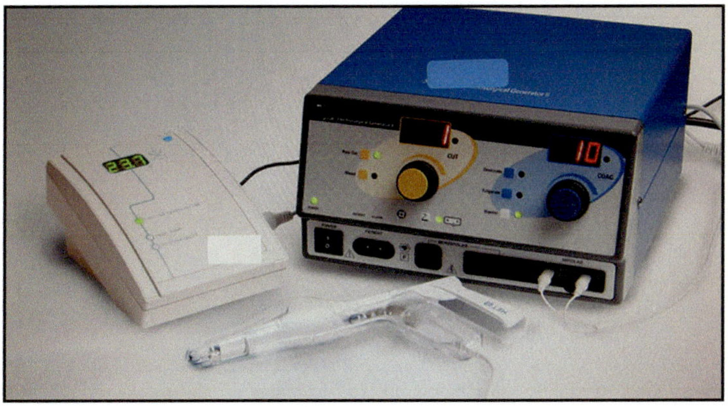

Figure 2-14. The HET bipolar device by Medtronic/Covidien.

SCLEROTHERAPY

Morgan in Dublin first described sclerotherapy in 1869. Although still performed today, it is reserved for first- and second-degree hemorrhoids. A submucosal injection of 2 mL 5% phenol in almond or vegetable oil or a sclerosant such as sodium tetradecyl sulfate is injected just proximal to the internal hemorrhoid column. It is performed through an anoscope under direct vision using a long 25- or 30-gauge needle and takes only minutes. A raised bleb confirms the proper depth of injection. This causes thrombosis of the vessels, shrinkage through scarring, and fixation to the rectal wall, decreasing blood flow and prolapse. Although effective, the symptoms seem to recur in about 3 years.[28] Although the procedure is minimally invasive, discomfort or pain is reported in 12% to 70% of patients and may last up to 48 hours.[29-31] Transient bacteremia is reported in 8%, suggesting antibiotic prophylaxis in high-risk individuals.[32] Rare but potentially serious complications include prostatic or hepatic abscess, retroperitoneal sepsis, and the dreaded necrotizing fasciitis.[33-35] Impotence, urinary retention, and anaphylactic shock have been reported.[35,36]

CRYOTHERAPY

A freezing cryoprobe ablates the hemorrhoidal tissue in this procedure. Although the procedure is not painful, it is associated with prolonged discomfort, a foul-smelling discharge, and a persistent hemorrhoidal mass.[37] Therefore, it has gone out of favor.

COMPARISON OF THE IN-OFFICE HEMORRHOID TREATMENT DEVICES

The studies are few, but 2 meta-analyses comparing RBL with IRC found that, although RBL was more effective, patients seemed to prefer IRC because it was less likely to cause discomfort or pain. In a meta-analysis of 18 randomized prospective studies comparing in-office treatments, banding was more effective, requiring fewer sessions and a lower need for retreatment, compared with sclerotherapy or IRC.[16,38] In another study, when a combination of RBL and IRC was used, symptoms had resolved at the 1-month follow-up.[39] In that study, there was no preference for IRC over RBL.

RBL is probably the most effective of the nonsurgical in-office techniques for grades I, II, and III internal hemorrhoids that have failed conservative treatment.[40] As expected, banding proved less effective and less painful and had fewer complications than surgery.[41] Operative hemorrhoidectomy is indicated for large third- and fourth-degree hemorrhoids, mixed hemorrhoids with prominent external hemorrhoids, and incarcerated hemorrhoids.

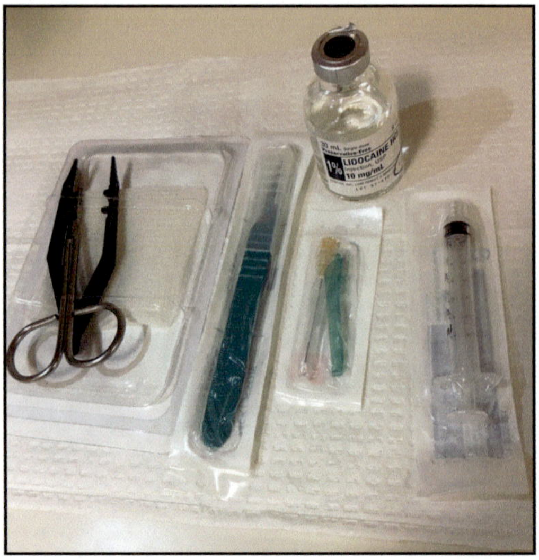

Figure 2-15. Office kit for incision clot removal in thrombosed hemorrhoids.

Treatment of Thrombosed External Hemorrhoids

Hemorrhoids cause pain usually only when they undergo acute thrombosis. Patients present with acute-onset anal pain and a palpable exquisitely tender lump at the anal orifice. Thrombosis occurs more commonly in external hemorrhoids than internal ones. Pain onset is usually sudden and intense. Diagnosis is easily confirmed by inspection of the perineum and digital rectal examination if the patient will allow it. If the patient presents within 72 hours of onset, excision or incision and drainage of the clot will produce immediate relief.[42] After this time, the clot is likely beginning to resolve, and conservative treatment with analgesia, sitz baths, and perhaps nitroglycerin for the associated sphincter spasm will help with pain as symptoms slowly settle. Thrombosed hemorrhoids are common, and one should keep an incision and drainage kit in the office (Figure 2-15). This would consist of a scalpel, 1% lidocaine, forceps, and 4 × 4 gauze.

References

1. Johanson JF, Sonnenberg A. The prevalence of hemorrhoids and chronic constipation. An epidemiologic study. *Gastroenterology*. 1990;98(2):380-386.
2. Johanson JF, Sonnenberg A. Temporal changes in the occurrence of hemorrhoids in the United States and England. *Dis Colon Rectum*. 1991;34(7):585-591.
3. Johanson JF. Hemorrhoids. In: Everhart JE, ed. *Digestive Diseases in the United States: Epidemiology and Impact*. US Department of Health and Human Services, Public Health Service, National Institutes of Health, National Institute of Diabetes and Digestive and Kidney Diseases. Washington, DC: US Government Printing Office; 1994:273-298; NIH Publication No. 94-1447.
4. Thomson WH. The nature of haemorrhoids. *Br J Surg*. 1975;62(7):542-552.
5. Morgado PJ, Suárez JA, Gómez LG, Morgado PJ Jr. Histoclinical basis for a new classification of hemorrhoidal disease. *Dis Colon Rectum*. 1988;31(6):474-480.
6. Stankevicius E, Kevelaitis E, Vainorius E, Simonsen U. [Role of nitric oxide and other endothelium-derived factors]. *Medicina (Kaunas)*. 2003;39(4):333-341.
7. Bleday R, Pena JP, Rothenberger DA, Goldberg SM, Buls JG. Symptomatic hemorrhoids: current incidence and complications of operative therapy. *Dis Colon Rectum*. 1992;35(5):477-481.
8. Beck DE, Perry WB. History and physical examination. In: Beck DE, ed. *Handbook of Colorectal Surgery*. 2nd ed. New York, NY: Marcel Dekker Inc; 2003:31-42.
9. Alonso-Coello P, Mills E, Heels-Ansdell D, et al. Fiber for the treatment of hemorrhoids complications: a systematic review and meta-analysis. *Am J Gastroenterol*. 2006;101(1):181-188.

10. Alonso-Coello P, Guyatt G, Heels-Ansdell D, et al. Laxatives for the treatment of hemorrhoids. *Cochrane Database Syst Rev*. 2005;4:CD004649.
11. Sardinha TC, Corman ML, Hemorrhoids. *Surg Clin North Am*. 2002;82:1153-1167.
12. Johannsson HO, Graf W, Pahlman L. Bowel habits in hemorrhoid patients and normal subjects. *Am J Gastroenterol*. 2005;100:401-406.
13. Johanson JF. Nonsurgical treatment of hemorrhoids. *J Gastrointest Surg*. 2002;6(3):290-294.
14. Godeberge P. Daflon 500 mg in the treatment of hemorrhoidal disease: a demonstrated efficacy in comparison with placebo. *Angiology*. 1994;45(6, pt 2):574-578.
15. Cospite M. Double-blind, placebo-controlled evaluation of clinical activity and safety of Daflon 500 mg in the treatment of acute hemorrhoids. *Angiology*. 1994;45(6, pt 2):566-573.
16. MacRae HM, McLeod RS. Comparison of hemorrhoidal treatment modalities. A meta-analysis. *Dis Colon Rectum*. 1995;38(7):687-694.
17. Albuquerque A. Rubber band ligation of hemorrhoids: a guide for complications. *World J Gastrointest Surg*. 2016;8(9):614-620.
18. Bat L, Melzer E, Koler M, Dreznick Z, Shemesh E. Complications of rubber band ligation of symptomatic internal hemorrhoids. *Dis Colon Rectum*. 1993;36(3):287-290.
19. Walker AJ, Leicester RJ, Nicholls RJ, Mann CV. A prospective study of infrared coagulation, injection and rubber band ligation in the treatment of haemorrhoids. *Int J Colorectal Dis*. 1990;5(2):113-116.
20. Jutabha R, Jensen DM, Chavalitdhamrong D. Randomized prospective study of endoscopic rubber band ligation compared with bipolar coagulation for chronically bleeding internal hemorrhoids. *Am J Gastroenterol*. 2009;104(8):2057-2064.
21. Johanson JF, Rimm A. Optimal nonsurgical treatment of hemorrhoids: a comparative analysis of infrared coagulation, rubber band ligation, and injection sclerotherapy. *Am J Gastroenterol*. 1992;87(11):1600-1606.
22. Russell TR, Donohue JH. Hemorrhoidal banding. A warning. *Dis Colon Rectum*. 1985;28(5):291-293.
23. Sim HL, Tan KY, Poon PL, et al. Life-threatening perineal sepsis after rubber band ligation of haemorrhoids. *Tech Coloproctol*. 2009;13:161-164.
24. Poen AC, Felt-Bersma RJ, Cuesta MA, Devillé W, Meuwissen SG. A randomized controlled trial of rubber band ligation versus infra-red coagulation in the treatment of internal haemorrhoids. *Eur J Gastroenterol Hepatol*. 2000;12(5):535-539.
25. Kantsevoy SV, Bitner M. Nonsurgical treatment of actively bleeding internal hemorrhoids with a novel endoscopic device (with video). *Gastrointest Endosc*. 2013;78(4):649-653.
26. Randall GM, Jensen DM, Machicado GA, et al. Prospective randomized comparative study of bipolar versus direct current electrocoagulation for treatment of bleeding internal hemorrhoids. *Gastrointest Endosc*. 1994;40(4):403-410.
27. Yang R, Migikovsky B, Peicher J, Laine L. Randomized, prospective trial of direct current versus bipolar electrocoagulation for bleeding internal hemorrhoids. *Gastrointest Endosc*. 1993;39(6):766-769.
28. Tokunaga Y, Sasaki H, Saito T. Evaluation of sclerotherapy with a new sclerosing agent and stapled hemorrhoidopexy for prolapsing internal hemorrhoids: retrospective comparison with hemorrhoidectomy. *Dig Surg*. 2010;27(6):469-472.
29. Cocorullo G, Tutino R, Falco N, et al. The non-surgical management for hemorrhoidal disease. A systematic review. *G Chir*. 2017;38(1):5-14.
30. Kanellos I, Goulimaris I, Vakalis I, et al. Long-term evaluation of sclerotherapy for haemorrhoids. A prospective study. *Int J Surg Investig*. 2000;2:295-298.
31. Crawshaw BP, Russ AJ, Ermlich BO, Delaney CP, Champagne BJ. Prospective case series of a novel minimally invasive bipolar coagulation system in the treatment of grade I and II internal hemorrhoids. *Surg Innov*. 2016;23(6):581-585.
32. Adami B, Eckardt VF, Suermann RB, Karbach U, Ewe K. Bacteremia after proctoscopy and hemorrhoidal injection sclerotherapy. *Dis Colon Rectum*. 1981;24(5):373-374.
33. Yoshikawa K, Kawashima R, Hirose Y, et al. Liver injury after aluminum potassium sulfate and tannic acid treatment of hemorrhoids. *World J Gastroenterol*. 2017;23(27):5034-5040.
34. Suh YJ, Ha HK, Oh HK, Shin R, Jeong SY, Park KJ. Rectal perforation caused by anal stricture after hemorrhoid treatment. *Ann Coloproctol*. 2013;29:28-30.
35. Murray-Lyon IM, Kirkham JS. Hepatic abscesses complicating injection sclerotherapy of haemorrhoids. *Eur J Gastroenterol Hepatol*. 2001;13:971-972.
36. Pilkington SA, Bateman AC, Wombwell S, Miller R. Anatomical basis for impotence following haemorrhoid sclerotherapy. *Ann R Coll Surg Engl*. 2000;82(5):303-306.
37. Smith LE, Goodreau JJ, Fouty WJ. Operative hemorrhoidectomy versus cryodestruction. *Dis Colon Rectum*. 1979;22:10-16.
38. Marques CF, Nahas SC, Nahas CS, Sobrado CW Jr, Habr-Gama A, Kiss DR. Early results of the treatment of internal hemorrhoid disease by infrared coagulation and elastic banding: a prospective randomized cross-over trial. *Tech Coloproctol*. 2006;10(4):312-317.

39. Linares Santiago E, Gómez Parra M, Mendoza Olivares FJ, Pellicer Bautista FJ, Herrerías Gutiérrez JM. Effectiveness of hemorrhoidal treatment by rubber band ligation and infrared photocoagulation. *Rev Esp Enferm Dig.* 2001;93(4):238-247.

40. Poen AC, Felt-Bersma RJ, Cuesta MA, Devillé W, Meuwissen SG. A randomized controlled trial of rubber band ligation versus infra-red coagulation in the treatment of internal haemorrhoids. *Eur J Gastroenterol Hepatol.* 2000;12(5):535-539.

41. Shanmugam V, Thaha MA, Rabindranath KS, Campbell KL, Steele RJ, Loudon MA. Rubber band ligation versus excisional haemorrhoidectomy for haemorrhoids. *Cochrane Database Syst Rev.* 2005;3:CD005034.

42. Greenspon J, Williams SB, Young HA, Orkin BA. Thrombosed external hemorrhoids: outcome after conservative or surgical management. *Dis Colon Rectum.* 2004;47(9):1493-1498.

3

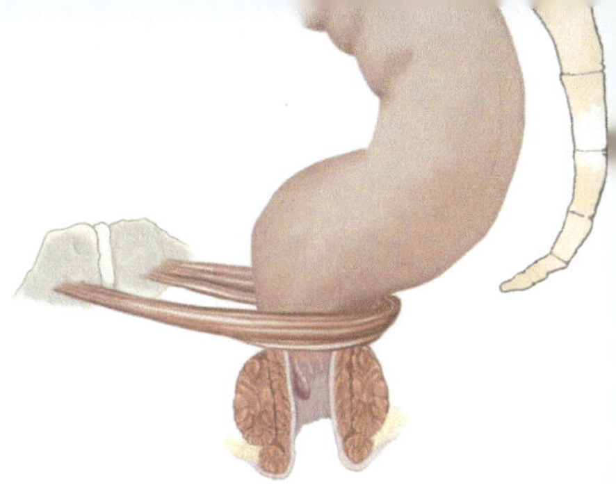

Anal Fissures

Mitchel Guttenplan, MD, FACS

Key Points

- At least 20% of patients complaining of hemorrhoids have coexistent anal fissures.
- Fissures are located in the posterior midline 80% to 90% of the time and in the anterior midline 10% to 20% of the time.
- Women have more anterior fissures than men, but they still have posterior fissures more often than they have anterior fissures.
- Many patients with fissures have mild or intermittent symptoms.
- The diagnosis of a fissure is a clinical one because most cannot be visualized.
- Nonsurgical treatment includes diet and behavioral measures, topical medications, and, for persistent disease and resistant patients, botulinum toxin.
- Surgery should be reserved for patients failing nonsurgical treatment.

Perianal issues, including hemorrhoids and fissures, are very common in Western cultures. The vast majority of these issues can be successfully treated without surgery, and many of these patients will present to their primary care provider, their gynecologist, or their gastroenterologist[1] looking for care. Many postgraduate training programs do not include the evaluation and treatment of many of these perianal problems in their curriculum,[2] so patients are all too often referred for surgical care.

It is the goal of this chapter to provide some clarity on the evaluation and treatment of patients with anal fissures because, in our experience, fissures are frequently overlooked and are commonly responsible for patients' residual symptoms after treatment of another perianal issue fails to resolve all of their symptoms.

Qureshi W, ed. *Diagnosis and Management Guide for Anorectal Disease: A Clinical Reference* (pp 27-35).

Figure 3-1. Classic findings with a chronic anal fissure. (Reprinted with permission from Iain Cleator, MD and CRH Medical Corp.)

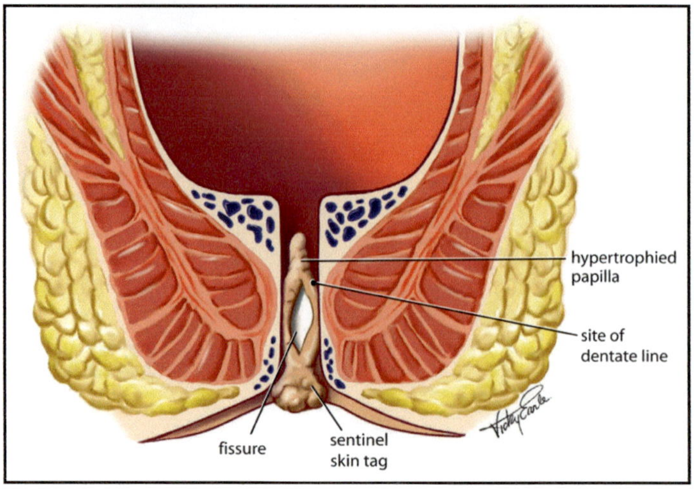

Anatomy

The anal canal is approximately 4 cm in length, extending from the anal verge to the levator complex. The so-called *dentate line* is located approximately 2 cm from the verge and represents the junction of the squamous anoderm and columnar mucosa.[3] The internal anal sphincter (IAS) has been described as the continuation of the longitudinal smooth muscle of the rectum and is contracted while "at rest," helping to maintain continence. The IAS relaxes during defecation, allowing for the passage of stool.[4] The external anal sphincter (EAS), on the other hand, is composed of striated muscle, which extends in an anterior-posterior direction, dividing around the anus and providing more support laterally than it does posteriorly and anteriorly (which may come into play when we talk about the pathogenesis of an anal fissure).[5]

As demonstrated in Figure 3-1, anal fissures are linear breaches of the anoderm, generally distal to the dentate line, which may or may not extend past the anal verge. Secondary signs of a fissure can include a bit of hypertrophic tissue at the introitus known as a *sentinel tag* or *sentinel pile*. Similarly, a "hypertrophic papilla" can be noted at the proximal margin of the fissure. In the case of a deeper, chronic fissure, transverse fibers of the internal sphincter may be noted, serving as the base of the fissure (see Figure 3-1). Anal fissures are classically found in the midline, with approximately 90% occurring posteriorly and 10% anteriorly. Women tend to have anterior fissures more commonly than men, but they still have many more fissures posteriorly than anteriorly.

Approximately 1% of fissures are "atypical" and, therefore, not in the midline. These atypical fissures can occur in patients with anorectal carcinoma, Crohn's disease, immunodeficiency syndromes such as AIDS, tuberculosis, and a number of sexually transmitted diseases.[6] The treatment of these "atypical" fissures requires treatment of the underlying disease rather than the treatments discussed in this chapter.

Etiology and Pathophysiology

An anal fissure is an extremely common ailment; in one colorectal clinic's experience, the prevalence of fissures among its patients was 10%.[7] In addition, at least 20% of patients with symptomatic hemorrhoids also have anal fissures,[8] and the prevalence rate of hemorrhoids has been stated to be as low as 4.4%[9] and as high as 40%.[10] It is our contention that fissures occur much more frequently than many expect and, therefore, are often overlooked by practitioners.

There are a number of factors that have been described as being involved in the development of anal fissures, including trauma to the anoderm by the passage of a large, hard stool or the passage of multiple diarrheal stools.[5] Initial minor tears likely occur often, healing spontaneously rather than progressing to an acute or chronic fissure.[11]

POSTERIOR ANAL FISSURES

As noted previously, approximately 90% of symptomatic fissures are located in the posterior midline because it seems that "tears" tend to occur here more commonly as well as the fact that an injury in the posterior midline is much less likely to heal than one anywhere else around the circumference of the anorectum. These nonhealing superficial "tears" then progress to become more classic fissures.

Tears are most likely to occur in the posterior midline, in part because the supporting musculature of the external sphincter is weakest at the posterior commissure,[5] and, according to Perry,[12] forces created during defecation are the strongest at the posterior midline because of the anorectal angle, causing the breach of the anoderm in this location.

Although most tears heal spontaneously, those occurring in the posterior midline have more difficulty doing so. Postmortem angiography has revealed that in 85% of subjects, there is a paucity of blood vessels in the posterior midline, and Doppler studies confirm that the area is poorly perfused in these patients.[13] In addition, patients with posterior fissures tend to have a hypertonic IAS (as do patients with symptomatic hemorrhoids). Although it is not completely clear whether the hypertonic sphincter predisposes the patient to the development of a fissure (and/or symptomatic hemorrhoids) or if it is caused by the disease, the relationship is clear.[14-16] Studies have shown that the contraction of the EAS is similar in both anal fissure patients and controls, so it seems as if the IAS is solely responsible for this phenomenon.[17] This hypertonic sphincter further reduces blood flow to the affected area, and it is this hypertonia that is so often the target of both medical and surgical treatment of fissure disease.

ANTERIOR ANAL FISSURES

Approximately 10% of anal fissures occur in the anterior midline. Women tend to have these more often than men, and they often occur without increased anal pressures. These cases have been said to be associated with a vaginal delivery, a complicated episiotomy, a rectocele, rectoanal intussusception, and EAS dysfunction or injury.[18]

ACUTE VERSUS CHRONIC ANAL FISSURES

Acute fissures appear as simple breaches or tears of the anoderm, whereas chronic fissures are characterized by the presence of fibrosis and often the secondary signs of an anal fissure (ie, sentinel pile, hypertrophic papillae, and visible internal sphincter fibers in the base of the wound). From a time perspective, chronicity has been described as being symptomatic for a certain length of time, generally considered anywhere from 4 to 12 weeks, depending on the author.[19,20]

DIAGNOSIS

The classic presentation of an anal fissure includes complaints of severe pain on defecation, the "passing of razor blades," postdefecation pain,[5] a visible open wound of the anoderm (Figure 3-2) in the posterior position, and severe pain when attempting to perform an anorectal examination; the diagnosis is a relatively easy one to reach. Many to most cases of anal fissures are far more subtle in their presentation, and the symptoms are so often wrongly attributed to "hemorrhoids" that many fissures are not diagnosed.[21]

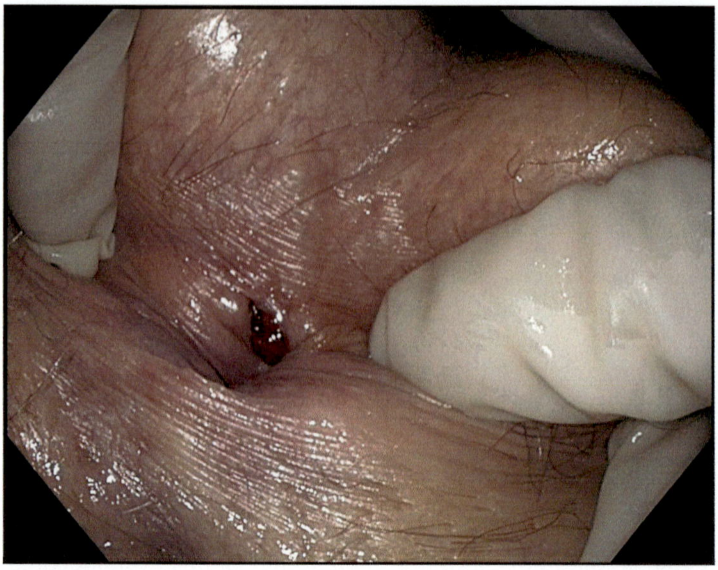

Figure 3-2. Physical examination showing a posterior anal fissure. (Reprinted with permission from Waqar Qureshi, MD.)

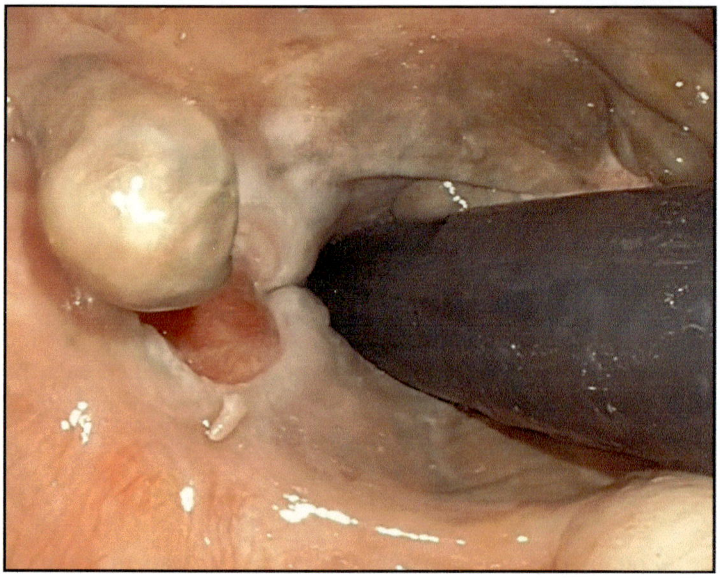

Figure 3-3. An endoscopic view of a posterior anal fissure and the accompanying hypertrophic papilla.

Because an anal fissure extends distally from the dentate line, much or all of it resides within the anal canal, so external visual inspection will only identify those fissures running to and past the anal verge. A flexible endoscope may help us to see the proximal-most aspect of a fissure or the hypertrophic papilla, which extends proximally from a chronic fissure (Figure 3-3); however, a flexible endoscope is generally a poor tool to use in order to identify anorectal issues. Kelly[22] noted that a flexible scope in retroflexion missed almost half of the anorectal issues present in the patients examined as opposed to an anoscope, which identified 99% of the issues.

In addition to the value of anoscopy, digital rectal examination is an invaluable tool in the evaluation of these patients. Tenderness in the midline, regardless of the severity, or palpation of a scar or induration in the midline of the distal anal canal may well represent a fissure that is partially healed and extremely difficult to see, even when using anoscopy.[21] In light of all of this, we recommend that the diagnosis of an anal fissure is a clinical one, and the proper evaluation of these patients requires the use of an anoscope and digital rectal examination.

Medical Treatment

Although surgical approaches are more reliable in their ability to treat anal fissures, their cost and potential for postoperative complications compel us to attempt more conservative treatments first, reserving surgical options for those who fail conservative treatments.

DIETARY AND BEHAVIORAL MODIFICATION

It has been estimated that adults should consume 25 to 30 g of dietary fiber daily along with sufficient fluid intake in order to create a large, soft, bulky stool. Western diets are typically lacking in dietary fiber, so supplemental fiber is recommended, along with sitz baths or application of heat. Soft, bulky stools result in a "physiologic dilatation," both helping with the healing of the fissure as well as limiting its recurrence, and the heat encountered when taking sitz baths relieves sphincter spasms, which are responsible for most patients' pain.[23-25] There have also been longstanding recommendations to limit one's time on the commode as a part of these recommendations.

TOPICAL MEDICATIONS

Topical Anesthetics

Topical anesthetics may well provide symptomatic relief, but they do not affect the healing of the fissure[26] and, if used, should be used alongside other measures.

Topical Nitroglycerin

Topical nitrates used intra-anally have been shown to be helpful in the healing of anal fissures. In smooth muscle cells (found in the IAS), nitrates are metabolized into nitric oxide, which causes relaxation of the sphincter.[27,28] This relaxation leads to increased anodermal blood flow, and although a *Cochrane Review*[29] concluded that nitrates are only marginally better than placebo in the treatment of fissures, there are a number of individual studies demonstrating superior results.[30]

The use of topical nitrates has been associated with postadministration headaches in up to 70% of patients,[26] severe enough in up to 20% of patients to cause them to discontinue treatment.[31] The side effects seem to be dose dependent whereas efficacy is not, according to a study looking at fissure patients receiving 0.1%, 0.2%, or 0.4% nitroglycerin ointment. Each group had similar pain relief and rates of fissure healing, but patients receiving the more concentrated compounds had increasing rates of headaches.[32] With this information in mind, our own practice is to use a "pea-sized" amount of a compound of 0.125% nitroglycerin ointment intra-anally 3 times per day for 8 to 12 weeks. If compounding is not available, then others will use a pea-sized amount of the commercially available 0.4% nitroglycerin ointment with a bit of lubricant as the dose,[33] as opposed to the prescribing recommendation of using 1 inch of the ointment per dose. It is this 1-inch dose that has been associated with very high rates of headaches.[34]

Patients taking erectile dysfunction medications should not be given topical nitrates because of the potential of developing acute hypotension.[35-37] It has been suggested that this should not be a concern if it has been at least 24 hours since the last dose of sildenafil[38] or 48 hours after a dose of tadalafil.[39,40]

Topical Calcium Channel Blockers

In order to avoid the headaches that can accompany the administration of higher concentrations of nitroglycerin ointment, many advocate the use of topical calcium channel blockers (eg, nifedipine and diltiazem), which also lower IAS pressures.[41] There have been individual studies showing healing rates of up to 95% when using diltiazem[42]; however, the same *Cochrane Review*[29] cited previously noted that, although these medications caused fewer adverse effects (headaches), it could not be concluded whether they offered any advantage over placebo. For these reasons, we typically use these medications with our patients failing or not tolerating an initial course of nitroglycerin ointment or those taking erectile dysfunction medications, as the safety profile of calcium channel blockers seems to be superior to nitroglycerin when taking erectile dysfunction medications.[43]

With the exception of 0.4% nitroglycerin ointment, the use of the remainder of these topical medications is "off-label." We have found that a number of insurers will not cover the cost of the 0.4% ointment, which can exceed $600.[44] Many insurers will also not cover the cost of compounded medications, causing difficulty for a number of patients to obtain these medications. We have spoken with some physicians who, as a "work-around," will prescribe nifedipine capsules for their patients, which are covered. The patient then cuts the capsules open, using the liquid within the capsule for their dose. We have no personal experience with this technique, but it presents an interesting alternative to accommodate the needs of some patients.

BOTULINUM TOXIN A

Botulinum toxin (BT) is a neurotoxin produced by the bacterium *Clostridium botulinum*. Its mechanism of action in striated muscle is to bind to the presynaptic terminal at the neuromuscular junction, prohibiting the release of acetylcholine and causing muscular paralysis. However, in the smooth muscle of the IAS, the mechanism of action is likely different because blockage of acetylcholine release would actually increase IAS tone rather than decrease it.[28] In the IAS, BT is believed to act on the postganglionic sympathetic nerves to release norepinephrine, which, in turn, blocks sympathetic output and, by doing so, relaxes the internal sphincter. These changes persist for 2 to 3 months until reinnervation occurs.[45] This has often been referred to as a *temporary chemical sphincterotomy*.

The clinical data have been somewhat mixed with BT, but a large meta-analysis[29] has confirmed that BT is superior to placebo, and a double-blind, randomized study[46] comparing 20 U BT with placebo not only demonstrated a healing rate of 73% for BT versus 13% with placebo, but also 70% of the placebo failures were healed when subsequently treated with BT. BT has also been shown to be effective in patients failing topical therapy.[47]

There have been innumerable suggested protocols for the use of BT in the treatment of anal fissures without any real consensus as to the dosage of BT to be used or the number and location(s) of injections. BT has been used in doses ranging from 5 to 100 U and has been injected into the IAS, the EAS, and the intersphincteric groove, each with varying numbers of injection sites.[6,20] We follow one of the more commonly used protocols of 25 U divided into 2 injections into the IAS on either side of the midline because it is technically very simple to perform and has excellent response rates with minimal complaints of postinjection incontinence.[46] Reports of incontinence of flatus in up to 18% of patients and of stool in up to 5% of patients have been described,[48] but using the techniques recommended previously, we have not seen this to be a problem. Cost is another issue because BT is considered "off-label" when used for anal fissures and, therefore, is not covered by many insurers.[49] For these reasons, it seems reasonable to use BT as a second-line treatment if topical medications fail. Of note, the use of topical nitroglycerin has been shown to potentiate the actions of BT,[50] so we continue recommending topical therapy even if a BT injection is performed on a resistant patient.

SURGICAL TREATMENT

In cases in which more conservative treatment options fail, surgical care should be considered.

ANAL DILATION

Anal dilation for the treatment of anal fissures was first described in the 1860s and became more popular in the 1960s,[6] in and around the same time that Dr. Lord described what became known as the *Lord's stretch* for the treatment of symptomatic hemorrhoids.[51] The initial dilation techniques were quite extreme because the procedure was performed with progressive force so that 4 fingers could be inserted into the canal, and outward pressure was held for several minutes.[52] The technique has been criticized for its lack of uniformity in technique and dilation pressures and the fact that disruption of the IAS and/or EAS may occur.[53] A *Cochrane Review*[54] noted that a lateral internal sphincterotomy offers better efficacy, lower recurrence rates, and, most importantly, fewer cases of postprocedural incontinence than manual dilation.

There have been efforts to help standardize the dilation of the internal sphincter using pneumatic balloons, and these results have been promising with good clinical results but without significant incontinence numbers.[55,56]

INTERNAL SPHINCTEROTOMY

Historically, there have been references to some form of sphincterotomy for anal fissures dating back to the 1800s, but in 1959, an evaluation of the anatomy and physiology led to the description of what was a posterior internal sphincterotomy by Eisenhammer.[57] Although the procedure was helpful in the healing of chronic anal fissures, it also caused what became known as a *keyhole deformity* at the anal opening, resulting in an unsatisfactory rate of incontinence issues. Later work demonstrated that these issues did not occur if the sphincterotomy was performed laterally, so this became the procedure of choice in most centers because the rate of incontinence issues seemed to be less than 6%.[23]

Lateral internal sphincterotomy has become the surgical treatment of choice for patients failing medical management because the procedure provides results superior to dilation, posterior fissurectomy/sphincterotomy, BT, etc. The procedure can be performed either "open" or "closed" with similar results,[20] and in one guideline piece,[58] it was suggested that it may be offered as a first-line treatment as well.

ANOPLASTY WITH A LOCAL ADVANCEMENT FLAP

A number of authors have achieved excellent results by creating a local advancement flap and suturing it in place over the fissure site without affecting the IAS, thus limiting the risk of postsurgical incontinence.[59,60] These procedures may be especially valuable in the subset of fissure patients without significant IAS spasms because there is reasonable concern that dividing a nonhypertonic IAS may leave the patient more prone to developing incontinence than healing the fissure. As noted earlier, anterior fissures may be associated with EAS damage rather than with hypertonia; these procedures may offer significant advantages in these circumstances.

CONCLUSION

The prevalence rate of perianal symptoms is quite high in Western cultures. Patients tend to "blame" all of these symptoms on their hemorrhoids when, in fact, associated anal fissures (which are very common) are often responsible for at least a portion of these issues. The textbook presentation of a patient with a symptomatic anal fissure (searing pain, visible fissure, and severe pain on examination) is a relatively uncommon one because the majority of fissure patients have had at least some healing of the fissure by the time they present for treatment. The diagnosis should be a clinical one because many to most fissures are not visible due to the location in the anal canal or partial healing.

The treatment of anal fissures consists of dietary and behavioral recommendations (supplemental fiber, increased fluid intake, sitz baths, and minimal time on commode), topical therapy with nitrates, or calcium channel blockers. For those who are resistant to these treatments, consideration should be given to injection of the IAS with BT, and if problems persist, surgical intervention should be considered. Lateral internal sphincterotomy is very effective but has a small chance of causing problems with continence, so it should be held in reserve for patients resistant to more conservative treatments.

References

1. Guttenplan M, Ganz RA. Hemorrhoids: office management and review for gastroenterologists. https://www.crhsystem.com/assets/pdfs/Touch_Gastroenterology_Guttenplan_Ganz.pdf. Accessed June 13, 2019.
2. Di Palma JA. Introducing comprehensive non-surgical anorectal care to the gastroenterology fellowship training curriculum: The University of South Alabama Experience. *Pract Gastroenterol.* 2011;5:31-36.
3. Wexner SD, Jorge JMN. Anatomy and embryology of the anus, rectum, and colon. In: Corman ML, ed. *Colon and Rectal Surgery*. Philadelphia, PA: Lippincott-Raven; 1998.
4. Shawki S, Sands DR. Anorectal physiology. In: Sands LR, Sands DR, eds. *Ambulatory Colorectal Surgery*. New York, NY: Informa Healthcare; 2008:21-44.
5. Corman ML. Anal fissure. In: Corman ML, ed. *Colon and Rectal Surgery*. 4th ed. Philadelphia, PA: Lippincott-Raven; 1998.
6. Zaghiyan KN, Fleshner P. Anal fissure. *Clin Colon Rectal Surg.* 2011;24(1):22-30.
7. Pescatori M, Interisano A. Annual report of the Italian coloproctology units. *Tech Coloproctol.* 1995;3:29-30.
8. Schubert MC, Sridhar S, Schade RR, Wexner SD. What every gastroenterologist needs to know about common anorectal disorders. *World J Gastroenterol.* 2009;15(26):3201-3209.
9. Johanson JF, Sonnenberg A. The prevalence of hemorrhoids and chronic constipation. An epidemiologic study. *Gastroenterology*. 1990;98:380-386.
10. Janicke DM, Pundt MR. Anorectal disorders. *Emerg Med Clin North Am.* 1996;14:757-788.
11. Poritz LS. Anal fissure. *Medscape*. https://emedicine.medscape.com/article/196297-overview. Accessed November 20, 2017.
12. Perry GG. Fissure in ano—a complication of anusitis. *South Med J.* 1962;55:955-957.
13. Klosterhalfen B, Vpogel P, Rixen H, Mittermayer C. Topography of the inferior rectal artery: a possible cause of chronic, primary anal fissure. *Dis Colon Rectum.* 1989;32:43-52.
14. Deutsch AA, Moshkovitz M, Nudelman I, et al. Anal pressure measurements in the study of hemorrhoid etiology and their relation to treatment. *Dis Colon Rectum.* 1987;30:855-857.
15. Sun WM, Read NW, Shorthouse AJ. Hypertensive anal cushions as a cause of the high anal canal pressures in patients with haemorrhoids. *Br J Surg.* 1990;77:458-462.
16. Sardinha TC, Corman ML. Hemorrhoids. *Surg Clin North Am.* 2002;82:1153-1167.
17. Gibbons CP, Read NW. Anal hypertonia in fissures: cause or effect? *Br J Surg.* 1986;73:443-445.
18. Jenkins JT, Urie A, Molloy RG. Anterior anal fissures are associated with occult sphincter injury and abnormal sphincter function. *Colorectal Dis.* 2008;10(3):280-285.
19. Gavin J, Cuffy M, Abir F, Longo WE. Benign anorectal disease: an update on diagnosis and management. *JAAPA*. 2006;19(6):28-33.
20. Perry WB, Dykes SL, Buie WD, Rafferty JF; Standards Practice Task Force of the American Society of Colon and Rectal Surgeons. Practice parameters for the management of anal fissures (3rd revision). *Dis Colon Rectum.* 2010;53(8):1110-1115.
21. Guttenplan M. Anal fissures: diagnosis and management for the gastroenterologist. *Gastro Endo News.* 2015;66:10.
22. Kelly SM, Sanowski RA, Foutch PG, et al. A prospective comparison of anoscopy and fiberendoscopy in detecting anal lesions. *J Clin Gastroenterol.* 1986;8(6):658-660.
23. Shawki S, Costedio M. Anal fissure and stenosis. *Gastroenterol Clin North Am.* 2013;42(4):729-758.
24. Hananel N, Gordon PH. Reexamination of the clinical manifestations and responses to therapy of fissure-in-ano. *Dis Colon Rectum.* 1997;40:229-233.
25. Jensen SL. Maintenance therapy with unprocessed bran in the prevention of acute anal fissure recurrence. *J R Soc Med.* 1987;80:296-298.
26. Lacy BE, Weiser K. Common Anorectal disorders: diagnosis and treatment. *Curr Gastroenterol Rep.* 2009;11:413-419.
27. Loder PB, Kamm MA, Nicholls RJ, et al. 'Reversible chemical sphincterotomy' by local application of glyceryl trinitrate. *Br J Surg.* 1994;81(9):1386-1389.
28. American Society of Cataract and Refractive Surgery. (n.d.). Hemorrhoids & fissure-in-ano. https://physicians.crhsystem.com/wp-content/uploads/ASCRS-Hemorrhoids-and-Fissure-in-ano.pdf
29. Nelson R. Non surgical therapy for anal fissure. *Cochrane Database Syst Rev.* 2006;4:CD003431.
30. Lund JN, Scholefield JH. A randomised, prospective, double-blind, placebo controlled trial of glyceryl trinitrate ointment in treatment of anal fissure. *Lancet.* 1997;349(9044):11-14.
31. Bailey HR, Beck DE, Billingham RP, et al; Fissure Study Group. A study to determine the nitroglycerin ointment dose and dosing interval that best promote the healing of chronic anal fissures. *Dis Colon Rectum.* 2002;45:1192-1199.
32. Scholefield JH, Bock JU, Marla B, et al. A dose finding study with 0.1%, 0.2%, and 0.4% glyceryl trinitrate ointment in patients with chronic anal fissures. *Gut.* 2003;52:264-269.

33. Henderson PK, Cash BD. Common anorectal conditions: evaluation and treatment. *Curr Gastroenterol Rep.* 2014;16(10):408.
34. Rectiv [package insert]. Bridgewater, NJ: Aptalis Pharma US, Inc; 2013.
35. Viagra [package insert]. New York, NY: Pfizer Inc; 2015.
36. Levitra [package insert]. Whippany, NY: Bayer Healthcare Pharmaceuticals, Inc; 2014.
37. Cialis [package insert]. Indianapolis, IN: Lilly USA, LLC; 2014.
38. Kloner RA, Mitchell M, Emmick JT. Cardiovascular effects of tadalafil. *Am J Cardiol.* 2003;92:37M-46M.
39. Kloner RA, Hutter AM, Emmick JT, Mitchell MI, Denne J, Jackson G. Time course of the interaction between tadalafil and nitrates. *J Am Coll Cardiol.* 2003;42(10):1855-1860.
40. Kloner RA. Erectile dysfunction and hypertension. *Int J Impot Res.* 2007;19(3):296-302.
41. Bhardwaj R, Vaizey CJ, Boulos PB, Hoyle CH. Neuromyogenic properties of the internal anal sphincter: therapeutic rationale for anal fissures. *Gut.* 2000;46(6):861-868.
42. Shrivastava UK, Jain BK, Kumar P, et al. A comparison of the effects of diltiazem and glyceryl trinitrate ointment in the treatment of chronic anal fissure: a randomized clinical trial. *Surg Today.* 2007;37:482-485.
43. Webb DJ, Freestone S, Allen MJ, Muirhead GJ. Sildenafil citrate and blood-pressure-lowering drugs: results of drug interaction studies with an organic nitrate and a calcium antagonist. *Am J Cardiol.* 1999;83:21C-28C.
44. GoodRx. Rectiv. https://www.goodrx.com/rectiv. Accessed January 15, 2018.
45. Jones OM, Brading AF, Mortensen NJ. The mechanism of action of botulinum toxin on the internal anal sphincter. *Br J Surg.* 2004;91:224-228.
46. Maria G, Cassetta E, Gui D, Brisinda G, Bentivoglio AR, Albanese A. A comparison of botulinum toxin and saline for the treatment of chronic anal fissure. *N Engl J Med.* 1998;338:217-220.
47. Lindsey I, Jones OM, Cunningham C, George BD, Mortensen NJ. Botulinum toxin as second-line therapy for chronic anal fissure failing 0.2 percent glyceryl trinitrate. *Dis Colon Rectum.* 2003;46:361-366.
48. Wald A, Bharucha AE, Cosman BC, Whitehead WE. ACG clinical guideline: management of benign anorectal disorders. *Am J Gastroenterol.* 2014;109(8):1141-1157.
49. Johnson EK, Steele SR. Anal fissure. In: Bailey HR, Billingham RP, Stamos MJ, et al. *Colorectal Surgery*. New York, NY: Elsevier; 2013:117-128.
50. Lysy J, Israelit-Yatzkan Y, Sestiery-Ittah M, Weksler-Zangen S, Keret D, Goldin E. Topical nitrates potentiate the effect of botulinum toxin in the treatment of patients with refractory anal fissure. *Gut.* 2001;48:221-224.
51. Lord PH. A new regime for the treatment of haemorrhoids. *Proc R Soc Med.* 1968;61(9):935-936.
52. Watts JM, Bennett RC, Goligher JC. Stretching of anal sphincters in treatment of fissure-in-ano. *Br Med J.* 1964;2(5405):342-343.
53. Speakman CT, Burnett SJ, Kamm MA, et al. Sphincter injury after anal dilatation demonstrated by endosonography. *Br J Surg.* 1991;78:1429-1430.
54. Nelson RL. Operative procedures for fissure in ano. *Cochrane Database Syst Rev.* 2010;1:CD002199.
55. Sohn N, Eisenberg MM, Weinstein MA, Lugo RN, Ader J. Precise anorectal sphincter dilatation—its role in the therapy of anal fissures. *Dis Colon Rectum.* 1992;35(4):322-327.
56. Renzi A, Izzo D, Di Sarno G, et al. Clinical, manometric, and ultrasonographic results of pneumatic balloon dilatation vs. lateral internal sphincterotomy for chronic anal fissure: a prospective, randomized, controlled trial. *Dis Colon Rectum.* 2008;51(1):121-127.
57. Eisenhammer S. The evaluation of the internal anal sphincterotomy operation with special reference to anal fissure. *Surg Gynecol Obstet.* 1959;109:583-590.
58. Orsay C, Rakinic J, Perry WB, et al. Practice parameters for the management of anal fissures (revised). *Dis Colon Rectum.* 2005;47(12):2003-2007.
59. Giordano P, Gravante G, Grondona P, et al. Simple cutaneous advancement flap anoplasty for resistant chronic anal fissure: a prospective study. *World J Surg.* 2009;33:1058-1063.
60. Nyam DC, Wilson RG, Stewart KJ, et al. Island advancement flaps in the management of anal fissures. *Br J Surg.* 2005;82(3):326-328.

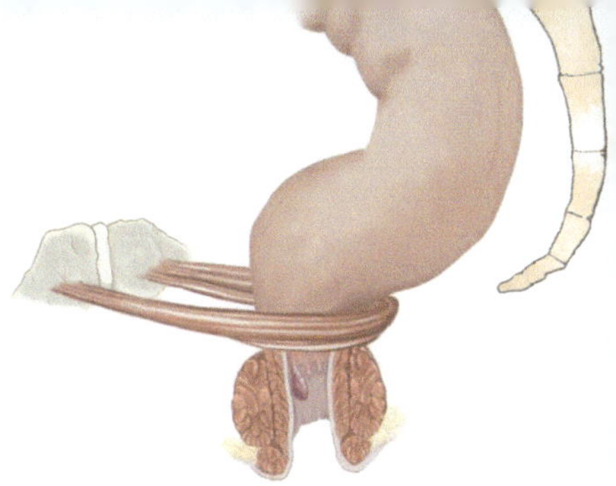

4

Abscesses and Fistulas of the Anorectum

Lisa M. Haubert, MD, MS, FASCRS and Lisa S. Brubaker, MD

Key Points

- Obstruction of the anal cryptoglandular unit causes abscesses (acutely) and fistulas (chronically).
- Symptoms of anorectal abscesses include fever, swelling, and a constant anal pain that is not necessarily associated with bowel movements.
- About 30% of patients with a perianal abscess will develop an anal fistula.
- The Parks classification is most commonly used to classify a fistula-in-ano.
- The Parks classification categorizes fistulas based on the relationship of the fistula tract to the external sphincter and puborectalis muscle; this allows the physician to determine whether either of these muscles of continence may be affected by surgical treatment of the fistula.
- The anorectal muscles are organized as 2 cylinders, the internal and external sphincters. Anorectal abscesses/fistulas and their associated surgical interventions can disrupt these cylinders and cause fecal incontinence.
- Diagnosis of an anorectal abscess can be based on history and physical examination alone.
- A fistula-in-ano can be diagnosed by performing a history and physical examination with anoscopy, sigmoidoscopy, and/or examination under anesthesia.
- Patients with anorectal fistulas are less likely to have fevers and swelling and more likely to have chronic purulent or sanguineous drainage.

Qureshi W, ed. *Diagnosis and Management Guide for Anorectal Disease: A Clinical Reference* (pp 37-47).

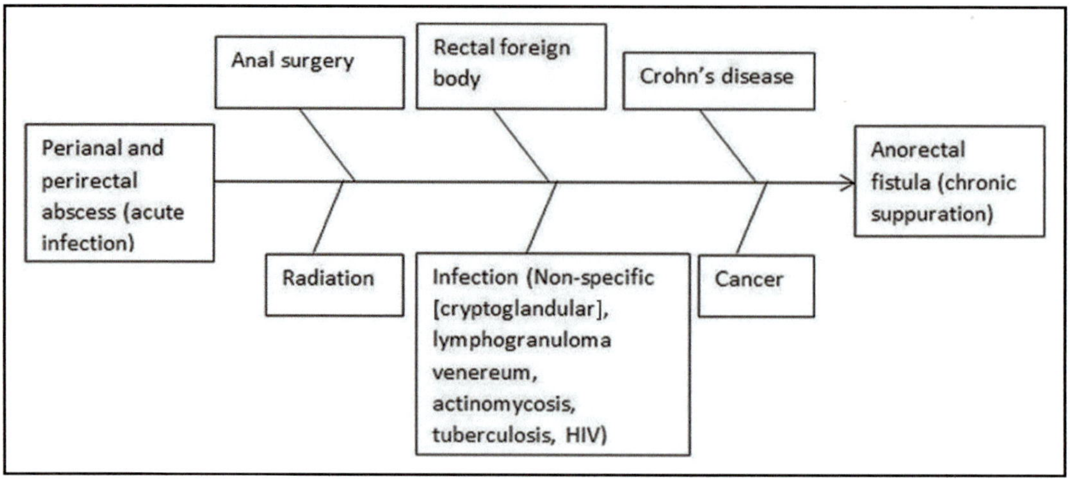

Figure 4-1. Etiology: anorectal abscesses and fistulas represent different stages on a common pathogenic spectrum.

- In the absence of symptoms suggestive of Crohn's disease, HIV, malignancy, or a serious underlying medical problem, laboratory evaluation and imaging studies are not necessary in the diagnosis of anorectal abscesses/fistulas.
- Timely surgical treatment is indicated for both anorectal abscesses and fistulas unless the patient has Crohn's disease, HIV, or malignancy.
- Patients with Crohn's disease, HIV, or malignancy can develop complex anorectal abscesses/fistulas. These patients require additional diagnostic evaluations and are often primarily treated with medications (antibiotics and immune-modulating agents) rather than with surgery.
- Fistulotomy, endoanal advancement flaps, noncutting setons, and ligation of the intersphincteric fistula tract (LIFT) are the procedures recommended to treat anorectal fistulas. Fibrin glue, fistula plugs, and cutting setons are not recommended.
- Anorectal abscesses and fistulas can be debilitating and difficult to treat; the goal of surgical operations is to eradicate infectious foci and preserve continence.

Pathophysiology

The pathogenesis of anorectal abscesses and fistulas is a continuum of the same anorectal infectious process[1] (Figure 4-1). Abscesses represent the acute phase of infection and are caused by obstruction of the anal cryptoglandular unit.[2] This obstruction results in stasis, infection, and acute abscess formation.[2,3] Chronic infections can track from the inciting anal gland through the anorectal region to form a persistently discharging fistula.[4] Although an acute abscess may resolve completely, ~30% of patients with perianal abscesses develop anal fistulas.[5,6] Inflammatory, traumatic, and malignant conditions are notable but rare causes of abscesses and fistulas.[7] Inflammatory abscesses caused by Crohn's disease, tuberculosis, actinomycosis, and lymphogranuloma venereum may be explained by reactivity of the lymphoid tissue surrounding the glands in the intersphincteric zone.[8] Impalement, foreign bodies, and surgeries, such as episiotomies, hemorrhoidectomies, and prostatectomies, are traumatic causes of anorectal abscesses.[9] Anal carcinoma, leukemia, lymphoma, and radiation may also predispose to anorectal abscesses.[10]

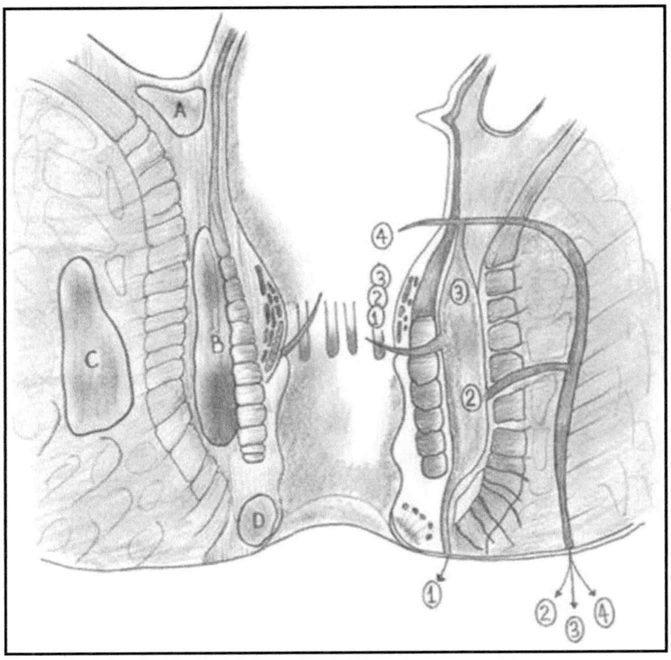

Figure 4-2. Locations of anorectal abscesses: (A) supralevator; (B) intersphincteric; (C) ischiorectal; (D) perianal. The direction of fistula spread: (1) intersphincteric; (2) transsphincteric; (3) suprasphincteric; (4) extrasphincteric.

Anorectal abscesses are classified based on their location within the potential anorectal spaces (ie, perianal, intersphincteric, ischiorectal, supralevator, and horseshoe; Figure 4-2).[1,11] The most common type of abscess, a perianal abscess, forms when an anorectal abscess traverses distally in the intersphincteric groove into the perianal skin.[1] An intersphincteric abscess is defined as an abscess that does not spread out of the intersphincteric space.[1] Lateral and superior spread of the infection results in ischiorectal and supralevator abscesses, respectively.[1] A horseshoe abscess results from circumferential spread through the supralevator, ischioanal, or intersphincteric spaces.[12] Although pain, fever, and swelling are common symptoms of all abscesses, additional clinical signs and symptoms may vary depending on the anatomic location of the abscess (Table 4-1).[13,14] Compared with other anorectal pathologic processes (ie, hemorrhoids and anal fissures), the pain associated with anorectal abscesses is often constant and not necessarily associated with a bowel movement.[14]

Once an abscess has ruptured or is drained, an epithelialized track (fistula) can form between the abscess cavity and the perianal/perirectal skin.[1,15] The internal opening of a fistula is most often at the dentate line (ie, the site of anal crypts) because these crypts represent the internal openings of the anal glands.[1] The external opening of a fistula often corresponds with the drainage site of a previous abscess.[1] Parks et al[8] classified fistulas based on the relationship of the fistula track to the external anal sphincter and puborectalis muscles. This anatomic classification of fistulas is critical because it allows the physician to quickly determine whether either of these muscles of continence may be affected by surgical treatment of the fistula.[8]

Parks et al[8] found that all fistulas could be classified into 1 of 4 main groups based on their involvement of the external anal sphincter and/or puborectalis muscles (Figure 4-3). Intersphincteric fistulas arise from perianal abscesses. Intersphincteric fistulas open in the perianal skin and do not involve the external sphincter muscle. The fistula tract passes within the intersphincteric space. Transsphincteric fistulas arise from ischioanal abscesses, and the tract extends through the external anal sphincter into the ischiorectal fossa. The tract of these fistulas remains distal to the puborectalis and terminates in the skin overlying the buttock. Suprasphincteric fistulas arise from supralevator abscesses. The tract extends over the entire external sphincter, including the puborectalis, before traveling through the puborectalis/levator ani into the ischiorectal fossa. Suprasphincteric fistulas

Table 4-1

Clinical Symptoms Associated With Different Types of Anorectal Abscesses

ABSCESS LOCATION	SYMPTOM	OTHER
Perianal abscess	Tender, erythematous, swollen region at anal verge	Most common anorectal abscess
Intersphincteric abscess	Asymptomatic or may present as pain out of proportion to physical exam. Can be palpated during digital rectal exam as a fluctuant mass protruding into the lumen. No visible external manifestations.	Account for 2% to 5% of anorectal abscesses
Ischiorectal abscess	Abscess may become quite large before appearance of physical exam findings. Pain and fever may develop before detection of obvious tender, indurated, or fluctuant mass in the buttocks.	Induration can be felt above the anorectal ring through the rectal wall.
Supralevator abscess	Vague pelvic or abdominal discomfort, gluteal pain, urinary retention, tenesmus, fever. Digital exam: induration or fluctuation felt above the level of the anorectal ring. In general, lack of external manifestations.	Originates from superior spread of cryptoglandular infection or from pelvic infectious processes, such as diverticulitis or Crohn's disease; most rare form of anorectal abscess.
Horseshoe abscess	Perianal swelling, pain, or drainage; fever, leukocytosis, or sepsis.	The nature and extent of these lesions frequently fail to be recognized; rigid anatomic boundaries force the abscess to extend laterally into one or both ischiorectal spaces.

exit via the skin overlying the buttock. Extrasphincteric fistulas pass from perineal/buttock skin through ischiorectal fat and levator muscles into the rectum; they may or may not be associated with a transsphincteric tract. Extrasphincteric fistulas due to trauma (ie, foreign body penetration of the perineum with subsequent tracking through the rectal wall or foreign body penetration of the rectal wall with subsequent tracking through the perineum) are not associated with a transsphincteric tract. Extrasphincteric fistulas arise from trauma to the rectum, Crohn's disease, or carcinoma.[8] Intersphincteric fistulas are the most common type of fistula and occur with a frequency of 70%.[8] The frequency distribution of transsphincteric, suprasphincteric, and extrasphincteric fistulas is 23%, 5%, and 2%, respectively.[8] Using this anatomic classification to diagnose fistulas allows the surgeon to surmise whether or not the muscles of continence will be affected during surgical management of the fistula.

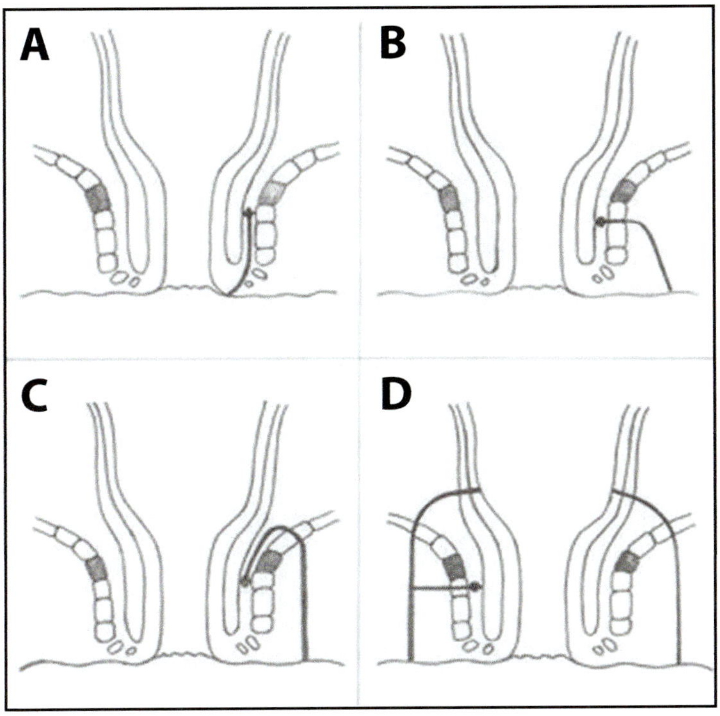

Figure 4-3. The classification of fistula-in-ano based on the involvement of external anal sphincter and puborectalis muscles: (A) intersphincteric; (B) transsphincteric; (C) suprasphincteric; (D) extrasphincteric.

The symptoms of an anorectal fistula include chronic purulent drainage associated with a pustule-like lesion in the perianal/buttock region.[4] Patients may recount a history of a "nonhealing" abscess, especially after abscess drainage.[16] Unlike the chronic pain and chance of fever associated with anorectal abscesses, patients with anorectal fistulas often have intermittent pain associated with defecation, may have bleeding secondary to the granulation tissue within the fistula track, and are less likely to report fevers.[15]

Pertinent Anatomy

ANATOMIC RELATIONS OF THE ANAL CANAL AND ANORECTAL SPACES

Understanding anorectal anatomy and the relationship of the anus to the surrounding structures is pivotal in the evaluation and management of anorectal abscesses and fistulas because both of these diseases are classified according to anatomic location. Anorectal abscesses are classified according to their location in anorectal spaces, and fistulas are classified in relationship to the anorectal musculature.[1,8,15] Anteriorly, the anal canal is attached by dense connective tissue to the perineal body. The perineal body separates the anal canal from the membranous urethra and penile bulb in males and from the lower vaginal wall in females. Laterally, the anal canal is surrounded by loose adipose tissue within the ischiorectal fossa. The posterior anus is attached to the coccyx by the anococcygeal ligament.

The anorectal spaces are potential spaces where anorectal abscesses and fistulas form and spread, respectively[1,15] (Figure 4-4). The perianal space is located deep to the anal verge, and it is continuous with the ischioanal fat laterally and with the intersphincteric space superiorly. The intersphincteric space lies between the internal and external sphincter muscles and travels superiorly until the level of the levator ani. Lateral to the external anal sphincter is the ischioanal fossa. The ischioanal fossa

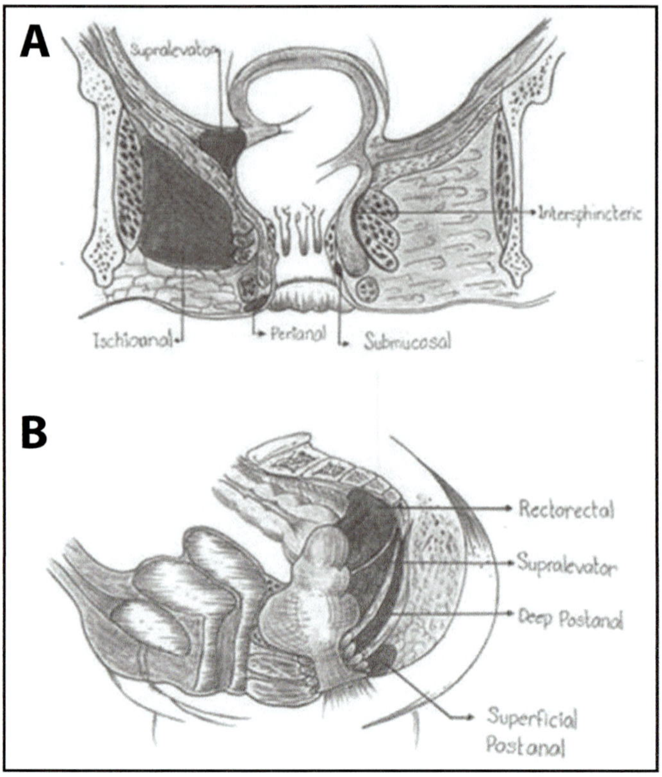

Figure 4-4. Anorectal spaces (sites of anorectal abscess formation): (A) coronal; (B) sagittal.

extends from the levator ani to the perineum; it is bound anteriorly by the transverse perineal muscles, superiorly by the levator ani, medially by the external anal sphincter, posteriorly by the gluteus maximus and sacrotuberous ligament, and laterally by the obturator internus. The supralevator space extends from the levator ani to the peritoneum; the rectal wall and the pelvic wall form the medial and lateral borders, respectively. The deep postanal space exists between the anococcygeal ligament (inferior border) and the levator ani (superior border).

MUSCLES OF THE ANAL CANAL

The muscles of the anal canal play a crucial role in continence, and the anatomy is critical because fistulas are classified in relationship to these muscles.[8] According to Parks et al,[8] the anorectal muscles can be thought of as 2 cylinders, one within the other. Deep to the mucosa and submucosa is the internal anal sphincter. The internal sphincter is a continuation of the inner circular muscle of the rectum. Deep to the internal sphincter is the intersphincteric plane, which contains the conjoined longitudinal muscle (a continuation of the outer longitudinal muscle layer of the rectum mixed with fibers of the levator ani muscle). The mucosa, submucosa, internal sphincter, and conjoined longitudinal muscle represent the inner cylinder of the anorectal muscles. Deep to the intersphincteric plane is the external anal sphincter. The external sphincter joins the puborectalis and the levator ani to form a continuous, funnel-shaped sheet of striated muscle. The levator ani divides the abdominal cavity from the perineum. The external anal sphincter, puborectalis, and levator ani represent the outer cylinder of anorectal muscles. This outer cylinder is attached to the coccyx posteriorly by the anococcygeal ligament and to the urethra (in men) and vaginal wall (in women) anteriorly by the perineal body.

THE EPITHELIUM OF THE ANAL CANAL

The epithelium of the surgical anal canal will be emphasized because the surgical anal canal extends from the anal verge to the levator ani and is, therefore, longer than the anatomic anal canal, which only extends from the anal verge to the dentate line.[3,17] This distinction is important because many complex fistulas exist within the surgical anal canal. From the most distal end of the rectum to the dentate line is the proximal anal canal. The epithelium in this region of the anal canal represents the anal transition zone (ie, the area between the rectal [simple columnar] and anal [squamous] epithelium).[17] The internal hemorrhoidal plexus is deep to the anal transition zone and imparts a purple hue to the epithelium. The dentate line separates the anal transition zone from the anal epithelium and represents the location of the anal valves and anal sinuses.[18]

The anal sinuses serve as the openings for the anal glands.[2,3] From their openings at the anal sinuses, the anal gland ducts travel deep to enter the submucosa. The majority of the anal gland ducts continue to travel deep through the internal anal sphincter before terminating in the intersphincteric plane.[3] Within the intersphincteric plane, the glandular structures are surrounded by lymphoid tissue; this may account for the frequency with which tuberculosis and Crohn's disease affect this region.[8] The anal glands are visceral structures that do not extend beyond the intersphincteric plane into the external sphincter group of muscles.[8] As described previously, obstruction of these ducts is the primary mechanism in the formation of perianal abscesses and fistulas.[1,2]

Distal to the dentate line is the anatomic anal canal. The anal epithelium in this region is a modified squamous epithelium that is devoid of hair follicles, sweat, or sebaceous glands. Normal skin begins at the anal verge and contains hair and apocrine sweat glands.

CONSERVATIVE TREATMENT OPTIONS

The American Society of Colon and Rectal Surgeons has issued practice parameters for the treatment of perianal abscesses and fistulas.[19] Based on these guidelines, a conservative approach is recommended for the evaluation of anorectal abscesses and fistulas. A disease-specific history and physical examination are appropriate to distinguish anorectal abscesses from other perianal suppurative processes. If a fistula is suspected based on the patient's history, anoscopy and sigmoidoscopy can be used to visualize the internal opening of a fistula. In the absence of clinical features or systemic symptoms suggestive of Crohn's disease, malignancy, or a serious underlying medical problem, laboratory evaluation and imaging studies are not necessary. If the diagnosis is unclear, magnetic resonance imaging with or without endoanal coils and endoanal ultrasound have higher rates of sensitivity and accuracy than fistulography or a computed tomographic scan.[20] Alternatively (or additionally), fistula tracts can be identified by performing an examination under anesthesia.

Once an anorectal abscess is diagnosed, the American Society of Colon and Rectal Surgeons strongly recommends timely surgical treatment.[19] Conservative management with antibiotics is ineffective and can result in sepsis, necrotizing infection, or the formation of a more complicated abscess, which can injure the sphincter muscles.[21] The mainstay of fistula treatment is also surgical; specific goals of fistula surgery include preventing recurrence and preserving sphincter function.[8]

A major caveat to contemporary abscess/fistula therapy is in patients with Crohn's disease or HIV. Upon initial presentation, these patients require additional preoperative evaluations (endoanal ultrasound or magnetic resonance imaging) to delineate the fistulous tracts[19,22]; a computed tomographic scan may be necessary to delineate fistulas and abscesses from rectal inflammation.[19,22] Additionally, the primary treatment of perianal Crohn's disease is medical rather than surgical.[19,22] Medical management (antibiotics and immune-modulating agents) is attempted primarily because patients with Crohn's disease experience poor wound healing, a higher risk of sphincter injury, and a high frequency of disease relapse subsequent to surgical intervention.[22] Patients with HIV more often have incomplete anal fistulas, leading to blind sinus tracts.[23] Similar to patients with Crohn's

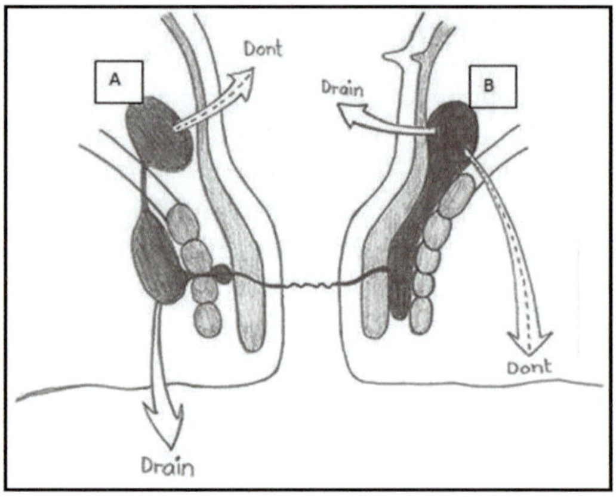

Figure 4-5. The technique of supralevator abscess drainage depends on the origin of the abscess. (A) Supralevator abscesses with ischioanal origins should be drained through the perianal skin. (B) Supralevator abscesses with intersphincteric origins should be drained through the rectum.

disease, patients with HIV also suffer from impaired wound healing. In these populations, it is generally recommended to manage fistulizing disease with antibiotics.[23] Long-term draining setons are recommended for patients with complex fistulas or sepsis who require surgery.[19,23,24]

Surgical Options

SURGICAL TREATMENT OF ANORECTAL ABSCESSES

Although the treatment of anorectal abscesses is incision and drainage, variations of the procedure are required to adequately treat the different types of anorectal abscesses.[21] Perianal and ischioanal abscesses can be drained via a cruciate or elliptical incision located as close to the anal side of the abscess as possible (this minimizes the complexity of a subsequent fistula).[21] It is not necessary to pack the abscess cavity after incision and drainage.[19] A prospective, randomized, controlled trial comparing packing with nonpacking of the abscess cavity revealed that the rate of abscess recurrence, the postoperative fistula rate, and pain scores at the first dressing change were similar between patients who packed versus those who did not pack the abscess cavity.[25]

Intersphincteric abscesses should be drained into the rectum by making a mucosal incision below the dentate line and dividing the internal sphincter up to the dentate line.[21] The abscess cavity remains open to drain.

Supralevator abscesses are drained differently depending on their origin. Supralevator abscesses that are upward extensions of ischioanal abscesses should be drained through a skin incision (similar to ischioanal abscesses), whereas those that are extensions of intersphincteric or pelvic abscesses should be drained through the rectum to avoid creating an extrasphincteric fistula[8,26] (Figure 4-5).

Adequately draining postanal and horseshoe abscesses requires gaining access to the deep postanal space.[12] To enter the postanal space, an incision is made between the coccyx and anus. The superficial external sphincter and anococcygeal ligament can be divided to drain the posterior infection. An opening is also made in the internal sphincter in order to drain the gland in which the infection originated. Because postanal abscesses also spread laterally into the ischioanal spaces (ie, horseshoe abscesses), counter incisions can be made in the skin over the ischioanal fossa to allow additional drainage[12] (Figure 4-6).

There is active debate about whether fistulotomy should be performed in conjunction with incision and drainage in patients who have anorectal abscesses with observed fistula tracts. Although a meta-analysis published in 2006[27] and a *Cochrane Review* published in 2010[28] both concluded that sphincter-cutting procedures (fistulectomy or fistulotomy) performed concurrently with incision and drainage resulted in a statistically significant reduction in recurrence rate and a nonsignificant

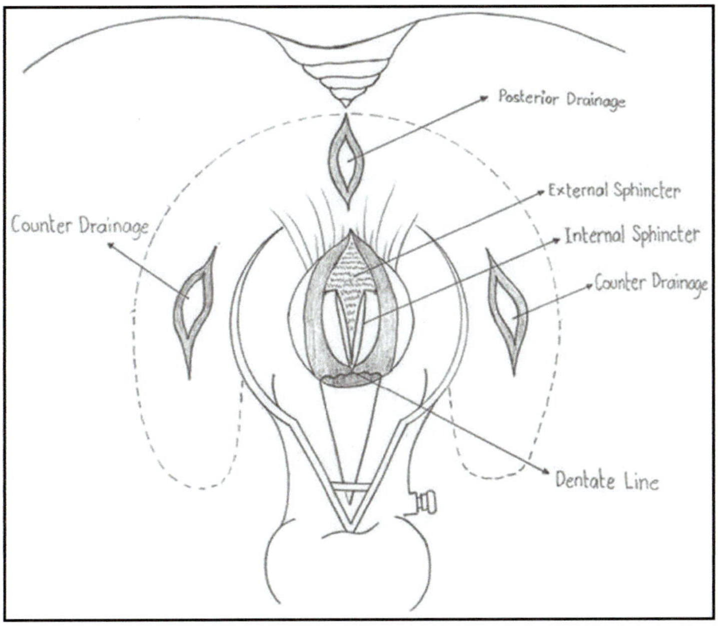

Figure 4-6. Drainage of a horseshoe abscess.

increased risk of fecal incontinence, there are still no guidelines that definitively recommend concomitant fistulotomy.[19] Therefore, clinicians should weigh the benefits of fistulectomy/fistulotomy (eg, a decreased rate of persistent fistula/abscess, abscess recurrence, and subsequent surgery) against the risks (eg, incontinence) for each patient. Delayed fistulotomy (ie, 6-12 weeks after treatment of the initial anorectal abscess) is often cited as a favorable option because it provides time for edema and inflammation to subside, facilitating identification of the fistula track.[21]

SURGICAL TREATMENT OF FISTULA-IN-ANO

Surgical treatment of a fistula-in-ano aims to obliterate all fistula openings and tracts while minimizing sphincter division to preserve fecal continence.[8,11] This can be accomplished by identifying the internal fistula opening and all tracts relative to the sphincter muscles preoperatively in the clinic or with imaging. The tract is identified during surgery by careful insertion of a fistula probe through the entire tract. If further evaluation of the tract is needed despite preoperative digital examination, imaging, and anoscopy/sigmoidoscopy, intraoperative measures including hydrogen peroxide/methylene blue injection of the external opening can be used to identify the tract origin.[20] It is also important to consider that no single operation can be used to treat all anorectal fistulas. Similar to the treatment of anorectal abscesses, the appropriate procedure depends on the location of the fistula.[8]

Intersphincteric and low transsphincteric fistulas have long been treated by the fistulotomy/lay open technique.[8] In this procedure, a probe is inserted from the external opening along the tract to the internal opening at the dentate line.[15] The tissue overlying the probe is then incised and the granulation tissue curetted. The edges of the incision can then be sewn to the tract (marsupialized). This procedure only causes the lower half of the internal sphincter to be divided; therefore, there is minimal risk of incontinence.[8] The American Society of Colon and Rectal Surgeons strongly recommends that simple anal fistulas be treated by fistulotomy with marsupialization.[19]

There are several surgical procedures used to treat complex anal fistulas. Complex fistulas are defined as those that are suprasphincteric; are extrasphincteric; encompass >30% of the external sphincter; have high tracks proximal to the dentate line; are rectovaginal or anterior fistulas in women; are fistulas with multiple tracts; are recurrent fistulas; are fistulas in patients with inflammatory bowel disease, infectious disease (tuberculosis/HIV), or a history of radiation; or are fistulas in patients with anal incontinence.[15] The American Society of Colon and Rectal Surgeons strongly recommends endoanal advancement flaps or the use of a seton and/or staged fistulotomy for complex fistulas. According to these guidelines, the data on the LIFT are too preliminary to formally recommend this procedure as a treatment for complex anal fistulas.[19]

Endoanal advancement flaps, setons, and LIFT are the procedures recommended to treat complex fistulas.[19] These procedures are recommended because they allow the surgeon to preserve the anal sphincter muscles.[19,29,30] In the advancement flap procedure, a mobilized flap of healthy mucosa and submucosa is mobilized to close off the internal opening of the fistula. This allows the tract to heal and close. A noncutting seton can be placed for drainage and is used to eradicate the septic focus and to promote maturation of the tract before eradication of the fistula.[15] Cutting setons (ie, a seton that is placed through the fistula tract and tightened at regular intervals) are no longer recommended because they are associated with a high risk of anal incontinence.[31] LIFT is another sphincter-sparing procedure. In this procedure, the intersphincteric tract is identified and isolated by dissection between the internal and external anal sphincter muscles. The fistula tract is identified within the intersphincteric plane, ligated, and divided. A meta-analysis[32] has been performed to evaluate LIFT. Compared with an anorectal advancement flap, LIFT has similar results in regard to success rate, incontinence status, and complications, but has significantly better results regarding operative time and time to return to normal activity.[32] Furthermore, there was no association between the placement of a pre-LIFT drainage seton and the success of LIFT, indicating that LIFT can be performed as a standalone treatment.[32] Regardless of the surgical technique used, it is important to provide long-term follow-up for the patient to evaluate for incontinence and recurrence.

Of note, fibrin glue injections and anal fistula plugs are not recommended for the treatment of simple or complex anal fistula disease.[19] Although these treatments offer advantages such as ease of use, low morbidity, and repeatability, the rate of healing is decreased compared with fistulotomy, especially when patients are evaluated for longer follow-up periods.[19]

Anorectal abscesses and fistulas can be potentially debilitating, difficult to treat, and associated with high rates of recurrence or complications. Fortunately, an appreciation for the complexity of this disease has kindled advancements in the evaluation and management of patients with anorectal abscesses and fistulas. Surgical operations that aim to eradicate infectious foci and preserve continence remain paramount in the management of anorectal abscesses and fistulas.

References

1. Eisenhammer S. A new approach to the anorectal fistulous abscess on the high intramuscular lesion. *Surg Gynecol Obstet.* 1958;106(5):595-599.
2. Hill MR, Shryock EH, ReBell FG. Role of the anal glands in the pathogenesis of ano-rectal disease. *JAMA.* 1943;121(10):742-746.
3. Tucker CC, Hellwig C. Anal ducts: comparative and developmental histology. *Arch Surg.* 1935;31(4):521-530.
4. Parks AG, Morson BC. The pathogenesis of fistula-in-ano. *Proc R Soc Med.* 1962;55:751-754.
5. Vasilevsky CA, Gordon PH. The incidence of recurrent abscesses or fistula-in-ano following anorectal suppuration. *Dis Colon Rectum.* 1984;27:126-130.
6. Pearce L, Newton K, Smith SR, et al. Multicentre observational study of outcomes after drainage of acute perianal abscess. *Br J Surg.* 2016;103(8):1063-1068.
7. Rizzo JA, Naig AL, Johnson EK. Anorectal abscess and fistula-in-ano: evidence-based management. *Surg Clin North Am.* 2010;90(1):45-68.
8. Parks AG, Gordon PH, Hardcastle J. A classification of fistula-in-ano. *Br J Surg.* 1976;63(1):1-12.
9. Cash DJ, Sadat MM, Abu-Own AS. Anorectal abscess and fistula caused by an ingested chicken bone. *Am J Gastroenterol.* 2004;99:1617-1618.
10. Chen CY, Cheng A, Haung SY, et al. Clinical and microbiological characteristics of perianal infections in adult patients with acute leukemia. *PLoS One.* 2013;8(4):e60624.
11. Parks AG. Pathogenesis and treatment of fistula-in-ano. *BMJ.* 1961;1(5224):463-469.

12. Hamilton C. Anorectal problems: the deep postanal space—surgical significance in horseshoe fistula and abscess. *Dis Colon Rectum.* 1975;18(8):642-645.
13. Parks AG, Thomson JP. Intersphincteric abscess. *Br Med J.* 1973;2(5865):537-539.
14. Schubert MC, Sridhar S, Schade RR, Wexner SD. What every gastroenterologist needs to know about common anorectal disorders. *World J Gastroenterol.* 2009;15(26):3201-3209.
15. Lilius HG. Fistula-in-ano, an investigation of human foetal anal ducts and intramuscular glands and a clinical study of 150 patients. *Acta Chir Scand Suppl.* 1968;383:7-88.
16. Thompson H. The orthodox conception of fistula-in-ano and its treatment. *Proc R Soc Med.* 1962;55:754.
17. Dujovny N, Quiros RM, Saclarides TJ. Anorectal anatomy and embryology. *Surg Oncol Clin N Am.* 2004;13(2):277-293.
18. Milligan ET, Morgan CN. Surgical anatomy of the anal canal with special reference to anorectal fistule. *Lancet.* 1934;2:1213-1217.
19. Steele SR, Kumar R, Feingold DL, Rafferty JL, Buie WD; Standards Practice Task Force of the American Society of Colon and Rectal Surgeons. Practice parameters for perianal abscess and fistula-in-ano. *Dis Colon Rectum.* 2011;54(12):1465-1474.
20. Saranovic D, Barisic G, Krivokapic Z, Masulovic D, Djuric-Stefanovic A. Endoanal ultrasound evaluation of anorectal diseases and disorders: technique, indications, results and limitations. *Eur J Radiol.* 2007;61(3):480-489.
21. Goligher J. *Surgery of the Anus, Rectum and Colon.* Springfield, IL: Charles C Thomas; 1961.
22. Lightner AL, Faubion WA, Fletcher JG. Interdisciplinary management of perianal Crohn's disease. *Gastroenterol Clin North Am.* 2017;46:547-562.
23. Aleali M, Gottesman L. Anorectal disease in HIV-positive patients. *Clin Colon Rectal Surg.* 2001;14:265-273.
24. Pearl RK, Andrews JR, Orsay CP, et al. Role of the seton in the management of anorectal fistulas. *Dis Colon Rectum.* 1993;36(6):573-577.
25. Tonkin DM, Murphy E, Brooke-Smith M, et al. Perianal abscess: a pilot study comparing packing with nonpacking of the abscess cavity. *Dis Colon Rectum.* 2004;47(9):1510-1514.
26. Prasad ML, Read DR, Abcarian H. Supralevator abscess: diagnosis and treatment. *Dis Colon Rectum.* 1981;24(6):456-461.
27. Quah HM, Tang CL, Eu KW, Chan SY, Samuel M. Meta-analysis of randomized clinical trials comparing drainage alone vs primary sphincter-cutting procedures for anorectal abscess–fistula. *Int J Colorectal Dis.* 2006;21(6):602-609.
28. Malik AI, Nelson RL, Tou S. Incision and drainage of perianal abscess with or without treatment of anal fistula. *Cochrane Database Syst Rev.* 2010;7:CD006827.
29. van Koperen PJ, Wind J, Bermelman WA, Slors JF. Fibrin glue and transanal rectal advancement flap for high transphincteric perianal fistulas: is there any advantage? *Int J Colorectal Dis.* 2008;23:697-701.
30. Shanwani A, Nor AM, Amri N. Ligation of the intersphincteric fistula tract (LIFT): a sphincter-saving technique for fistula-in-ano. *Dis Colon Rectum.* 2010;53(1):39-42.
31. Hamalainen KP, Sainio AP. Cutting seton for anal fistulas: high risk of minor control defects. *Dis Colon Rectum.* 1997;40(12):1443-1446.
32. Hong KD, Kang S, Kalaskar S, Wexner SD. Ligation of intersphincteric fistula tract (LIFT) to treat anal fistula: systemic review and meta-analysis. *Tech Coloproctol.* 2014;18(8):685-691.

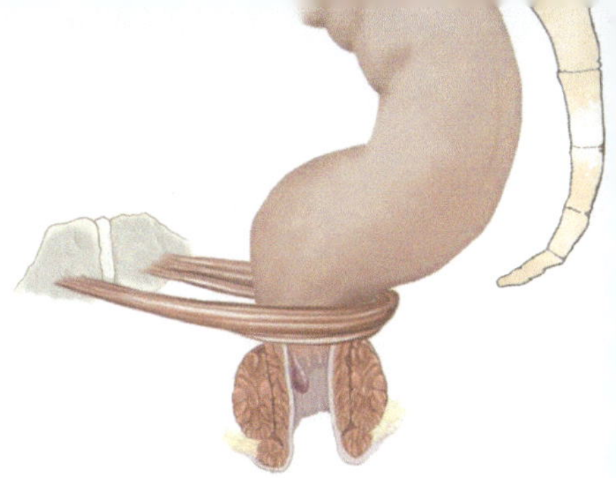

5

Stool Incontinence

Treatment and Outcomes

Ihsan Al-Bayati, MD; Sarah Al-Obaidi, MD; and Richard McCallum, MD, FACP, FRACP (AUST), FACG, AGAF

Key Points

- Fecal incontinence (FI) is the uncontrolled, involuntary loss of liquid and solid stool. Physicians need to focus on the etiology of the disease when performing the history and physical, looking for signs and symptoms of systemic diseases like diabetes and scleroderma; neurologic diseases like myasthenia gravis, Parkinson disease, and stroke; and gastrointestinal diseases like dumping syndrome, irritable bowel syndrome, inflammatory bowel disease, and surgical history.
- Endoscopy is an important initial step in the workup. Anorectal manometry (ARM) is key, and it gives valuable information about rectal sensation, resting, and squeeze pressure of the anal sphincter. Endoscopic ultrasound (EUS) is a great tool to identify the structural integrity of the anal sphincter, quantify the amount of damage, and open the door for these patients in whom a sphincter repair is the first step in treatment.
- In patients with mild disease (ie, not having daily FI episodes), supportive care needs to be stressed as a major part in the initial therapy. A high-fiber diet, Imodium (loperamide hydrochloride), and Kegel exercises are the initial cornerstones of therapy. Biofeedback helps improve the strength of the external anal sphincter and increase rectal sensation to distension in nonresponding patients.
- The injection of dextranomer stabilized in hyaluronic acid is a safe and efficacious method to improve FI in patients who failed initial therapy and biofeedback.
- In patients who still have at least daily FI events, sacral nerve stimulation is a well-established and effective next step, which is minimally invasive and well tolerated for the remainder of FI patients.
- Colostomy has been used with good results in patients who fail or are not candidates for the aforementioned treatments.

Qureshi W, ed. *Diagnosis and Management Guide for Anorectal Disease: A Clinical Reference* (pp 49-61).

Definition

FI is defined as the uncontrolled, involuntary loss of liquid and solid stool. This includes soiling underwear with stains or mucus, even if it is not a significant amount of stool.[1] The term *anal incontinence* extends the definition of *stool incontinence* to include the uncontrolled passage of flatus besides liquid and solid stool. Based on the mechanism, FI can be described as "urge incontinence" when patients feel the need to defecate, but, despite efforts to retain stool or seek a bathroom setting in a timely fashion, incontinence still occurs. The other described situation is when patients do not get a warning sensation for the need to defecate before the incontinence accident takes place; this is referred to as *passive incontinence*.

As much as the term *FI* is commonly used among physicians, it is usually substituted with accidental bowel leakage when communicating with patients to avoid social embarrassment and misunderstanding. Because FI has a large social and economic impact, it impairs quality of life significantly, leads to the loss of the ability to live independently, and causes social isolation because of the perceived "stigma" of losing fecal control along with the loss of self-esteem and depression.[2]

Epidemiology

It is obvious that studies underestimate the prevalence of FI because patients are reluctant to report it.[3] In a large review examining 38 studies with a sample size up to 20,000 people, the average prevalence of FI was found to range from 2% to 21%, with a median of 7.7%.[4] It was observed that FI increased with advancing age. The rates were shown to be similar between men and women. Our large referral practice at an academic gastroenterology setting indicates female predominance with a 2:1 ratio. Many concomitant factors are identified in FI including diarrhea, old age, urine incontinence, and previous pelvic surgeries.

As stated previously, the frequency of FI does increase with age, which may be explained by many factors such as decreased mobility, a weakened anal sphincter muscle, impaired anorectal sensation, and the effects of longstanding diabetes mellitus. Severe constipation and fecal impaction can be associated with the phenomenon of "overflow" incontinence, a problem that is more common in the elderly and in the setting of neurologic disease (eg, Parkinson disease and dementia).

Basic Anatomy and Pathophysiology

FI is multifactorial, as summarized in Table 5-1. Because there are many mechanisms that maintain continence, the loss of one may be compensated by the others. A change in stool consistency, abnormal rectal compliance, decreased rectal sensation, anal sphincter abnormality, or a combination of any of these, may lead to FI.

The functional anatomy of the anorectal area plays a major role in maintaining continence (Figure 5-1). The rectum, being a muscular tube with peculiar muscular configuration (a continuous longitudinal layer that interlaces with an inner circular layer), hence the terms *external* and *internal sphincters*, serves the purpose of both a reservoir and a pump to store and empty stool, respectively.[5] The anus is another muscular tube 2- to 4-cm long. It forms an angle with the rectum, and the transition zone is called the *dentate line*. This angle is 90 degrees at rest, becomes more acute with voluntary squeeze (70 degrees), and becomes more obtuse during defecation (110 to 130 degrees).

The anal sphincter consists of 2 muscles: the internal anal sphincter (IAS), which is the thin (0.3 to 0.5 cm), circular smooth muscle, and the external anal sphincter (EAS), which is a thicker layer (0.6 to 1.0 cm) expanding distally from the levator ani muscles[6] (see Figure 5-1). The IAS is the major contributor to anal continence at rest, providing 70% to 85% of resting anal sphincter pressure,

Table 5-1

MULTIPLE ETIOLOGIES OF FECAL INCONTINENCE

ANAL SPHINCTER WEAKNESS	• Traumatic: obstetric, surgical (eg, fistulotomy, internal sphincterotomy) • Nontraumatic: scleroderma, internal sphincter degeneration of unknown etiology
NEUROPATHY	Peripheral (eg, pudendal) or generalized (eg, diabetes mellitus)
DISTURBANCES OF PELVIC FLOOR	Rectal prolapse, descending perineum syndrome
INFLAMMATORY CONDITIONS	Radiation proctitis, Crohn's disease, ulcerative colitis
CENTRAL NERVOUS SYSTEM DISORDERS	Dementia, stroke, brain tumors, multiple sclerosis, spinal cord lesions
DIARRHEA	Irritable bowel syndrome, postcholecystectomy diarrhea
OTHER	Fecal retention with overflow, behavioral disorders

This table summarizes the causes of FI and the different mechanisms related to the anal sphincter, rectal sensation, systemic causes, neurologic causes, and miscellaneous etiologies.

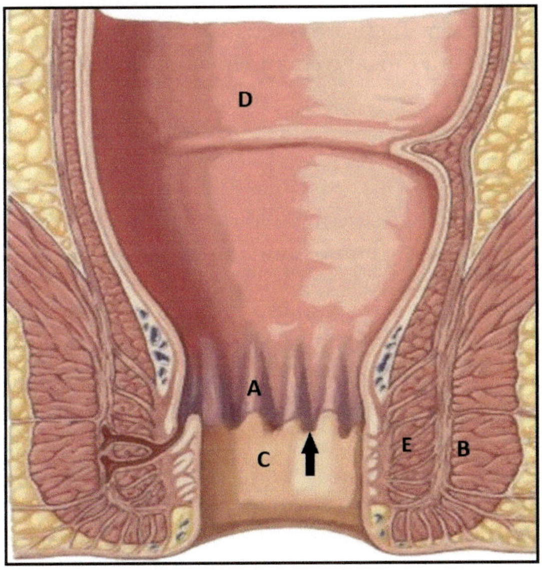

Figure 5-1. An illustration showing the anatomy of the anal canal and rectum. The dentate line is identified as the transition from squamous anal mucosa to columnar rectal mucosa (arrow). The anal sphincter is shown around the anal canal. (A) The area above the dentate line where columnar mucosa starts; (B) the EAS; (C) the anoderm; (D) the rectum; (E) the IAS.

40% of the pressure if there was sudden distension, and 65% of the pressure in case of constant rectal distension. The remainder of resistance is provided by the EAS and the puborectalis muscle.[7] The puborectalis muscle creates a flaplike valve that provides a forward pull that reinforces the anorectal angle.

The pudendal nerve supplies the EAS with both motor and sensory fibers. It arises from the S2, S3, and S4 sacral nerves. Pudendal nerve block leads to a loss of sensation in the perianal and genital skin and weakness to the anal sphincter muscles but does not cause loss of rectal sensation. The parasympathetic fibers of S2, S3, and S4 transmit the sensation to rectal distension.

Passive distension of the rectum by stool and contraction of the rectal smooth muscles activate the afferent nerve endings that trigger rectal sensation. The sensation of an intolerable urge to defecate happens when a large amount of stool causes the rectal smooth muscles to contract reflexively. It is critical to be able to feel the rectal distension so that a warning is transmitted to the central nervous system to voluntarily contract the pelvic floor muscles, particularly the EAS. This leads to the prevention of FI. When this sensation is absent or decreased because of spinal cord transection or peripheral nerve injury (rectal hyposensitivity), these patients do not receive any early or adequate warning and are likely to develop passive FI.

The IAS normally maintains a resting pressure of 40 to 70 mm Hg, which is higher than the resting rectal pressure of 10 mm Hg. This gradient is a barrier to the passage of gas and stool. In response to increased rectal distension, IAS contraction is reflexively inhibited; this is called the *rectoanal inhibitory reflex*. This reflex is normally countered voluntarily by the individual by contracting the EAS, delaying the need to defecate until there is an appropriate time or setting available. The loss of rectoanal inhibitory reflex is specific for Hirschsprung's disease.

The EAS is a voluntary striated muscle that contracts in response to the perception of rectal distension and is a major mechanism of continence. The puborectalis muscle together with the ileorectalis and coccygeus muscles form the levator ani group. These muscles contract in conjunction with the EAS to increase the anorectal angle and maintain continence. Surgical damage is an example of disrupted functionality of these groups of muscle.

Steps for Making the Diagnosis

The approach to FI starts with a careful medical history and then thorough physical examination. This helps initiate a plan for further workup and evaluation. There are several tests that may be performed to further understand the etiology and severity of FI in a given individual including ARM, EUS, and magnetic resonance imaging (MRI).

History

The first step when approaching a patient with FI is to make sure to build strong trust and establish a rapport with the patient. It is important to understand the onset, duration, frequency of events including the number of days having incontinence per week (this is applied in a scoring system that assists in communicating the severity of the condition), and the amount leaking (whether a small stain or a full bowel movement). Accidents occurring during both day and night indicate a more severe setting. It is also important to know if the leaking is solid, liquid, or only gas. Questions about the presence or absence of an urge are important to remember. Diarrhea and medication use as well as long-term constipation should be focused on during the history taking. Back pain, urine incontinence, and sensory or motor weakness in the lower extremities can point to neurologic causes. Asking about previous pelvic surgeries; traumatic childbirth including prolonged labor, episiotomy, or forceps use; diabetes mellitus; systemic sclerosis; myasthenia gravis; radiotherapy; or a history of stroke is a key to making the diagnosis.

Differentiating between nonfecal, mucous, watery, small material discharge staining underwear, which is seen in rectal prolapse, from cases of real FI with true fecal material is also very important because the treatment approaches are very different. Mobility issues may also be a major issue during patient assessment when evaluating etiologies of FI as well as in planning further treatment and understanding the limitations that may interfere with the desired outcomes.

PHYSICAL EXAMINATION

Inspecting the perianal area may show dermatitis from prolonged exposure and contact with fecal material, suggesting chronic FI. The presence of a fistula may point to the etiology of soiling in the absence of true FI and a normal continence mechanism. Hemorrhoids and rectal prolapse should be paid attention to; the patient is asked to bear down to induce prolapsed rectal mucosa, which has to be differentiated from internal hemorrhoids that also can occur with bearing down. Bearing down during the digital rectal examination also allows the examiner to document normal descent of the pelvic floor over the inserted finger. A decreased sphincter tone at rest and impaired squeeze pressure will provide early evidence for FI. If the sphincter tone and squeeze are good, then the spectrum of not sensing stool is more likely the explanation for FI (passive incontinence). The maneuver of stroking the skin around the anal area and observing contraction of the EAS is referred to as the *anocutaneous reflex*. Neurologic damage is suspected if there is a lack of reflex on either side. A fecal mass may be felt during the digital rectal examination, raising the question of underappreciated constipation. Cases of constipation refractory to medical management should be evaluated for pelvic floor dysfunction with ARM.[8] A colonoscopy is indicated if a mass other than an internal hemorrhoid is felt during the examination. Also, the EAS and resting anal tone are evaluated when the examiner inserts his or her finger and requests the patient to squeeze and relax, respectively. During the general examination, focus on systemic disease that can contribute to FI. Look for signs that may point to scleroderma, ptosis caused by myasthenia gravis, peripheral neuropathy caused by diabetes, the patient's mobility and neurologic status, and others.

LABORATORY STUDIES AND COLONOSCOPY

The next step in evaluation when diarrhea is present should include laboratory testing of the stool for infectious versus inflammatory causes; small and large bowel imaging; and, in selective cases, testing for vasoactive intestinal peptide, serum gastrin, and stool electrolytes to differentiate secretory from osmotic diarrhea.[9] Postcholecystectomy diarrhea can also be an explanation, which can be easily treated. The spectrum of "dumping syndrome" associated with postprandial diarrhea must also be considered when there is a history of gastric or esophageal surgeries and diabetes. Small intestine bacterial overgrowth can explain diarrhea, particularly nocturnal FI, and here one needs to consider a history of surgical procedures such as obesity surgery, Billroth II, Roux-en-Y, or intestinal resections as well as longstanding diabetes with peripheral neuropathy and scleroderma involving the intestine.

A colonoscopy or flexible sigmoidoscopy is performed to exclude tumors, inflammatory bowel diseases, and strictures or to make the diagnosis of microscopic colitis, particularly when there is nocturnal diarrhea.

SPECIALIZED STUDIES

After the initial gastroenterology evaluation, further specialized motility and structural evaluations are warranted. ARM and EUS are performed next. If patients continue to be refractory to treatment, barium defecography or magnetic resonance defecography may be considered if concerns about pelvic floor anatomy are present.

Anorectal Manometry

This test helps evaluate the function of the IAS, EAS, and rectal sensation and compliance. Minimal preparation is required with 2 to 3 fleet enemas. A tube that has pressure sensors measures the anal canal pressures, whereas a balloon attached to the tip measures the sensation thresholds (Figure 5-2). High-resolution ARM and high-definition ARM are novel, solid-state manometric systems with good correlation to water-perfused manometry and greater anatomic detail. The baseline

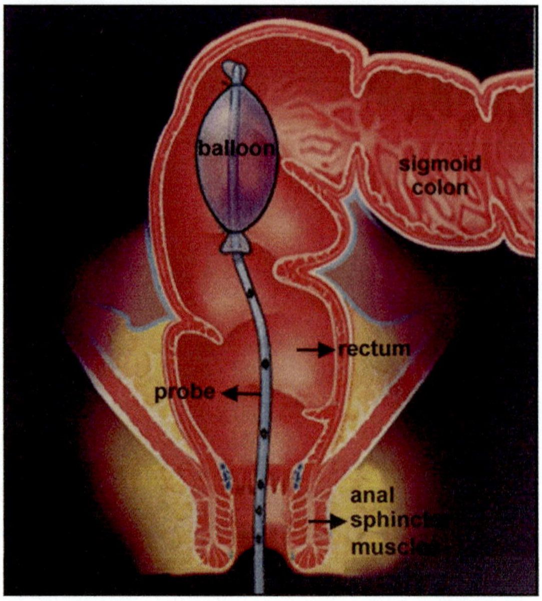

Figure 5-2. ARM is a very important tool in the diagnosis of FI. This method gives essential information about the IAS and EAS. The resting and squeeze status are evaluated based on pressure measurements from transducers embedded in the catheter pressures as well as the rectal sensation. Rectal sensation is assessed by introducing increasing volumes into a balloon positioned in the rectal vault.

and maximum resting sphincter pressure as well as the sphincter length are measured. This evaluates the function of the IAS. The maximum squeeze should result in an incremental increase in pressure of at least 50 mm Hg above the baseline, the sustained squeeze pressure is held for at least 15 seconds, and the squeeze length is measured to evaluate the function of the EAS. (Figure 5-3 shows normal and abnormal sphincter responses.) Then, the rectal balloon is inflated at increments of 10 mL until the first sensation (normal is 20 to 25 mL, >40 mL is definitely abnormal) and then further increments up to 250 to 320 mL. The preferred method is inflating with syringe boluses. With increasing inflation comes a desire to have a bowel movement that lasts more than 15 seconds, called the *desire to defecate* or *urge to go*. This sensation is what the patient experiences at home before having to go to the bathroom. In some cases, the patient does not make it to the bathroom after experiencing this "urge to go."

Endoscopic Ultrasound and Magnetic Resonance Imaging

Abnormalities in the IAS, EAS, and pelvic muscle structure are best evaluated with EUS and MRI. EUS is superior for evaluating both the IAS and EAS (Figure 5-4). MRI colpocystography provides dynamic evaluation using ultrasound gel as a contact agent. The patient squeezes while MRIs are being captured.[10] Combined EAS and IAS damage is always an indication of severe cases of FI. If >30% of the EAS is damaged or there is combined IAS and EAS involvement, further medical therapy may not be considered until the defect is repaired.

Defecography

This study is performed in refractory cases and in patients undergoing surgery. Barium is introduced to the rectum, and radiographic images are taken at rest and during defecation. It is good for evaluating the length of the anal sphincter, the anorectal angle, and pelvic descent. It can also detect enteroceles, rectoceles, and rectal prolapse.[11] Nowadays, this study has essentially been replaced with pelvic MRI for the assessment of pelvic anatomy because rectal prolapse as well as the anatomy of the urinary bladder and female organs can be better appreciated.

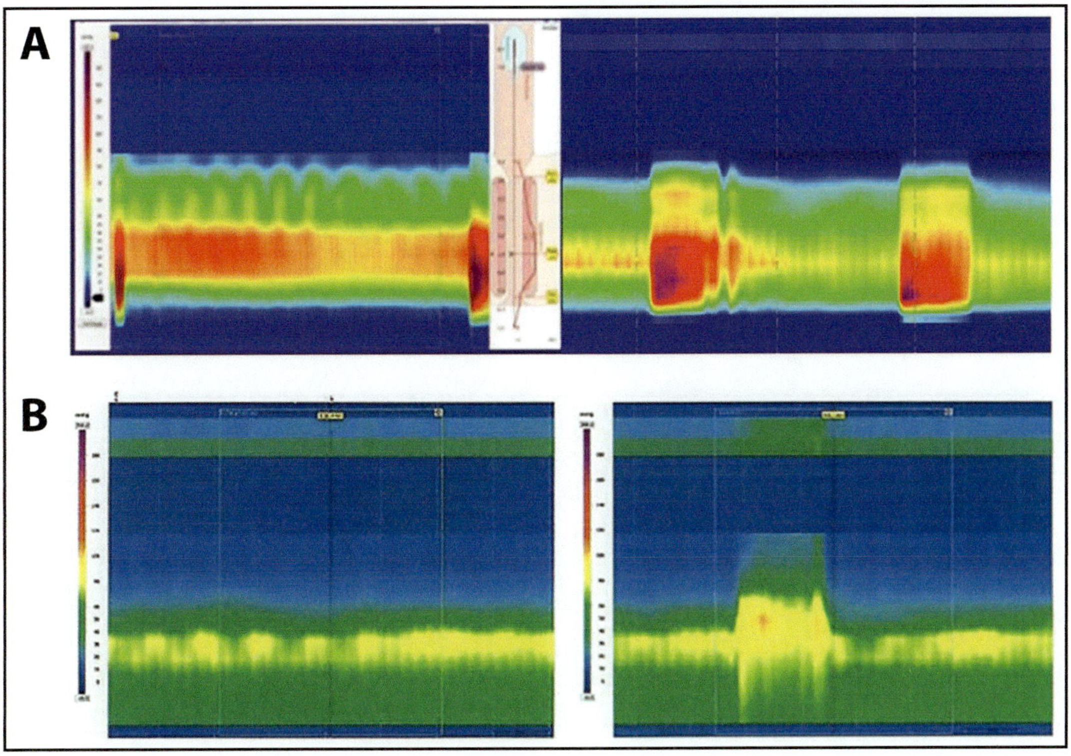

Figure 5-3. High-resolution ARM. (A) Normal ARM with good sphincter tone at rest (left) and a strong squeeze (right). (B) A decreased anal sphincter tone at rest (left) and a weak squeeze response (right).

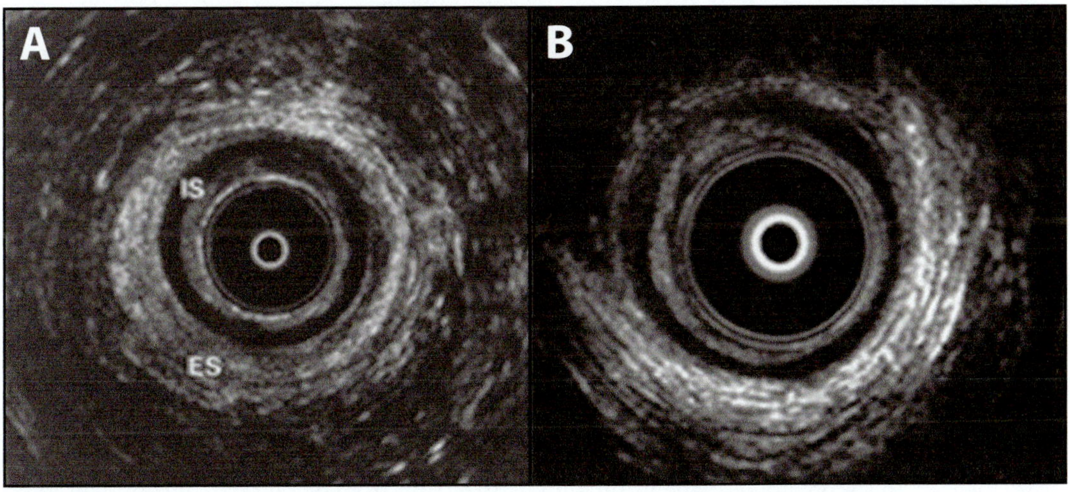

Figure 5-4. EUS showing the anal sphincter. (A) Both the internal anal sphincter (IS) and external anal sphincter (ES) have normal shape and continuity. (B) There is obvious damage to both the IS and ES, evident by thinning and loss of continuity.

Balloon Expulsion Test

This test is used to evaluate patients in whom there is a definite strong history of constipation to address the possibility of dyssynergic defecation and fecal impaction. A non-latex balloon filled with 50 mL warm water is introduced to the rectum. If the patient is unable to expel the balloon within 2 minutes, the test is considered abnormal.[12]

Table 5-2

The Wexner Scoring Scale for Grading the Severity of Fecal Incontinence

TYPE OF INCONTINENCE	FREQUENCY				
	Never	*Rarely*	*Sometimes*	*Usually*	*Always*
Solid	0	1	2	3	4
Liquid	0	1	2	3	4
Gas	0	1	2	3	4
Wears pad	0	1	2	3	4
Lifestyle alteration	0	1	2	3	4

Never, 0; rarely, < 1 per month; sometimes, < 1 per week and ≥ 1 per month; usually, < 1 per day and ≥ 1 per week; always, ≥ 1 per day.

The type of incontinence (whether incontinent to solid, liquid, or gas) is weighed with the frequency of events. Wearing pads and lifestyle alteration are taken into consideration as well, and the total score is calculated. When a patient's score is 20, he or she is considered to have complete FI, whereas a score of 0 means no FI.

Electromyography

A probe with multiple stainless steel electrodes is placed in the anal canal to measure the average electromyographic activity of the striated muscles surrounding the anal canal. This provides better indication of the pelvic floor muscle than ARM. Electromyography is complimentary but does not replace ARM because it does not measure sensation or compliance, but it can separate neurologic from morphologic causes of decreased squeeze pressure.[13]

Pudendal Nerve Terminal Motor Latency

Markers for pudendal nerve terminal motor latency have been used widely. They can identify pudendal nerve injury, but they are inaccurate and in general are not recommended for evaluating patients with FI.[14]

Grading the Severity of Fecal Incontinence

There are many scales used to create a unified communication language between physicians to quantify the severity of FI in objective terms. One of the most commonly used scales is the Wexner score for FI.[15] This score grades patients on a linear spectrum from being rarely incontinent to being completely incontinent (Table 5-2). Other scores like the Douglas Wong, Pescatori, American Medical Systems, and Vaizey scores have similarities and differences in some aspects in defining the severity of FI.

In our experience, patients with FI events less than daily can usually be successfully managed and treated with supportive care, medical management, biofeedback, and intrarectal injection of a bulking agent. Patients with advanced FI (ie, having daily or even more than once daily events) may require the next step, which is sacral nerve stimulation. There are infrequent patients in whom sphincter replacement surgery or colostomy is the last choice.

Treatment

The management of FI starts initially with supportive care and medical therapy, and the goal of treatment is to improve quality of life and increase continence.

Supportive Care

Supportive care involves regulating or scheduling bowel movement timing and avoiding foods that provoke diarrhea or incontinence. Patients may be asked to keep a diary of food and bowel movements. It is important to keep the perianal area clean and dry. Hygienic measures include changing undergarments, cleaning the area soon after soiling events using wet wipes, and using zinc oxide cream and calamine lotion as a barrier to prevent skin excoriation. Managing patients' general well-being and treating perianal fungal infections are essential. Recommending a high-fiber diet is one of the first steps in managing FI. This may include adding Metamucil (psyllium fiber) to maximize fiber intake.

Some cases of FI may respond to these measures. The short-term success rate for these measures has been shown to be up to 60% in one case series.[16] Dietary modification includes avoiding caffeine intake, which is known to increase the gastrocolic reflex and colonic motility. It also causes increased fluid secretion from the small bowel. Lactose and fructose are avoided because they may be malabsorbed. Physical activity immediately after meals is also limited because it may enhance colonic motility.

Pharmacologic Therapy

Imodium and Lomotil (diphenoxylate and atropine sulfate) are the mainstays for initial stool control in FI.[17] Imodium is initially given in a standard dose, 2 mg daily or even every other day based on patients' sensitivity to these agents. The final goal is to induce "pseudoconstipation," meaning a frequency of 1 stool every day or every other day. Imodium will need to be titrated to reach this goal. Up to 4 to 12 mg daily in divided doses to improve urgency, reduce incontinence events, increase colonic transit time, and increase anal resting sphincter pressure may be required. Careful dose monitoring might be required to avoid adverse events including abdominal pain, cramping, and difficult evacuation. Cholestyramine and colestipol are used to treat cases of bile salt malabsorption that could be causing diarrhea and FI, typically postcholecystectomy.[18] The physician should also be aware of the immediate postmeal urgency that could signal dumping syndrome and consider a gastric emptying study in these cases. Diarrhea in the clinical setting suggesting small intestinal bacterial overgrowth will need glucose breath testing to confirm this suspicion and initiate antibiotic therapy. Kegel exercises are usually taught to patients to be performed on a daily basis for many sessions per day at home to strengthen the pelvic floor muscles. With this combination of diet, Imodium, and Kegel exercises, essentially most cases with FI events less than daily will be successfully managed.

Biofeedback Therapy

Also known as *neuromuscular training*, biofeedback works by improving symptoms of incontinence, quality of life, and anorectal function. When patients have a weak sphincter or impaired rectal sensation and are not responding adequately to the previously described measures, then biofeedback is an important step in the treatment of FI. With repeated reinforcement and feedback, patients acquire new behavior by conditioning techniques. The aims of biofeedback or neuromuscular training are to increase anorectal sensory perception, enhance anal sphincter strength, and improve the synchrony of the abdominal, sphincter, and gluteal muscles while patients voluntarily squeeze. This treatment modality must be individualized based on each case, and the etiology of incontinence usually guides the therapy.

A manometry probe is inserted in the rectum. The patient is asked to squeeze, and the increase in anal sphincter pressure is visualized, presenting instant feedback to the patient. Rectoanal coordination training aims to achieve the maximum voluntary squeeze pressure within 2 seconds from balloon inflation. This process simulates stool arrival to the rectum and trains the patient to use the muscle groups that should contract to voluntarily retain stool. With high-resolution ARM equipment, biofeedback is now more patient friendly because the patient can watch the screen and see a weak sphincter (yellow-green column) change to red as the pressure increases with squeezing.

Repetition of balloon inflation and deflation is used to improve patients' ability to perceive lower volumes of rectal distension. With continuing sensory training, patients start to feel lower volumes of balloon distension but with the same intensity they felt it with higher volumes.

The first 1 or 2 sessions are performed in the motility center and then practiced at home. It is largely restricted to specialized centers. In some cases, continuing biofeedback requires a pelvic floor therapist available only in pelvic pain centers, typically gynecologic more than gastroenterologic centers. Patient motivation, the enthusiasm of the therapist, and the severity of incontinence play major roles in the response to treatment.

Kegel exercises are very important to be performed to strengthen the pelvic floor at the same time of biofeedback training. Usually, no less than 4 to 6 training sessions are required.[19] The number of treatments are best titrated to the patient's response to therapy.

PLUGS

Because diapers are unsatisfactory in general to give enough comfort or sense of security and are not helpful in skin protection and hiding odor, other similar methods like anal plugs have been made to help occlude the anal canal temporarily.[20] Unfortunately, the inconvenience of device insertion makes lots of patients unable to tolerate insertion for a long time. This plug is helpful for patients with neurologic disease or impaired anal canal sensation, immobilized and institutionalized patients, some patients with fecal seepage, and those who are mentally challenged. It is recommended not to wear it for more than 12 hours.[19] For minor soiling between the buttocks, small anal dressings may be helpful.

BULKING AGENTS

This is another tactic to contract the rectal vault, hence making it more sensitive to the presence of stool. Bulking agents have been used to inject submucosally to achieve a reduction in the rectal volume. These include glutaraldehyde-treated collagen, autologous fat, and synthetic macromolecules.[21,22] Dextromer beads are injected at least 1 cm above the dentate line. This approach can be efficacious in patients with FI refractory to conventional medical therapy.[23] We conducted a study on 17 patients with FI. We injected stabilized hyaluronate approximately 1 cm above the dentate line so there was no pain involved; the injection was submucosal under direct anoscopic visualization (see Figure 5-1). Four quadrants were injected with 1-mL increments. After the first injection, 82% of patients had a successful outcome, defined as more than a 50% reduction in FI events when followed over 12 months. The remaining 18% (3 patients) had a second injection 3 months after the first treatment and responded to therapy. During the follow-up period, 7 out of 17 patients did not have any FI events; the other 10 patients had a significant reduction in FI events from baseline (ie, 6.4 to 2.8 episodes per week). However, there is still limited experience in this technique, and randomized, controlled studies with long-term follow-ups are needed to demonstrate strong evidence for the benefit of this kind of treatment. Pain is the main side effect of this therapy. The physician needs to be aware of the anatomy of the area and inject at least 1 cm above the dentate line to avoid pain.

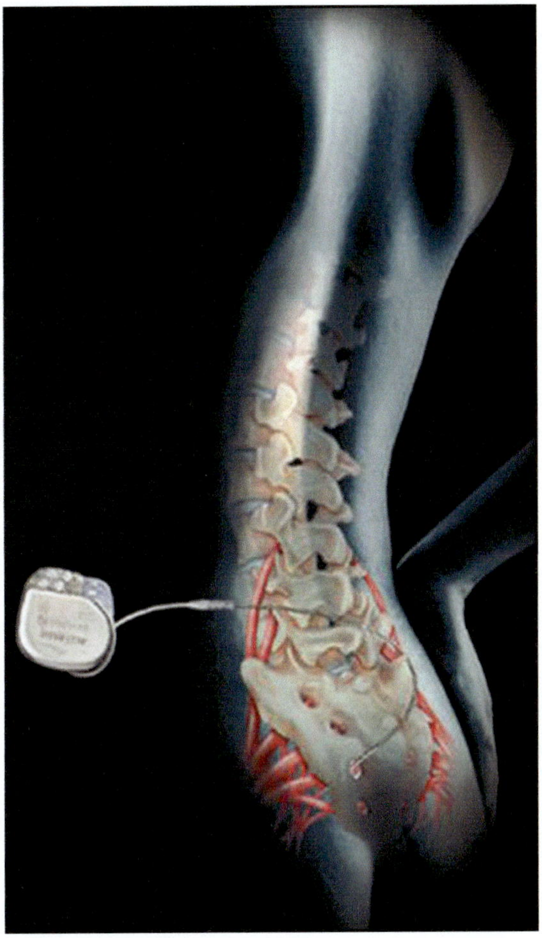

Figure 5-5. Sacral nerve stimulation. The lead is implanted at level S3 or S4. The stimulator is placed in a subcutaneous pocket. This minimally invasive procedure is safe and is generally done on an outpatient basis.

SACRAL NERVE STIMULATION

A guideline to the stepwise approach in surgical therapies suggests supportive measures, medical therapy, and then biofeedback and injecting bulking agents.[24] Sacral nerve stimulation is to be considered in patients with moderate to severe symptoms who do not respond to the aforementioned treatments for at least 3 months. Patients with daily FI or at least >1 per week may be considered nonresponders. The treatment was initially tried only on patients with intact anal sphincters, but later studies showed success in patients with EAS and IAS defects.[25,26] The proposed mechanism of action of sacral stimulation is through a direct peripheral effect on colorectal sensory or motor function or an effect on the central nervous system, although more data suggest the effect is not on increasing the sphincter tone but rather on enhancing rectal sensation. The treatment involves 2 stages. In the beginning, a temporary electrode is placed in the sacral foramen and implanted in the second or third sacral nerve roots. If in 2 weeks patients respond to the trial, they then move to the permanent stage of placing a subcutaneous electrode connected to an embedded stimulator (Figure 5-5). In this method, fecal continence is enhanced by improving the resting and squeeze pressure and rectal sensation.

This treatment has shown good outcomes. In a study of 120 patients with FI (110 females) with at least daily FI events and a duration of FI of about 7 years, therapeutic success was achieved in 85% of patients at 24 months. This was seen after a significant decrease in FI events from baseline of 9.4 per week to 2.9 at 2 years.[27] Actually, 41% of patients achieved 100% continence. Infection of the implantation site was reported in 10% of patients and required surgical intervention in only about 6% of patients; the others were successfully treated medically.

Surgical Therapy

In cases of obstetric trauma, overlapping sphincter repair may be a sufficient treatment strategy. This is often triggered by EUS detecting > 30% sphincter damage. After sphincter repair, other treatment modalities can be pursued.

Dynamic graciloplasty is another surgical treatment that is used in severe structural damage. The gracilis muscle is transposed around the anal canal. An implantable pulse generator provides continuous electric stimulation. An external magnetic device is used to temporarily stop the pacemaker. The average rate of improvement from this approach is 67%.[28]

Artificial bowel sphincter is another approach to make a neosphincter. Here, an inflatable cuffed device is implanted. When filled with fluid from an implanted reservoir controlled by a subcutaneous pump, defecation can be controlled upon the patient's desire. The major drawback from this technique is device explantation. Both these major surgeries also have a high revision rate, reaching up to 50% in some reports. Overall, it is fair to comment that these surgical "creations" are rarely done. In this chapter, we cannot recommend any specific one.

Colostomy

Colostomy is the last resort for patients who fail all other treatment modalities or are not candidates for the aforementioned approaches, specifically patients with substantial mental limitations, paralysis, or mobility issues.[29] Although not always acceptable from a cosmetic or convenience standpoint, it remains a safe option for such patients. It is mostly used for patients with uncontrolled skin damage, neurologic impairment, spinal cord injury, or extensive colon surgery (eg, breakdown of ileorectal anastomosis) and immobilized patients. It is an effective option that can be well maintained.

Conclusion

FI is the passage of fecal matter (solid or liquid) involuntarily through the anus. The severity of incontinence ranges from soiling underwear to having large bowel movements. The problem carries a great social burden on patients and can lead to poor quality of life, isolation, and depression. It is more prevalent in the elderly. Incontinence occurs mainly in the setting of diarrhea but can present with constipation as well. Damage of the anal sphincter from surgeries or related to traumatic vaginal delivery; neurologic disease including stroke, spinal cord injury, multiple sclerosis, myasthenia gravis, and diabetic neuropathy; physical restraints; and loss of mobility are all different etiologic factors of incontinence. The diagnostic process starts with a detailed history and thorough physical examination with careful attention to the rectal examination. Endoscopy, ARM, and EUS are used for defining the exact mechanism of loss of continence. Treatment starts with supportive care and trying to identify the treatable etiologies of diarrhea and constipation and reducing stool frequency with the aggressive use of Imodium (loperamide hydrochloride). Other therapies can then be initiated including Kegel exercises, biofeedback, and intrarectal injection of bulking agents. For the subset of patients not adequately responding to these regimens (eg, daily incontinence events), sacral nerve stimulation is the usual solution. Very rarely, surgical repair or creating neosphincters may be considered. Colostomy is needed in some cases, especially with neurologic and mobility-related clinical settings.

References

1. Nelson R, Norton N, Cautley E, Furner S. Community-based prevalence of anal incontinence. *JAMA*. 1995;274(7):559-561.
2. Rothbarth J, Bemelman WA, Meijerink WJ, et al. What is the impact of fecal incontinence on quality of life? *Dis Colon Rectum*. 2001;44(1):67-71.
3. Johanson JF, Lafferty J. Epidemiology of fecal incontinence: the silent affliction. *Am J Gastroenterol*. 1996;91(1):33-36.
4. Ng K-S, Sivakumaran Y, Nassar N, Gladman MA. Fecal incontinence: community prevalence and associated factors—a systematic review. *Dis Colon Rectum*. 2015;58(12):1194-1209.
5. Rao SS. Pathophysiology of adult fecal incontinence. *Gastroenterology*. 2004;126:S14-S22.
6. Matzel KE, Schmidt RA, Tanagho EA. Neuroanatomy of the striated muscular anal continence mechanism. *Dis Colon Rectum*. 1990;33(8):666-673.
7. Frenckner B, Euler C. Influence of pudendal block on the function of the anal sphincters. *Gut*. 1975;16(6):482-489.
8. Wald A, Bharucha AE, Cosman BC, Whitehead WE. ACG clinical guideline: management of benign anorectal disorders. *Am J Gastroenterol*. 2014;109(8):1141-1157.
9. Eherer AJ, Fordtran JS. Fecal osmotic gap and pH in experimental diarrhea of various causes. *Gastroenterology*. 1992;103(2):545-551.
10. Lienemann A, Anthuber C, Baron A, Reiser M. Diagnosing enteroceles using dynamic magnetic resonance imaging. *Dis Colon Rectum*. 2000;43(2):205-212.
11. Mahieu P, Pringot J, Bodart P. Defecography: II. Contribution to the diagnosis of defecation disorders. *Gastrointest Radiol*. 1984;9(1):253-261.
12. Rao SS, Hatfield R, Soffer E, Rao S, Beaty J, Conklin JL. Manometric tests of anorectal function in healthy adults. *Am J Gastroenterol*. 1999;94(3):773-783.
13. Remes-Troche JM, Rao SS. Neurophysiological testing in anorectal disorders. *Expert Rev Gastroenterol Hepatol*. 2008;2(3):323-335.
14. Diamant N, Kamm M, Wald A, Whitehead W. AGA technical review on anorectal testing techniques. *Gastroenterology*. 1999;116(3):735-760.
15. Vaizey C, Carapeti E, Cahill J, Kamm M. Prospective comparison of faecal incontinence grading systems. *Gut*. 1999;44(1):77-80.
16. Chassagne P, Jego A, Gloc P, et al. Does treatment of constipation improve faecal incontinence in institutionalized elderly patients? *Age Ageing*. 2000;29(2):159-164.
17. Rao SS. Diagnosis and management of fecal incontinence. *Am J Gastroenterol*. 2004;99(8):1585.
18. Remes-Troche JM, Ozturk R, Philips C, Stessman M, Rao SS. Cholestyramine—a useful adjunct for the treatment of patients with fecal incontinence. *Int J Colorectal Dis*. 2008;23(2):189-194.
19. Norton C. Fecal incontinence and biofeedback therapy. *Gastroenterol Clin North Am*. 2008;37(3):587-604.
20. Chan CL, Lunniss PJ, Wang D, Williams NS, Scott SM. Rectal sensorimotor dysfunction in patients with urge faecal incontinence: evidence from prolonged manometric studies. *Gut*. 2005;54(9):1263-1272.
21. Shafik A. Perianal injection of autologous fat for treatment of sphincteric incontinence. *Dis Colon Rectum*. 1995;38(6):583-587.
22. Shafik A. Polytetrafluoroethylene injection for the treatment of partial fecal incontinence. *Int Surg*. 1993;78(2):159-161.
23. Al-Bayati I, Saadi M, Elhanafi S, McCallum RW. Effectiveness of bulking agent (Solesta) therapy in fecal incontinence in patients refractory to conventional therapies. *Am J Med Sci*. 2017;354(5):476-479.
24. Bharucha AE, Rao SS, Shin AS. Surgical interventions and the use of device-aided therapy for the treatment of fecal incontinence and defecatory disorders. *Clin Gastroenterol Hepatol*. 2017;15(12):1844-1854.
25. Melenhorst J, Koch S, Uludag Ö, Van Gemert W, Baeten C. Is a morphologically intact anal sphincter necessary for success with sacral nerve modulation in patients with faecal incontinence? *Colorectal Dis*. 2008;10(3):257-262.
26. Vitton V, Gigout J, Grimaud J-C, Bouvier M, Desjeux A, Orsoni P. Sacral nerve stimulation can improve continence in patients with Crohn's disease with internal and external anal sphincter disruption. *Dis Colon Rectum*. 2008;51(6):924-927.
27. Wexner SD, Coller JA, Devroede G, et al. Sacral nerve stimulation for fecal incontinence: results of a 120-patient prospective multicenter study. *Ann Surg*. 2010;251(3):441.
28. Gladman MA, Knowles CH. Surgical treatment of patients with constipation and fecal incontinence. *Gastroenterol Clin*. 2008;37(3):605-625.
29. Stone J, Wolfe V, Nino-Murcia M, Perkash I. Colostomy as treatment for complications of spinal cord injury. *Arch Phys Med Rehabil*. 1990;71(7):514-518.

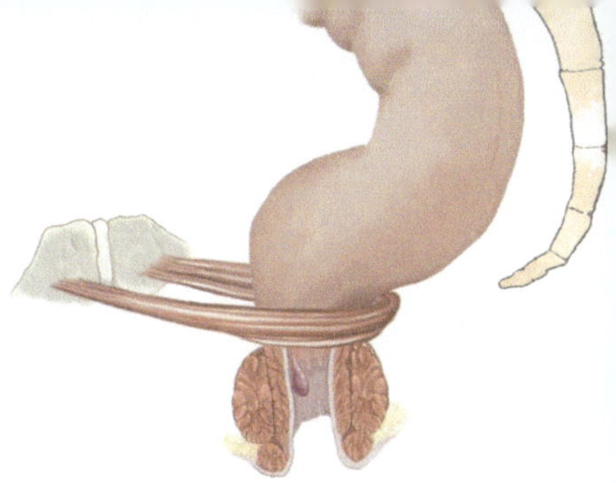

6

Pelvic Floor Disorders and Functional Anorectal Pain

Leila Neshatian, MD, MSc

Key Points

- Functional defecation disorders should be suspected in individuals with chronic constipation or constipation-predominant irritable bowel syndrome who are not responding to conservative management.
- Dyssynergic defecation and impaired propulsive forces are the 2 major subtypes of functional defecation disorders.
- Diagnosis is confirmed through 2 of 3 abnormal anorectal physiologic tests. These tests include an abnormal balloon expulsion test, anorectal manometry, electromyography (EMG), and dynamic imaging.
- The best evidence-based treatment is pelvic floor retraining with biofeedback.
- Functional anorectal pain disorders consist of 3 major subgroups: levator ani syndrome, nonspecific anorectal pain, and proctalgia fugax.
- Levator ani syndrome is characterized by chronic, intermittent rectal pain episodes that last more than 30 minutes and the presence of tenderness during posterior traction on the puborectalis muscle.
- In unspecified anorectal pain disorders, there is no tenderness during the rectal examination.
- Proctalgia fugax is defined by brief attacks of rectal pain that last between a few seconds and minutes and disappear spontaneously.
- Pelvic floor dyssynergia is believed to serve as the mechanism of pathology in levator ani syndrome.

Qureshi W, ed. *Diagnosis and Management Guide for Anorectal Disease: A Clinical Reference* (pp 63-77).

Table 6-1

Rome IV Diagnostic Criteria for Functional Defecation Disorders

- The patient must satisfy diagnostic criteria for functional constipation and/or irritable bowel syndrome with constipation.
- During repeated attempts to defecate, there must be features of impaired evacuation, as demonstrated by 2 of the following 3 tests:
  1. An abnormal balloon expulsion test
  2. An abnormal anorectal evacuation pattern with manometry or anal surface electromyography
  3. Impaired rectal evacuation by imaging

Functional Defecation Disorders: Inadequate Defecatory Propulsion and Dyssynergic Defecation

Functional defecation disorders and slow transit constipation are the 2 major subtypes of chronic constipation. Functional defecation disorders are characterized by impaired evacuation secondary to dyssynergic defecation or inadequate defecatory propulsion. Diagnosis is made using physiologic tests in the context of the clinical presentation. Despite the growing awareness of defecatory dysfunction, it remains an under-recognized condition in clinical practice.

Definition

Functional defecation disorders are characterized by impaired rectal evacuation in patients with chronic and intractable symptoms of constipation. Functional defecation disorders are often the result of abnormal anorectal function; however, structural abnormalities may coexist. Table 6-1 summarizes the Rome IV diagnostic criteria for functional defecation disorders. Based on Rome IV diagnostic criteria, patients with functional defecation disorders should fulfill the diagnosis of chronic constipation or constipation-predominant irritable bowel syndrome. The 2 major subtypes of functional defecation disorders are dyssynergic defecation and inadequate defecatory propulsion (Table 6-2).[1] Dyssynergic defecation is defined by paradoxical anal contraction or incomplete anal relaxation (<20%) during attempted defecation, while inadequate defecatory propulsion results from the inability to increase rectal/intra-abdominal pressures during attempted defecation.

Epidemiology

Although functional defecation disorders have been exceedingly recognized as the etiologies of chronic constipation in patients who are unresponsive to trials of laxatives, the true prevalence of the problem is not known. In tertiary referral centers, the prevalence of dyssynergia in patients with constipation has varied from 20% to 80% based on the methodology.[1] In one recent retrospective review from 2 major tertiary referral centers in Boston, MA, impaired evacuation apparent by an abnormal balloon expulsion test was noted in more than 50% of patients seen for chronic constipation.[2] The incidence rate for functional defecation disorders was found to be 19.3 per 100,000 person years in adults from Olmsted County, MN.[3] The prevalence of functional defecation disorders has

Table 6-2

Rome IV Subcategories of Patients With Functional Defecation Disorders

INADEQUATE DEFECATORY PROPULSION	DYSSYNERGIC DEFECATION
• Inadequate propulsive forces measured with manometry • With or without inappropriate contraction of the anal sphincter and/or pelvic floor muscles	• Inappropriate contraction of the pelvic floor as measured with anal surface electromyography or manometry • Adequate propulsive forces during attempted defecation
Criteria fulfilled for the last 3 months with symptom onset at least 6 months before diagnosis.	

been reported to be 3 times higher in women. Consistently, its incidence rate was found to be 4-fold higher in women compared with men.[3] However, this higher incidence rate does not correlate with the incidence of chronic constipation, which is 2 times higher in women than men. The reason for female predisposition is uncertain. Although there is a female sex predominance in health care utilization for functional gastrointestinal disorders, this is unlikely to explain the wide divergence. Despite the notion of obstetric trauma, the peak incidence rate of diagnoses of functional defecation disorders appears to be in young nulliparous women.[3] Indeed, a few studies inspecting the risk factors for functional defecation disorders have failed to support the role of obstetric risk factors in developing functional defecation disorders.

A history of abuse is reported in 18% to 31% of patients with functional defecation disorders from different studies.[4] Sexual abuse is especially a risk factor for developing functional defecation disorders in women.[5] Comorbid psychological disorders have been reported in as high as 50% to 65% of patients with functional defecation disorders. Depression consistently has been the most common diagnosis, and more than half of the patients with functional defecation disorders take antidepressants.[3] There is a strong correlation between psychological problems and symptoms of constipation, and both correlate with health-related quality of life.[6]

The impact of functional defecation disorders on quality of life is tremendous. They negatively affect individuals' social life as well as their personal life. Interestingly, this impairment in quality of life appears to be more prominent in patients with functional defecation disorders compared with patients with slow transit constipation.[6]

HEALTH CARE AND ECONOMIC BURDEN

In general, constipation represents an immense and expansive financial burden to the health care system. The cost is both direct through the accumulating costs associated with medical management and indirect through sufferers' loss of productivity.[7,8] Among patients with all causes of constipation, patients with functional defecation disorders are found to have significantly greater constipation-related visits and overall higher health care utilization compared with patients with slow transit constipation.[9] On the other hand, nearly 70% of patients with functional defecation disorders are reported to have interruption in their occupational productivity because of their condition.[5] This highlights the importance of proper diagnosis of the etiology of chronic constipation, which will direct medical management.

PATHOPHYSIOLOGY

Despite the advances in high-resolution anorectal manometry and a better understanding of anorectal function over the past decade, the pathophysiology of functional defecation disorders remains poorly understood. Although dyssynergic defecation, impaired rectal propulsion, or a combination of these are commonly seen in patients with functional defecation disorders, these features are not unique and could be commonly seen in healthy volunteers.[10] Functional defecation disorders are not conventionally known to result from neurologic pathologies but rather from a maladaptive learning process. The sensory and motor dysfunctions of the anorectum that may be seen in some patients with functional defecation disorders, such as rectal hyposensitivity, are thought to be acquired abnormalities secondary to chronic functional abnormalities.[11] Abnormal toileting behavior with neglecting the urge to defecate and stool withholding is suggested to be an important contributor to the development of functional defecation disorders. Indeed, one-third of adults with functional defecation disorders had reported symptoms going back to their early childhood.[5] By the same token, in adults with a history of abuse or pelvic trauma, functional defecation disorder is thought to be the result of an abnormal response to rectal stimuli.[4] This is supported by the fact that biofeedback is the only evidence-based treatment option for constipation caused by functional defecation disorders and emphasizes the habitual nature of the problem.

It is not clear if functional defecation disorders are caused by disturbances in motor and/or sensory function of the pelvic floor and rectum; there is often a suggestion of a learned or acquired problem, which may be the result of deferred stooling, "stress," or sometimes a history of physical or sexual abuse including anal intercourse.

CLINICAL PRESENTATION

Patients with functional defecation disorders often complain of less than 3 bowel movements per week, as well as hard stools, excessive straining, a sensation of anorectal blockage during defecation, incomplete evacuation, and the need for anal digitations. There is often a feeling of pressure on the vagina, with straining requiring digital manipulation of a rectocele through the vaginal canal. Although these symptoms suggest the presence of functional defecation disorders, they lack sensitivity to discriminate between slow transit and anorectal dysfunction.[5,12]

DIAGNOSTIC APPROACH

Functional defecation disorders should be suspected in patients with constipation who are not responsive to trials of laxatives. Digital rectal examination (DRE) is key to detecting pelvic floor descent over the finger and pressing toward the vagina to look for a rectocele. DRE is of significant value in detecting dyssynergia through the evaluation of abnormal contraction of the puborectalis and/or external anal sphincter muscle during simulated evacuation. The observation of perineal tenderness, anocutaneous reflexes, anal resting tone, and pelvic floor movements could also provide additional relevant information. When compared with anorectal manometry, expert examination is considered to have up to 93% sensitivity and 58% specificity for dyssynergia.[13] The high positive predictive value of DRE compared with anorectal manometry makes it a reliable bedside tool for screening dyssynergic defecation in patients with chronic constipation. For the diagnosis to be confirmed, further anorectal physiologic testing is required.

Anorectal Manometry

Anorectal manometry is the first recommended test for the evaluation of patients with constipation and suspected functional defecation disorders.[14] It provides unique information on anorectal pressures at rest, during squeeze, during cough, and during simulated evacuation. Other than motor function, it also assesses rectal sensory thresholds and rectoanal reflexes. Although conventional

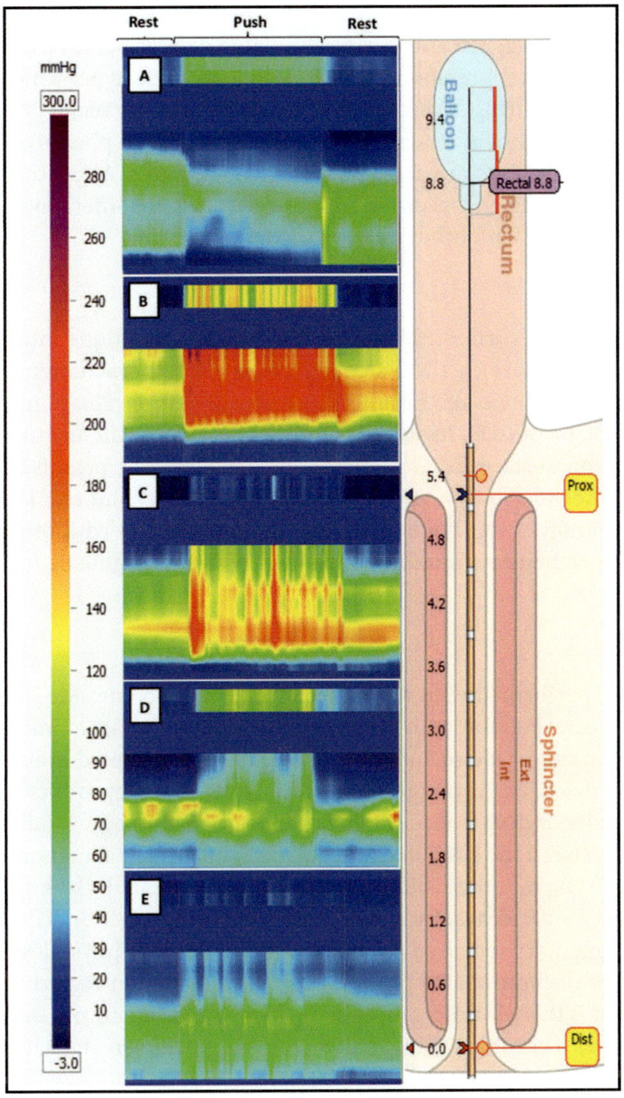

Figure 6-1. High-resolution abnormal anorectal manometry patterns during simulated defecation. Top panels show rectal pressures and lower panels show anal pressures. (A) A normal response consists of an increase in intrarectal pressure combined with a relaxation of the anal sphincter. (B) Type I dyssynergic defecation: an appropriate increase in intrarectal pressure but simultaneous paradoxical anal sphincter contraction. (C) Type II dyssynergic defecation: an inadequate increase in intrarectal pressure along with a paradoxical anal sphincter contraction. (D) Type III dyssynergic defecation: impaired anal sphincter relaxation despite a normal increase in intrarectal pressure. (E) Type IV dyssynergic defecation: impaired anal sphincter relaxation along with a diminished intrarectal pressure.

manometry with water-perfused, air-charged, or solid-state sensors has long been used, advances in high-resolution anorectal manometry techniques over the past decade have brought new dimensions to the test. High-resolution anorectal manometry has enhanced our understanding of anorectal function by providing a detailed assessment of the anal and rectal pressure profiles.

The following 4 manometric patterns have been defined in patients with functional defecation disorders (Figure 6-1)[15]: type I, a paradoxical increase in anal pressure with a normal increase in rectal pressure; type II, a paradoxical increase in anal pressure without an adequate increase in rectal pressure; type III, incomplete relaxation (< 20%) of anal pressure with normal rectal pressure; and type IV, anal pressure without an adequate increase in rectal pressure. However, a paradoxical contraction pattern is commonly seen in healthy controls during simulated evacuation on high-resolution anorectal manometry, questioning its diagnostic value. A recent study reported an adequate increase in rectal pressure accompanied by a simultaneous reduction in anal pressure during simulated evacuation, which is considered the normal pattern of defecation, in less than 10% of healthy individuals.[10]

In a large review of anorectal manometry patterns from patients with functional defecation disorder in comparison with healthy controls, 3 phenotypes discriminated between patients who had an abnormal balloon expulsion test from healthy controls.[12] These phenotypes included (1) a high anal phenotype characterized by elevated anal pressures at rest and during simulated defecation, (2) a low rectal phenotype characterized by diminished rectal pressures, and (3) a hybrid phenotype, which included low rectal and impaired anal relaxation during simulated evacuation. While low rectal profiles are more common among patients with functional defecation disorder, the hybrid phenotype appears to be the only phenotype that is useful for discriminating patients from controls. Altogether, although anorectal manometry cannot make the diagnosis of functional defecation disorders independently, its findings should be interpreted along with other physiologic tests.

Electromyography

EMG of the pelvic floor, by means of needle or surface EMG recordings, provides unique information about muscle behavior. A sustained increase in EMG activity on simulated evacuation is frequently seen in patients with dyssynergia. While needle EMG is more sensitive for evaluation of the external anal sphincter and the puborectalis muscle, its utility is limited because of the invasive nature of the test. The newer, high-resolution surface EMG methods have emerged as promising techniques that allow evaluation of the puborectalis muscle as well as the external anal sphincter less invasively.[16] Although the current EMG techniques can guide diagnosis in combination with other physiologic tests, they lack the sensitivity/specificity required to make it an optimal diagnostic tool for functional defecation disorder.

Balloon Expulsion Testing

The balloon expulsion test is commonly performed with the patient sitting on a commode in a private setting after expanding an inserted rectal balloon with 50 to 60 mL room temperature water. The inability to expel the water-filled balloon out of the rectum after 2 minutes of attempted evacuation is suggestive of functional defecation disorder. Although the test is shown to be reproducible in patients with functional defecation disorder, it does not reveal the underlying pathology. Studies have reported variable levels of agreement between the balloon expulsion test and anorectal manometry or EMG in patients with dyssynergia.[17] Overall, the balloon expulsion test appears to lack the sensitivity and specificity required to make it a suitable test for screening or excluding functional defecation disorder; rather, it is a good complimentary test used in conjunction with other physiologic tests to evaluate anorectal function. Balloon distention also provides useful information regarding rectal sensation. Rectal sensation is impaired if there is not a sensation at 40 mL or greater or no urge to go at greater than 100 mL. This also implies a chronically distended and less sensitive rectal vault.

Defecography

The need for imaging in the diagnosis of functional defecation disorder usually becomes apparent when the results of anorectal manometry and balloon expulsion tests are equivocal and do not confirm the diagnosis. Imaging studies also have the benefit of adding unique information about the pelvic floor structure and its real-time dynamic changes with motion. Barium studies allow dynamic fluoroscopic evaluation of defecation performed in the physiologic position (Figure 6-2), whereas magnetic resonance defecography (Figure 6-3), which is performed in the supine position, has the advantage of high-resolution imaging of the anal sphincter and soft tissues with minimal radiation.[16] There is reasonable diagnostic agreement between barium and magnetic resonance defecography and anorectal manometry in patients with obstructive defecation. The availability of the imaging techniques and expertise as well as the costs associated with these tests have made them of limited clinical utility. Nonetheless, Rome IV inclusion of abnormal evacuation based on imaging as a separate diagnostic criterion highlights the position of imaging in the diagnosis of functional defecation disorder and emphasizes the need for resources and a unified protocol. Defecography has largely been replaced by pelvic magnetic resonance imaging (MRI) without contrast.

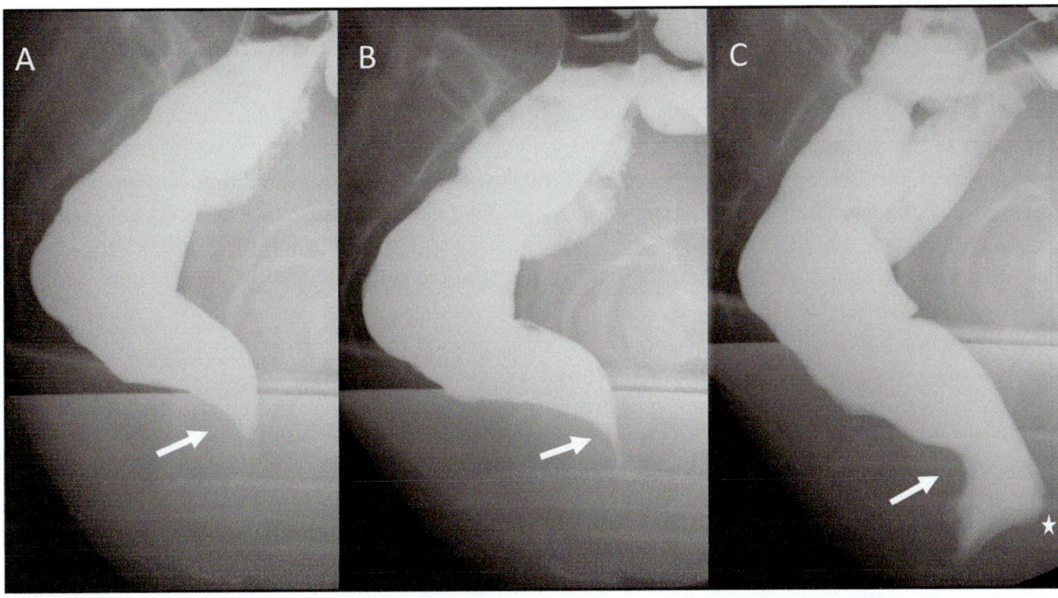

Figure 6-2. Barium defecography images obtained from a patient with functional defecation disorder during (A) resting, (B) straining, and (C) defecation with the arrow pointing to the puborectalis muscle. Note the persistent puborectalis impression and lack of pelvic floor descent during straining. During defecation, there is paradoxical contraction of puborectalis muscle, noted by the deep indentation in the posterior rectal wall, along with the prolonged and incomplete emptying of rectum. A small rectocele (star) is seen at the end of defecation.

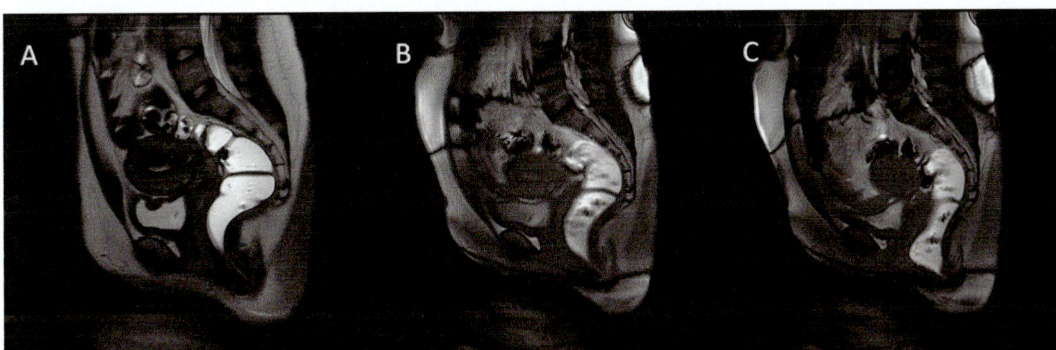

Figure 6-3. Magnetic resonance defecography. Midsagittal images from a patient with functional defecation disorder shows (A) the normal anorectal angle at rest. During (B) straining and (C) defecation, there is persistent prominent indentation of the puborectalis muscle on the posterior rectal wall, which prohibits the expected widening of the anorectal angle.

MANAGEMENT

Clinical Management

The management of patients with defecatory dysfunction often entails a multidisciplinary approach. Treatment should be individualized according to the etiology, underlying pathology, and patients' symptoms and preferences. While lifestyle modification with a healthy diet that contains abundant fiber and sufficient fluid and physical activity are to be emphasized for each individual, laxatives and newer prosecretory agents should be considered according to the symptoms. Nevertheless, avoiding hard stools and addressing constipation should be the major goals of any treatment plan for patients with pelvic floor dysfunction. Timed toilet training, prompt response to the call for stooling (urge for defecation), and avoidance of prolonged commode time are other important aspects of management. Stress management, mindfulness exercises, and cognitive behavioral therapy may be needed for some individuals. Regardless, the mainstay of treatment of functional defecation disorders remains pelvic retraining with biofeedback.

Biofeedback

Biofeedback is defined as device-based learning that enables an individual to modulate a targeted physiologic activity to improve its performance. The device allows translation of a physiologic activity, such as muscle activity, to visual, verbal, or auditory signals and, therefore, enables the user to use this feedback signal to correct to the desired physiologic state. Over time, this learned behavior will be independent of the device.

Biofeedback has emerged as the most effective approach in patients with functional defecation disorders over the past 2 decades.[18] Rao[19] defined 3 goals for biofeedback in patients with functional defecation disorders: (1) to restore the coordination of the abdominal and pelvic floor muscle and to correct dyssynergic defecation, (2) to facilitate normal defecation, and (3) to improve the rectal sensory threshold in patients with anorectal sensory dysfunction.

Biofeedback is offered in most centers by a trained nurse or physical therapist who may use a variety of instruments such as a rectal balloon and manometry or EMG systems to coach patients. In general, it is labor intensive, requiring multiple sessions followed by home exercises. Patients' willingness to participate is key, and it correlates directly with improvement in the bowel satisfaction score. Other clinical predictors of successful biofeedback therapy are harder stools and a shorter duration of laxative use.[18] A higher frequency of experiencing abdominal pain predicts a poor response to biofeedback. A prolonged balloon expulsion test is also associated with a good response to biofeedback therapy. However, the anorectal manometry parameters, except for rectal pressure during straining, neither predict nor mediate the response to treatment.[20] Biofeedback therapy has also been associated with an improvement in the quality of life of patients with functional defecation disorders.[18] However, it did not improve constipation symptoms or the satisfaction rate in patients with isolated slow transit constipation.[21]

There have been several clinical trials that have compared biofeedback with other therapies, such as laxatives, muscle relaxants, and sham feedback. In all of these studies, biofeedback was superior to the other interventions, with a 6-fold increase in the odds of treatment success compared with the other treatment options.[22] Overall, biofeedback for functional defecation disorders has a success rate of up to 80% in experienced centers. A sustained benefit has been reported at 44 months, although refresher courses may reinforce the success.[23]

The mechanism of action of biofeedback therapy is not quite clear. Nevertheless, biofeedback is associated with enhanced anorectal coordination through improved anal relaxation along with more effective abdominal pressures. Therapy is shown to be associated with changes in physiologic characteristics. Some have suggested that the effect of biofeedback is beyond its effect on the pelvic floor. In one study using laser Doppler flowmetry,[24] there was an increase in rectal mucosal blood flow after biofeedback therapy, which correlated with a decrease in colonic transit. The authors concluded that biofeedback is associated with enhanced activity of the autonomic nervous system.[24] More recently, cortical evoked potentials and transcranial magnetic stimulation tests have suggested a role for biofeedback in restoring the bidirectional brain-gut connections in patients with dyssynergic defecation.[25] In a study of patients with pelvic floor dysfunction and symptoms of urge urinary incontinence using functional MRI, researchers showed that biofeedback therapy was associated with changes in brain activation and deactivation patterns.[26] They noted different patterns of brain responses to bladder filling, which appeared to predict the success of biofeedback therapy. In patients who were nonresponders to biofeedback, the pattern of brain deactivation barely changed after therapy.[26] Whether biofeedback modulates the brain activation and deactivation pattern in patients with functional defecation disorders requires further study. It would also be helpful to know if there are different phenotypes of patients with functional defecation disorders based on brain activation patterns that predict the response to biofeedback.

Recently, the American Neurogastroenterology and Motility Society and the European Society of Neurogastroenterology and Motility convened a task force to examine the role of biofeedback therapy in patients with functional defecation disorders. The task force concluded that, based on the strength of evidence, biofeedback therapy is recommended for short- and long-term treatment of constipation with functional defecation disorders.[18] At present, biofeedback therapy is not widely available, except for at bigger academic centers. This is in part due to the lack of expertise and the costs associated with personnel and instruments that are required to deliver the therapy. In addition, reimbursements for biofeedback services have been notoriously uncertain and often low relative to the costs. These limitations emphasize the need for better selection of patients who will benefit from the therapy as well as a standardized protocol.

Botulinum Toxin A

There has recently been increasing interest in the use of botulinum toxin A in the treatment of pelvic floor disorders in patients with myofascial pain, detrusor sphincter dyssynergia, and dyssynergic defecation with varying results.[27,28] The toxin has been proven to be safe and effective for the treatment of pelvic muscle and sphincter hypertonicity. It has also gained interest for the management of functional defecation disorders in specific populations, such as patients with Parkinson disease[29] and pediatric patients.[30] Also, there might be an additional benefit for its use in conjunction with biofeedback for intractable patients. A recent systematic review of 7 trials of botulinum toxin injections in patients with functional defecation disorders estimated a median 77.4% symptomatic improvement initially, which declined to 46% at 4 months after injection.[31] Repeated injections might be of additional benefit in achieving long-term efficacy. Whether ultrasound-guided injection into the puborectalis muscle is advantageous over blind injections is unclear. The symptomatic improvement correlates with an improvement in the anorectal pressure profile as well as the balloon expulsion test, as shown in some studies. The major limitation of botulinum toxin is the need for repeated injections, and the most common complication is transient fecal incontinence, which is reversible. Although botulinum toxin appears to be of clinical significance in uncontrolled studies, its use is not endorsed by the most recent technical guidelines on the management of constipation.[14] Head-to-head randomized controlled trials are needed to prove its efficacy.

Surgery

Surgery is considered as the last resort for patients with refractory symptoms who have failed conservative measures. Although it may be conceivable, partial division of the puborectalis muscle has been disappointing with poor outcomes. Malone antegrade continence enemas, which are routinely used in children with a neurogenic bowel, create a skin fistula between the appendix or cecum and the abdominal wall and allow catheterization for the administration of enemas. They have been shown to be effective in the management of bowel symptoms in 65% of adults with functional defecation disorders in a small series.[32] Conduit stenosis requiring surgical interventions and infections were common. The effectiveness of this procedure in the management of functional defecation disorders requires further study. Sacral nerve stimulation has been tried in patients with functional defecation disorders who had significant rectal hyposensitivity in one small prospective trial. During the 4 weeks of temporary stimulation, there was significant improvement in rectal sensory thresholds and the percentage of successful bowel movements.[33] However, long-term results are not available to support the use of sacral nerve stimulation for the management of patients with functional defecation disorders.

Rectoceles and/or rectal intussusception are structural disorders that are commonly seen in the setting of functional defecation disorders. These structural abnormalities are believed to be secondary to the functional problem and will be best addressed by the management of the primary pathology or the correction of dyssynergia. Surgical interventions with stapled transanal rectal resection or ventral rectopexy are reserved only for clinically significant rectoceles and have been associated with high complications and unfavorable outcomes.[34]

Functional Anorectal Pain: Levator Ani Syndrome, Unspecified Functional Anorectal Pain, and Proctalgia Fugax

Functional anorectal pain disorders are characterized by chronic, recurrent anorectal pain in the absence of structural pathologies. The 3 types of functional anorectal pain disorders include levator ani syndrome, unspecified functional anorectal pain, and proctalgia fugax.[1] They are differentiated based on the duration of the pain and the presence or absence of anorectal tenderness on palpation.

LEVATOR ANI SYNDROME AND FUNCTIONAL ANORECTAL PAIN

Definition

Levator ani syndrome is defined by chronic, intermittent pain in the rectum that usually lasts more than 30 minutes and is associated with tenderness on palpation of the puborectalis muscle.[1] Patients with unspecified anorectal pain have similar pain symptoms without tenderness during the physical examination.

Epidemiology

A population-based survey of functional bowel disorder in the United States reported a prevalence of 11.6% for functional anorectal pain and 6.6% for levator ani syndrome.[35] The prevalence of anorectal pain and levator ani syndrome was higher in women and decreased by age.[35,36]

Functional anorectal pain disorders are shown to negatively impact the sufferers' quality of life[37] and productivity, with 8.3% of patients with functional anorectal pain and 11.5% with levator ani syndrome reporting the inability to work.[35]

Pathophysiology

The etiology of levator ani syndrome has been attributed to an elevated anal resting tone and increased muscle tension.[38] In a well-designed trial, the physiologic mechanisms responsible for levator ani syndrome were found to be similar to those of dyssynergic defecation, with the majority of patients with levator ani syndrome having evidence of paradoxical anal contraction at the time of simulated evacuation along with abnormal balloon expulsion tests.[39] The correction of dyssynergia being correlated with symptomatic improvement suggests that rectoanal incoordination may be a pathophysiological explanation for levator ani syndrome.[39] Interestingly, patients with unspecified anorectal pain do not share similar features and often have normal physiologic tests.[39] In a retrospective review of 170 patients with functional anorectal pain disorders, 35% of patients reported a chronic pain problem distinct from the anorectal pain, and 33% of the patients had a psychiatric history or symptoms of a psychological disturbance, with anxiety and depression being the most common problems.[36]

Clinical Presentation

Patients with levator ani syndrome often complain of a prolonged (more than 30 minutes), vague, aching pain high in the rectum.[1] The pain can be positional and worse with sitting than lying or standing.[38] Some patients will have increased pain during defecation. Although the symptoms are similar in levator ani syndrome and unspecified functional anorectal pain, a physical examination can distinguish between the two. There is distinct tenderness during posterior traction of the levator ani muscle in patients with levator ani syndrome during the rectal or pelvic examination.[1]

Table 6-3

Rome IV Diagnostic Criteria for Functional Anorectal Pain Disorders

I. DIAGNOSTIC CRITERIA FOR LEVATOR ANI SYNDROME
• Chronic or recurrent rectal pain or aching • Episodes last 30 minutes or longer • Tenderness during traction on the puborectalis
II. DIAGNOSTIC CRITERIA FOR UNSPECIFIED FUNCTIONAL ANORECTAL PAIN
• Symptom criteria for chronic levator ani syndrome • No tenderness during posterior traction on the puborectalis muscle
III. DIAGNOSTIC CRITERIA FOR PROCTALGIA FUGAX
• Recurrent episodes of pain localized to the rectum and unrelated to defecation • Episodes last from seconds to minutes, with a maximum duration of 30 minutes • There is no anorectal pain between episodes
* Other causes of rectal pain, such as inflammatory bowel disease, intramuscular abscess and fissure, thrombosed hemorrhoids, prostatitis, coccygodynia, and major structural alterations of the pelvic floor must be excluded. * All listed items must be present for each diagnosis. * Criteria must be fulfilled for 3 months with symptom onset at least 6 months before diagnosis.

Diagnostic Approach

Table 6-3 shows the Rome IV diagnostic criteria for unspecified anorectal pain and levator ani syndrome.[1] Diagnosis is clinical and based on symptoms and the physical examination after exclusion of other structural pathologies. Anoscopy and/or endoscopic evaluations may be indicated to rule out anal fissures and inflammatory etiologies such as Crohn's disease or ulcerative proctitis. Pelvic MRI will aid in detecting soft tissue pathologies such as perianal abscesses or fistulas. In patients with chronic constipation, functional defecation disorders should be ruled out by physiologic testing.

Management

A number of small, noncontrolled trials have evaluated a variety of options such as electrogalvanic stimulation, digital massage, and sitz baths for functional anorectal pain disorders with inconclusive results.[38] Belladonna suppositories containing opioids can be helpful. Muscle relaxants, including methocarbamol, diazepam, and cyclobenzaprine, are also commonly used with no evidence to support their efficacy in this condition.

In a prospective, randomized, controlled trial of 157 patients with anorectal pain, the efficacy of the 3 most common treatment approaches including biofeedback, electrogalvanic stimulations, and digital massage of the levator ani was compared.[39] The study showed unequivocal evidence that biofeedback is the most effective treatment in patients with levator ani syndrome, with 87% reporting adequate relief of rectal pain after biofeedback therapy compared with 45% after electrical stimulation and 22% after massage and sitz bath. Biofeedback improved the pain and discomfort by correcting the anorectal coordination during evacuation. This improvement was sustained at the 12-month follow-up.[39] Patients with levator ani syndrome who had paradoxical anal contraction and abnormal rectal balloon expulsion were more likely to respond to biofeedback therapy.[39]

In an uncontrolled study, a combination of steroid and local anesthetics was injected into the tender points in more than 100 patients with levator ani syndrome, up to 3 times at 2-week intervals. Close to 30% of patients reported a benefit in up to 6 months of follow-ups.[40] When compared with electrogalvanic stimulation twice per week, this injection showed better short-term results.[41] In another double-blind, placebo-controlled clinical trial, investigators failed to show efficacy for botulinum toxin injection over placebo in 12 patients with levator ani syndrome.[42] Higher doses of toxin might be of additional benefit in medically refractory patients as suggested by uncontrolled studies.[43] A pilot study of sacral nerve stimulation did not find it effective for the treatment of chronic anal pain.[44] Neither of these options have been proven to be effective in unspecified anorectal pain, and further clinical trials of neuromodulators and analgesics are currently unavailable.

The American Neurogastroenterology and Motility Society and the European Society of Neurogastroenterology and Motility task force recently recommended biofeedback therapy for patients with levator ani syndrome who (1) are unresponsive to standard therapies including antispasmodics and muscle relaxants, (2) have any structural or inflammatory causes of chronic anorectal and pelvic pain, or (3) have tenderness of the levator ani muscle on DRE.[18]

PROCTALGIA FUGAX

Definition

Proctalgia fugax is characterized by brief intermittent episodes of pain in the rectum that last seconds to minutes only and spontaneously resolve.

Epidemiology

The prevalence of proctalgia fugax in the general population is estimated to be between 4% and 18%.[35] A population-based study using the Rome II criteria in Australia reported the prevalence of proctalgia fugax at 6.5%.[45] Sex tendency for proctalgia fugax was not clear in earlier reports; however, a robust female predominance is reported in more recent studies.[45,46] It affects patients between 30 and 60 years of age and, while the majority of patients report the onset of symptoms postpuberty, there are a few anecdotal reports of proctalgia fugax in the pediatric population. Proctalgia fugax has been shown to be significantly associated with impaired quality of life by affecting the mental and physical functioning of the sufferer.[47]

Pathophysiology

Although the precise pathophysiology is not clear, abnormal smooth muscle contraction is suggested to be a potential pathology in some patients with proctalgia fugax.[47] An abnormal rise in the anal resting tone and an increase in slow wave amplitude have been reported during acute pain episodes and are thought to be driven from a sympathetic surge.[47] Increased sigmoid pressures as opposed to those in the rectal wall or anal sphincter during the attacks have been shown to correlate with pain attacks.[48] Proctalgia fugax was seen at a moderately increased rate in multiparous women with an advanced stage of pelvic organ prolapse,[49] and bilateral pudendal neuropathy due to perineal stretch has been suggested as a potential mechanism of pathology in some patients.[50]

Familial forms of proctalgia fugax associated with internal anal sphincter myopathy have also been described.[51-55] In these patients, the myopathy resulted in significant hypertrophy of the internal anal sphincter.[56]

Psychiatric comorbid conditions of perfectionism, anxiety, and hypochondriasis have been reported to be common in patients with proctalgia fugax in a case series.[57] Compared with patients with organic anorectal pathologies, patients with proctalgia fugax have greater neuroticism, psychoticism, depression, and pain,[58] suggesting a central pathology for this condition.

Clinical Presentation

Patients with proctalgia fugax typically experience erratic episodes of sudden-onset rectal pain that usually last less than 30 minutes and are completely self-remitting.[1] Pain is always at the same place in the rectum and is described as cramping, aching, gnawing, or stabbing and sharp. It could be so severe that some patients feel faint during the attacks. Pain attacks begin suddenly at irregular intervals during the day or night. Although most people do not have a trigger, the pain could be precipitated by intercourse, stress, defecation, or menstruation in some patients.[59] Pain attacks tend to be infrequent; they have been reported to occur up to once per month.[46]

Diagnostic Approach

Diagnosis is clinical and in the absence of structural pathologies. See Table 6-3 for a summary of the Rome IV diagnostic criteria for proctalgia fugax.

Management

Reassurance is an important and often sufficient aspect of the treatment of proctalgia fugax. In a majority of patients, the short episodes of pain impede any treatment, and no preventive measures are available for this condition to date. Nevertheless, frequent and/or prolonged pain attacks will warrant treatment. The use of a hot water enema or hot bath, digital dilatation, forceful evacuation, and positional changes have been reported to be beneficial in a small case series.[59] Topical treatment with antispasmodics and nitroglycerine may offer benefit in some patients based on uncontrolled reports.[59]

In a randomized, double-blind, placebo-controlled, crossover trial, inhalation of salbutamol during the attacks significantly reduced the duration of severe pain, especially in patients with prolonged pain attacks.[60] Belladonna suppositories containing opioids also can be helpful.

References

1. Rao SS, Bharucha AE, Chiarioni G, et al. Functional anorectal disorders. *Gastroenterology*. 2016. doi: 10.1053/j.gastro.2016.02.009. [Epub ahead of print]
2. Zakari M, Nee J, Hirsch W, Kuo B, Lembo A, Staller K. Gender differences in chronic constipation on anorectal motility. *Neurogastroenterol Motil*. 2017;29(4). doi: 10.1111/nmo.12980. Epub 2016 Nov 27.
3. Noelting J, Eaton JE, Choung RS, Zinsmeister AR, Locke GR 3rd, Bharucha AE. The incidence rate and characteristics of clinically diagnosed defecatory disorders in the community. *Neurogastroenterol Motil*. 2016;28(11):1690-1697.
4. Bharucha AE, Rao SS. An update on anorectal disorders for gastroenterologists. *Gastroenterology*. 2014;146(1):45.e2.
5. Rao SS, Tuteja AK, Vellema T, Kempf J, Stessman M. Dyssynergic defecation: demographics, symptoms, stool patterns, and quality of life. *J Clin Gastroenterol*. 2004;38(8):680-685.
6. Rao SS, Seaton K, Miller MJ, et al. Psychological profiles and quality of life differ between patients with dyssynergia and those with slow transit constipation. *J Psychosom Res*. 2007;63(4):441-449.
7. Sommers T, Corban C, Sengupta N, et al. Emergency department burden of constipation in the United States from 2006 to 2011. *Am J Gastroenterol*. 2015;110(4):572-579.
8. Sethi S, Mikami S, Leclair J, et al. Inpatient burden of constipation in the United States: an analysis of national trends in the United States from 1997 to 2010. *Am J Gastroenterol*. 2014;109(2):250-256.
9. Staller K, Barshop K, Kuo B, Ananthakrishnan AN. Resting anal pressure, not outlet obstruction or transit, predicts healthcare utilization in chronic constipation: a retrospective cohort analysis. *Neurogastroenterol Motil*. 2015;27(10):1378-1388.
10. Grossi U, Carrington EV, Bharucha AE, Horrocks EJ, Scott SM, Knowles CH. Diagnostic accuracy study of anorectal manometry for diagnosis of dyssynergic defecation. *Gut*. 2016;65(3):447-455.
11. Sharma A, Rao S. Constipation: pathophysiology and current therapeutic approaches. *Handb Exp Pharmacol*. 2017;239:59-74.
12. Ratuapli SK, Bharucha AE, Noelting J, Harvey DM, Zinsmeister AR. Phenotypic identification and classification of functional defecatory disorders using high-resolution anorectal manometry. *Gastroenterology*. 2013;144(2):322.e2.

13. Soh JS, Lee HJ, Jung KW, et al. The diagnostic value of a digital rectal examination compared with high-resolution anorectal manometry in patients with chronic constipation and fecal incontinence. *Am J Gastroenterol.* 2015;110(8):1197-1204.
14. American Gastroenterological Association, Bharucha AE, Dorn SD, Lembo A, Pressman A. American Gastroenterological Association medical position statement on constipation. *Gastroenterology.* 2013;144(1):211-217.
15. Rao SS, Mudipalli RS, Stessman M, Zimmerman B. Investigation of the utility of colorectal function tests and Rome II criteria in dyssynergic defecation (Anismus). *Neurogastroenterol Motil.* 2004;16(5):589-596.
16. Bharucha AE, Fletcher JG. Recent advances in assessing anorectal structure and functions. *Gastroenterology.* 2007;133(4):1069-1074.
17. Palit S, Thin N, Knowles CH, Lunniss PJ, Bharucha AE, Scott SM. Diagnostic disagreement between tests of evacuatory function: a prospective study of 100 constipated patients. *Neurogastroenterol Motil.* 2016;28(10):1589-1598.
18. Rao SS, Benninga MA, Bharucha AE, Chiarioni G, Di Lorenzo C, Whitehead WE. ANMS-ESNM position paper and consensus guidelines on biofeedback therapy for anorectal disorders. *Neurogastroenterol Motil.* 2015;27(5):594-609.
19. Rao SS. The technical aspects of biofeedback therapy for defecation disorders. *Gastroenterologist.* 1998;6(2):96-103.
20. Shim LS, Jones M, Prott GM, Morris LI, Kellow JE, Malcolm A. Predictors of outcome of anorectal biofeedback therapy in patients with constipation. *Aliment Pharmacol Ther.* 2011;33(11):1245-1251.
21. Chiarioni G, Salandini L, Whitehead WE. Biofeedback benefits only patients with outlet dysfunction, not patients with isolated slow transit constipation. *Gastroenterology.* 2005;129(1):86-97.
22. Koh CE, Young CJ, Young JM, Solomon MJ. Systematic review of randomized controlled trials of the effectiveness of biofeedback for pelvic floor dysfunction. *Br J Surg.* 2008;95(9):1079-1087.
23. Lee HJ, Boo SJ, Jung KW, et al. Long-term efficacy of biofeedback therapy in patients with dyssynergic defecation: results of a median 44 months follow-up. *Neurogastroenterol Motil.* 2015;27(6):787-795.
24. Emmanuel AV, Kamm MA. Response to a behavioural treatment, biofeedback, in constipated patients is associated with improved gut transit and autonomic innervation. *Gut.* 2001;49(2):214-219.
25. Remes-Troche JM, Tantiphlachiva K, Attaluri A, et al. A bi-directional assessment of the human brain-anorectal axis. *Neurogastroenterol Motil.* 2011;23(3):8.
26. Griffiths D, Clarkson B, Tadic SD, Resnick NM. Brain mechanisms underlying urge incontinence and its response to pelvic floor muscle training. *J Urol.* 2015;194(3):708-715.
27. Morrissey D, El-Khawand D, Ginzburg N, Wehbe S, O'Hare P 3rd, Whitmore K. Botulinum toxin A injections into pelvic floor muscles under electromyographic guidance for women with refractory high-tone pelvic floor dysfunction: a 6-month prospective pilot study. *Female Pelvic Med Reconstr Surg.* 2015;21(5):277-282.
28. Chai TC, Asfaw TS, Baker JE, et al. Future directions of research and care for urinary incontinence: findings from the National Institute of Diabetes and Digestive and Kidney Diseases Summit on Urinary Incontinence Clinical Research in Women. *J Urol.* 2017;198(1):22-29.
29. Rossi M, Merello M, Perez-Lloret S. Management of constipation in Parkinson's disease. *Expert Opin Pharmacother.* 2015;16(4):547-57.
30. Chumpitazi BP, Fishman SJ, Nurko S. Long-term clinical outcome after botulinum toxin injection in children with nonrelaxing internal anal sphincter. *Am J Gastroenterol.* 2009;104(4):976-983.
31. Emile SH, Elfeki HA, Elbanna HG, et al. Efficacy and safety of botulinum toxin in treatment of anismus: a systematic review. *World J Gastrointest Pharmacol Ther.* 2016;7(3):453-462.
32. Hirst GR, Arumugam PJ, Watkins AJ, et al. Antegrade continence enema in the treatment of obstructed defaecation with or without faecal incontinence. *Tech Coloproctol.* 2005;9(3):217-221.
33. Knowles CH, Thin N, Gill K, et al. Prospective randomized double-blind study of temporary sacral nerve stimulation in patients with rectal evacuatory dysfunction and rectal hyposensitivity. *Ann Surg.* 2012;255(4):643-649.
34. Madbouly KM, Abbas KS, Hussein AM. Disappointing long-term outcomes after stapled transanal rectal resection for obstructed defecation. *World J Surg.* 2010;34(9):2191-2196.
35. Drossman DA, Li Z, Andruzzi E, et al. U.S. householder survey of functional gastrointestinal disorders. Prevalence, sociodemography, and health impact. *Dig Dis Sci.* 1993;38(9):1569-1580.
36. Atkin GK, Suliman A, Vaizey CJ. Patient characteristics and treatment outcome in functional anorectal pain. *Dis Colon Rectum.* 2011;54(7):870-875.
37. Koloski NA, Talley NJ, Boyce PM. The impact of functional gastrointestinal disorders on quality of life. *Am J Gastroenterol.* 2000;95:67.
38. Bharucha AE, Lee TH. Anorectal and pelvic pain. *Mayo Clinic Proc.* 2016;91(10):1471-1486.
39. Chiarioni G, Nardo A, Vantini I, Romito A, Whitehead WE. Biofeedback is superior to electrogalvanic stimulation and massage for treatment of levator ani syndrome. *Gastroenterology.* 2010;138(4):1321-1329.
40. Kang YS, Jeong SY, Cho HJ, Kim DS, Lee DH, Kim TS. Transanally injected triamcinolone acetonide in levator syndrome. *Dis Colon Rectum.* 2000;43(9):1288-1291.

41. Park DH, Yoon SG, Kim KU, et al. Comparison study between electrogalvanic stimulation and local injection therapy in levator ani syndrome. *Int J Colorectal Dis.* 2005;20(3):272-276.
42. Rao SS, Paulson J, Mata M, Zimmerman B. Clinical trial: effects of botulinum toxin on levator ani syndrome—a double-blind, placebo-controlled study. *Aliment Pharmacol Ther.* 2009;29(9):985-991.
43. Bibi S, Zutshi M, Gurland B, Hull T. Is Botox for anal pain an effective treatment option? *Postgrad Med.* 2016;128(1):41-45.
44. Dudding TC, Thomas GP, Hollingshead JR, George AT, Stern J, Vaizey CJ. Sacral nerve stimulation: an effective treatment for chronic functional anal pain? *Colorectal Dis.* 2013;15(9):1140-1144.
45. Boyce PM, Talley NJ, Burke C, Koloski NA. Epidemiology of the functional gastrointestinal disorders diagnosed according to Rome II criteria: an Australian population-based study. *Intern Med J.* 2006;36(1):28-36.
46. de Parades V, Etienney I, Bauer P, Taouk M, Atienza P. Proctalgia fugax: demographic and clinical characteristics. What every doctor should know from a prospective study of 54 patients. *Dis Colon Rectum.* 2007;50(6):893-898.
47. Eckardt VF, Dodt O, Kanzler G, Bernhard G. Anorectal function and morphology in patients with sporadic proctalgia fugax. *Dis Colon Rectum.* 1996;39(7):755-762.
48. Harvey RF. Colonic motility in proctalgia fugax. *Lancet.* 1979;314(8145):713-714.
49. Jelovsek JE, Barber MD, Paraiso MF, Walters MD. Functional bowel and anorectal disorders in patients with pelvic organ prolapse and incontinence. *Am J Obstet Gynecol.* 2005;193(6):2105-2111.
50. Shafik A. Pudendal canal syndrome and proctalgia fugax. *Dis Colon Rectum.* 1997;40(4):504.
51. Celik AF, Katsinelos P, Read NW, Khan MI, Donnelly TC. Hereditary proctalgia fugax and constipation: report of a second family. *Gut.* 1995;36(4):581-584.
52. Kamm MA, Hoyle CH, Burleigh DE, et al. Hereditary internal anal sphincter myopathy causing proctalgia fugax and constipation. A newly identified condition. *Gastroenterology.* 1991;100(3):805-810.
53. de la Portilla F, Borrero JJ, Rafel E. Hereditary vacuolar internal anal sphincter myopathy causing proctalgia fugax and constipation: a new case contribution. *Eur J Gastroenterol Hepatol.* 2005;17(3):359-361.
54. Konig P, Ambrose NS, Scott N. Hereditary internal anal sphincter myopathy causing proctalgia fugax and constipation: further clinical and histological characterization in a patient. *Eur J Gastroenterol Hepatol.* 2000;12(1):127-128.
55. Zbar AP, de la Portilla, Borrero JJ, Garriques S. Hereditary internal anal sphincter myopathy: the first Caribbean family. *Tech Coloproctol.* 2007;11(1):60-63.
56. Guy RJ, Kamm MA, Martin JE. Internal anal sphincter myopathy causing proctalgia fugax and constipation: further clinical and radiological characterization in a patient. *Eur J Gastroenterol Hepatol.* 1997;9(2):221-224.
57. Pilling LF, Swenson WM, Hill JR. The psychologic aspects of proctalgia fugax. *Dis Colon Rectum.* 1965;8(5):372-376.
58. Magni G, de Bertolini C, Dodi G, Infantino A. Psychological findings in chronic anal pain. *Psychopathology.* 1986;19(4):170-174.
59. Jeyarajah S, Chow A, Ziprin P, Tilney H, Purkayastha S. Proctalgia fugax, an evidence-based management pathway. *Int J Colorectal Dis.* 2010;25(9):1037-1046.
60. Eckardt VF, Dodt O, Kanzler G, Bernhard G. Treatment of proctalgia fugax with salbutamol inhalation. *Am J Gastroenterol.* 1996;91(4):686-689.

7

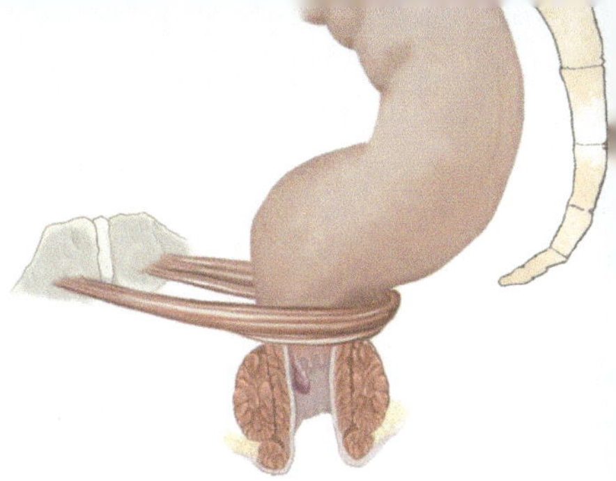

Anorectal Inflammatory Bowel Disease

Yezaz A. Ghouri, MD and Bo Shen, MD

Key Points

- Inflammatory bowel disease (IBD), especially Crohn's disease (CD), can present as fistulizing and nonfistulizing perianal disease. Most cases of fistulizing disease have a combination of a nonfistulizing lesion and an anal fissure, anal ulcer, anal stricture/stenosis, hemorrhoids, or skin tags.
- Perianal disease can be diagnosed with direct examination under anesthesia (EUA), pelvic magnetic resonance imaging (MRI), or lower endoscopic ultrasound (EUS). A combination of these modalities is superior to either one alone.
- Fistulas can be managed conservatively with systemic antibiotics, immunomodulators, and biological agents, but some form of endoscopic or surgical intervention is recommended.
- Endoscopic or surgical fistulotomy is recommended over a traditional surgical resection or diversion to assist in faster healing.
- Nonfistulizing disease is preferably managed with conservative treatment because surgical intervention frequently leads to poor wound healing and wound infection.
- Anal stricture/stenosis is frequently treated with endoscopic or surgical dilation.
- Fecal diversion with or without proctectomy is considered as a treatment of last resort.

IBD is a state of chronic gut inflammation that can sometimes involve the perianal area. It can present as fistulas, strictures, abscesses, sinuses, skin tags, and hemorrhoids.[1] CD is a segmental disease that commonly spares the rectum. The most common location of CD is the ileocecal area; about 15% of these cases develop perianal CD (PCD).[2] This number is lower than those who have isolated

Qureshi W, ed. *Diagnosis and Management Guide for Anorectal Disease: A Clinical Reference* (pp 79-87).

Table 7-1

Montreal Classification of Crohn's Disease[47]

AGE OF ONSET (A)	
A1	16 years or younger
A2	17 to 40 years
A3	Over 40 years
DISEASE LOCATION (L)	
L1	Terminal ileum
L2	Colon
L3	Ileocolon
L4	Upper gastrointestinal involvement
DISEASE BEHAVIOR (B)	
B1	Nonstricturing, nonpenetrating
B2	Stricturing
B3	Penetrating
p	Presence of perianal disease
Adapted from Satsangi J, Silverberg MS, Vermeire S, Colombel JF. The Montreal classification of inflammatory bowel disease: controversies, consensus, and implications. *Gut.* 2006;55(6):749-753.	

small bowel disease. In cases in which the colon and rectum are affected, about 92% develop PCD. In fact, the first description of CD by Dr. Crohn himself included a series of 3 patients with regional enteritis and perianal disease.[3] PCD mainly presents in the form of perianal fistulas, which in early stages may appear as blind sinus.

CD, because of its nature of extensive involvement in and outside the gastrointestinal tract and associated manifestations like fistulas and strictures, was initially classified into various phenotypes using the Greenstein and Vienna classification systems. These systems lost popularity because of the lack of applicability in clinical management and clinical research.[4,5] The Montreal classification is a revision of the Vienna classification system with excellent interobserver agreement for its classification of CD.[6] The system includes 3 main categories: age of onset (A), disease location (L), and disease behavior or nature of the disease (B). The presence of PCD as an independent entity complicating the progression of CD has been implemented in the Montreal classification system and is denoted by "p," as shown in Table 7-1. For example, a case of CD diagnosed at 21 years of age involving the terminal ileum and the cecum with perianal fistula formation would be classified as A2L3B3p using the Montreal system.

Classification

A perianal fistula develops in about 22% of patients suffering from CD.[7] By definition, a fistula is a communication tract between 2 hollow viscera or a connection between a hollow viscus and skin or a mucous membrane. In relation to the organs to which the tract connects, the fistula can be labeled

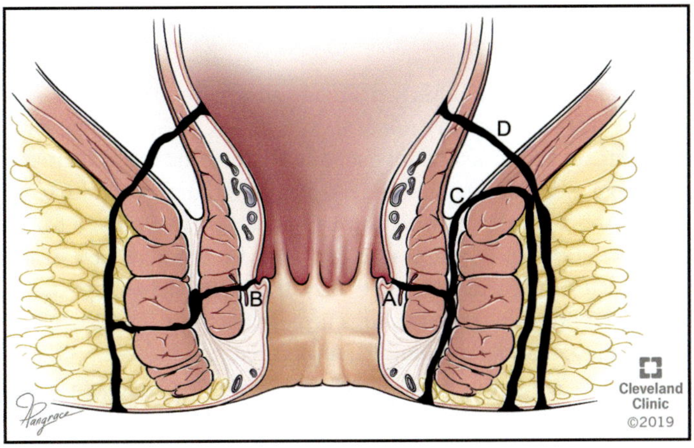

Figure 7-1. Park classification of perianal fistulizing CD: (A) intersphincteric fistula; (B) transsphincteric fistula; (C) suprasphincteric fistula; (D) extrasphincteric fistula. (Reproduced with permission, Cleveland Clinic Center for Medical Art & Photography © 2011-2019. All Rights Reserved.)

as a rectocutaneous fistula, rectovaginal fistula, or fistula-in-ano. In recent years, a global consensus has been reached to appropriately term perianal fistulas to avoid any confusion among experts regarding the anatomic appearance of the fistulous tract. Parks classification is used to divide fistulas into 4 main types, as shown in Figure 7-1. This was updated by adding a fifth type of fistula, which has been included in the following descriptions[8]:

1. Intersphincteric fistula: The tract begins between the internal and external sphincter muscles and opens close to the anal opening.
2. Transsphincteric fistula: The tract begins between the internal and external sphincter muscles. It then crosses the external sphincter and opens outside the anus.
3. Suprasphincteric fistula: The tract begins between the internal and external sphincter muscles and turns upward to above the puborectalis muscle, crosses this muscle, and then extends downward between the puborectalis and levator ani muscle and opens 1 or 2 inches outside the anus.
4. Extrasphincteric fistula: The tract begins in the rectum or sigmoid and then extends downward through the levator ani muscle and opens around the anus.
5. A fistula that does not involve the sphincter complex: The sphincter complex is composed of the external anal sphincter and the puborectalis muscle.

Clinical Presentation

A perianal fistula presents with symptoms such as perianal pain and drainage from the fistulous opening; the drainage can be purulent, mucoid, sanguineous, or mixed. Perianal fistulas tend to have a chronic relapsing course, and some develop anal incontinence because of involvement of the external anal sphincter. The fistulas frequently get infected, giving rise to perianal abscesses and cellulitis. This can have a significant impact on quality of life because of the symptoms and the associated risk of embarrassment, anxiety, and agoraphobia. Rarely, perianal fistulas can circumferentially extend on both sides of the anorectum, giving a horseshoe appearance and hence are termed *horseshoe fistulas*. In nearly 90% of cases, a high transsphincteric fistula leads to the development of horseshoe extensions.[9] Most of these types of fistulas develop because of unsuccessful medical therapy in patients with CD; they are effectively treated with deroofing and debridement or resection and ligation of the fistulous tract. The disease may be associated with active proctitis, which can affect their management; hence, it is necessary to establish if the patient has proctitis with flexible sigmoidoscopy and biopsies.

Diagnosis

Perianal fistulas in CD present with local symptoms, mainly drainage and pain or irritation. The physical examination must include a detailed rectal examination and, in females, an additional vaginal examination. Initially, the anus and perianal area must be inspected to determine the presence of drainage and, if present, the type of drainage (serous, purulent, or bloodstained) and to evaluate for visible fistulous tract openings. By performing a gentle examination using a lubricated gloved finger, one can appreciate the areas of stricture formation or compression of a tract that may release drainage. Some individuals may decline a finger examination because they may experience significant pain, and even a gentle examination with the little finger may cause unbearable pain. In such situations, perianal examination should be performed and a detailed EUA planned.

The assessment of perianal disease requires a 3-pronged approach that includes endoscopic imaging, radiologic imaging, and direct visualization or EUA. Abdominopelvic radiologic imaging is composed mainly of MRI. Endoscopic evaluation includes flexible sigmoidoscopy and rectal EUS. EUA is an effective approach to diagnose the disease and to determine its extent, but this technique is operator-dependent and can be considered a gold standard for diagnosing perianal fistulas in the hands of an experienced surgeon.[10] Broadly speaking, pelvic MRI, rectal EUS, and EUA are comparable with each other regarding the assessment of disease severity and the extent of CD. A combination of these techniques may actually be superior to relying on only one technique.[10] It is important to note that EUA gives the benefit of draining an abscess and control of infection. This may open doors to starting immunosuppressive or biological therapy early.

In a study comparing the pelvic MRI findings of patients with fistulas associated with CD and those without CD, there was no significant difference between the 2 groups in terms of the MRI appearance of fistulas, but the presence of rectal inflammation was primarily associated with CD-related fistulas.[11] MRI has also been shown to incidentally detect clinically silent luminal inflammation or abscess formation.[12] Studies have shown that pelvic MRI has some advantage over rectal EUS in diagnosing perianal fistulas, but the quality of the MRI reporting may be dependent on the expertise of the radiologist. Moreover, EUS provides the opportunity to perform biopsies and is more readily available for a gastroenterologist.[13] EUS can be used by a gastroenterologist to detect the disease course and to help guide therapy. It has been found to be reliable in guiding medical and surgical therapy and assessing response.[14] An IBD specialist may find it beneficial to be trained in the technique of diagnostic lower EUS.

Treatment

PCD has a chronic remitting course, and it takes months to several years in order to achieve complete control of inflammation. The goal of therapy in treating fistulas is to stop drainage and improve quality of life with partial or complete resolution of inflammation. This is approached using medical therapies like anti–tumor necrosis factor (TNF) agents, immunomodulators, and antibiotics, with a significant role of surgical intervention in managing this disease.[15] Medical treatment alone has some effect, but some sort of surgical (preferably minimal) intervention is usually needed to achieve adequate control of PCD.[16] Corticosteroids should be avoided in CD patients who have perianal fistulas.[17] The use of steroids can be detrimental by giving rise to abscess formation and nonhealing fistulas.[18] In fact, patients with PCD are usually refractory to therapy like aminosalicylates and corticosteroids, which are used for treating luminal CD. The management of PCD involves a multidisciplinary approach for best results.

MEDICAL THERAPY

The conventional therapeutic agents used for treating PCD are antibiotics and immunomodulators. The use of antibiotics like ciprofloxacin and metronidazole has been shown to be useful in controlling mild forms of the disease. In a meta-analysis of 3 clinical trials including a total of 123 patients, it was found that the use of ciprofloxacin or metronidazole was superior to placebo in treating PCD.[19] The study showed that there was a significant reduction in fistula drainage in the intervention group. Antibiotics can be used in the short term and help to control active symptoms. They can be used in combination with immunomodulators like azathioprine or 6-mercaptopurine for an early effect since azathioprine usually takes up to 4 weeks or so to start having an effect.[20] A combination of ciprofloxacin with adalimumab is superior to adalimumab therapy alone, and this may be the most practical use of antibiotics as a combination agent with biologicals.[21] The use of topical metronidazole ointment seems to have some effect on controlling symptoms and could be used as an adjunct to other therapies.[22]

The use of immunomodulators for treating PCD has not been studied in prospective randomized clinical trials. Retrospective data have been analyzed in a meta-analysis of studies in which azathioprine was compared with placebo.[23] The analysis showed that the clinical response rates were 54% and 21% for azathioprine and placebo, respectively. However, there may be disparity in the rates of fistula closure because the included studies did not have a standardized description of the outcome. There are insufficient data to support the use of methotrexate and cyclosporine in the treatment of PCD. In general, immunomodulators have a limited role as a monotherapy, and the increasing use of biologicals has minimized their use as an adjunct therapy in combination with anti-TNF agents.[24]

An aggressive top-down approach is generally recommended once fistulizing disease is detected. An initial assessment with flexible sigmoidoscopy, MRI of the pelvis, and EUS is performed to assess the extent and severity of the disease. Anti-TNF therapy alone is usually adequate in treating fistulizing CD. The serum trough levels for infliximab, which are associated with clinical remission of luminal ulcerative colitis or CD, are around 4 to 5 μg/mL. A higher trough level of >10 μg/mL showed better outcomes in healing perianal fistulas.[25] When infliximab was used in combination with surgical interventions, it was found to be more effective in treating fistulizing CD than when used as a single agent.[26-28] Surgical therapies that are used for the treatment of a fistula are fistulotomy, seton placement, plug closure or mucosal flap closure, and fecal diversion. A combination of surgical fistulotomy with anti-TNF therapy is an effective approach to managing PCD, which is generally difficult to treat with either of the therapies alone.[29]

There are insufficient data on the use of newer biological agents like vedolizumab (anti-integrin) and ustekinumab (anti-IL12/23) in treating PCD. Among other medical therapies, hyperbaric oxygen therapy has been shown to have a beneficial effect in the management of refractory PCD.[30] There is no standardization of the duration of treatment, but on an average, at least 15 to 20 sessions over a period of 2 months are recommended.

ENDOSCOPIC THERAPY

In recent years, endoscopic therapy for the treatment of PCD has become an alternative approach to surgery, especially in noncomplex cases. Fistulas in the perianal area may be endoscopically treated using an over-the-scope endoclip (Ovesco Endoscopy AG) in highly selected patients.[31] This can prevent a surgical fistulotomy or resection that in CD patients can lead to long-term healing and the development of new strictures or fistulas. However, this therapy has not shown consistent results, with the risk of forming an abscess and incomplete resolution of inflammation leading to chronicity of the disease. In recent years, Chidi and Shen[32] have been using needle knife electroincision to perform endoscopic fistulotomy, which follows the principle of adequate drainage of a fistula to help it heal faster. Further studies are needed to study the effectiveness of this technique. Injections of materials like doxycycline, 50% sucrose or honey, fibrin glue, and stem cells into the fistula have shown a variable effect and are currently being studied as alternative approaches in the management of fistulizing CD.[33]

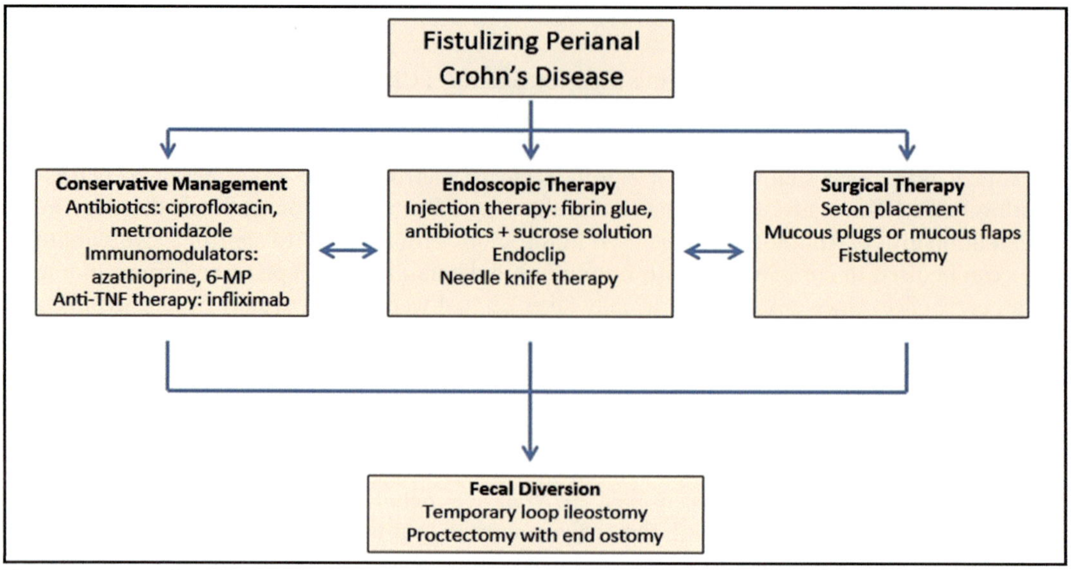

Figure 7-2. Algorithm showing approach to treating fistulizing PCD. Conservative, endoscopic, and surgical therapies are the initial frontline therapies. Fecal diversion is considered when there is no response to initial therapy or if there is disease progression.

SURGICAL THERAPY

Seton placement is a well-known treatment for perianal fistulas, and the placement of plugs has also been shown to be an effective therapy. The fistula heals once the seton is removed, and plug closure is not superior to treatment with a seton alone.[34] In an observational study, a combination of an anti-TNF agent, mainly infliximab, along with seton placement was successful in achieving complete perianal remission among 53% of cases of fistulizing PCD, of which only 9% had disease recurrence.[35] A consensus from multiple studies has shown that no single therapy is effective in treating perianal fistulas in CD; instead, a combination of seton placement with anti-TNF therapy with or without immunomodulator therapy has been found to be successful.[36] A study comparing fistula closure with a plug versus a mucosal flap showed no difference in outcome between the 2 techniques.[37] Mesenchymal stem cell–coated plugs are now being studied in the closure of fistulas in patients with PCD. The preliminary data from the studies have shown that such plugs have a promising benefit in perianal fistula closure, with formal clinical trials still underway to prove efficacy in response to this novel therapy.[38]

In refractory PCD, a fecal diversion usually in the form of a temporary ileostomy can be performed to achieve disease control.[1] However, in the majority of the cases, the temporary loop ileostomy ends up being a permanent end ileostomy due to chronicity of the inflammation in the rectal and perianal areas, making it difficult for a reanastomosis to heal. Using anti-TNF therapy has been shown to reduce the risk of a temporary fecal diversion leading to a permanent stoma.[39] Several studies have shown that there has been clear evidence of improvement in perianal disease when a combination of fecal diversion and the use of biologics has been utilized compared with either therapy alone.[1] A study of patients analyzing the outcomes of fecal diversion in the prebiological era and after the introduction of biologicals was performed by Coscia and colleagues,[40] comparing groups of patient populations between 1990 to 2002 and 2002 to 2010, respectively. A total of 96 patients were included in the review, with 23 of them in the prebiological era group who did not receive any biological therapy and 73 in the biological era group who received a biological agent after completion of a temporary ileostomy. The retrospective review showed that 60.8% of patients in the prebiological era group ended up with a permanent stoma, whereas only 19.2% of the cases required a permanent stoma in the group that received biologicals and underwent successful ileostomy reversal. The approach to management is summarized in Figure 7-2.

Inflammatory Bowel Disease–Associated Vaginal and Vesicular Fistula

These types of fistulas usually present with recurrent urinary tract infections (UTIs), hematuria, pneumaturia, or passage of feculent material in the urine. Initial antibiotic therapy is warranted to treat the UTI, and a long-term prophylactic antibiotic is commonly administered to those with recurrent UTIs. They are usually refractive to medical treatment and almost always require some sort of surgical intervention, usually primary closure using an advancement flap.[15] A combination of anti-TNF therapy with surgical closure is performed to improve the chances of recovery. Management should include the gynecologists, surgeons, and urologists and cannot be managed by the gastroenterologist alone.

Cancer Risk and Surveillance in Anorectal Inflammatory Bowel Disease

The presence of fistulas in CD puts one at risk of developing adenocarcinoma or squamous cell carcinoma arising from the fistula. The average time for the development of cancer from the time of fistula diagnosis is about 6 years.[41] Longstanding fistulas may undergo an adenomatous transformation from a squamous lining to an adenomatous rectal tissue type of lining. This adenomatous lining may then give rise to mucinous adenocarcinoma, which is more commonly encountered than the squamous cell variant.[42,43] The risk of developing carcinoma in a fistulous tract seems to be slightly more common in women and in those who have early development of a fistula after the diagnosis of CD.[43] Some experts suggest that patients with CD should undergo routine biopsies of the fistula to detect early cancer. An annual anoscopy or proctoscopy with biopsy of the fistulous tract should be adequate for this purpose. Although the incidence of fistula-related cancer is small at 0.74%, when feasible, a biopsy of the fistulous tract must be obtained.

Patients who develop anal CD or PCD have a higher risk of developing cancer in these areas.[44] Patients with IBD even without involvement of the anal canal are at increased risk of developing human papillomavirus–related cancer; therefore, vaccination against human papillomavirus is recommended.[45] The type of cancer seen in IBD patients can be squamous cell carcinoma or adenocarcinoma, which may arise in the anal canal or within the anal/perianal fistula. Neoadjuvant chemoradiation therapy (the "Nigro protocol") is the standard of care for the management of anal cancer, but in patients with CD, this protocol may be modified to fit the case at hand.[46] This may include performing surgery first to minimize or avoid radiation exposure because these patients are sensitive to radiotherapy.

Conclusion

PCD can present in the perianal area in the form of a fistula, sinus, abscess, or stricture. It is diagnosed using endoscopy (ie, flexible sigmoidoscopy and EUS), pelvic MRI, and direct EUA. A combination of these diagnostic modalities is superior than any of them alone. The approach to treatment can be conservative with oral antibiotics like ciprofloxacin, metronidazole, or tinidazole for a mild form of the disease, whereas a combination of immunomodulators with anti-TNF or anti-intergrin agents is recommended for more severe forms of the disease. Infected fistulas or the presence of perianal abscesses are managed by drainage. A combination of surgical interventions like seton placement, fistulotomy, or a mucosal flap with biological agents like infliximab or adalimumab is superior to any of the therapies alone. Fecal diversion can be offered as a treatment of last resort in severe forms of the disease, but it carries a risk of failure of reestablishment of fecal stream once the disease improves. This may lead to one having a permanent stoma. The use of biologics in combination with fecal diversion decreases the risk of failure of reanastomosis. Novel endoscopic therapies like the injection of certain solutions (antibiotics and 50% dextrose) into the sinuses and fistulas, needle knife fistulotomy, and endoclip closure of fistulas have offered a new dimension in managing fistulizing CD. Further studies are needed to establish the accuracy of these new therapeutic interventions in the management of PCD.

References

1. Harb WJ. Crohn's disease of the colon, rectum, and anus. *Surg Clin North Am.* 2015;95(6):1195-1210, vi.
2. Hellers G, Bergstrand O, Ewerth S, Holmström B. Occurrence and outcome after primary treatment of anal fistulae in Crohn's disease. *Gut.* 1980;21(6):525-527.
3. Penner A, Crohn BB. Perianal fistulae as a complication of regional ileitis. *Ann Surg.* 1938;108(5):867-873.
4. Greenstein AJ, Lachman P, Sachar DB, et al. Perforating and non-perforating indications for repeated operations in Crohn's disease: evidence for two clinical forms. *Gut.* 1988;29(5):588-592.
5. Gasche C, Scholmerich J, Brynskov J, et al. A simple classification of Crohn's disease: report of the Working Party for the World Congresses of Gastroenterology, Vienna 1998. *Inflamm Bowel Dis.* 2000;6(1):8-15.
6. Spekhorst LM, Visschedijk MC, Alberts R, et al. Performance of the Montreal classification for inflammatory bowel diseases. *World J Gastroenterol.* 2014;20(41):15374-15381.
7. Van Assche G, Dignass A, Reinisch W, et al. The second European evidence-based consensus on the diagnosis and management of Crohn's disease: special situations. *J Crohns Colitis.* 2010;4(1):63-101.
8. Gecse KB, Bemelman W, Kamm MA, et al. A global consensus on the classification, diagnosis and multidisciplinary treatment of perianal fistulising Crohn's disease. *Gut.* 2014;63(9):1381-1392.
9. de Parades V, Fathallah N, Blanchard P, Zeitoun JD, Bennadji B, Atienza P. Horseshoe tract of anal fistula: bad luck or an avoidable extension? Lessons from 82 cases. *Colorectal Dis.* 2012;14(12):1512-1515.
10. Schwartz DA, Wiersema MJ, Dudiak KM, et al. A comparison of endoscopic ultrasound, magnetic resonance imaging, and exam under anesthesia for evaluation of Crohn's perianal fistulas. *Gastroenterology.* 2001;121(5):1064-1072.
11. Oliveira IS, Kilcoyne A, Price MC, Harisinghani M. MRI features of perianal fistulas: is there a difference between Crohn's and non-Crohn's patients? *Abdom Radiol (NY).* 2017;42(4):1162-1168.
12. Bell SJ, Halligan S, Windsor AC, Williams AB, Wiesel P, Kamm MA. Response of fistulating Crohn's disease to infliximab treatment assessed by magnetic resonance imaging. *Aliment Pharmacol Ther.* 2003;17(3):387-393.
13. Wright EK, Novak KL, Lu C, Panaccione R, Ghosh S, Wilson SR. Transperineal ultrasonography in perianal Crohn disease: a valuable imaging modality. *Can J Gastroenterol Hepatol.* 2015;29(8):445-447.
14. Spradlin NM, Wise PE, Herline AJ, Muldoon RL, Rosen M, Schwartz DA. A randomized prospective trial of endoscopic ultrasound to guide combination medical and surgical treatment for Crohn's perianal fistulas. *Am J Gastroenterol.* 2008;103(10):2527-2535.
15. Schwartz DA, Ghazi LJ, Regueiro M, et al. Guidelines for the multidisciplinary management of Crohn's perianal fistulas: summary statement. *Inflamm Bowel Dis.* 2015;21(4):723-730.
16. Pescatori M, Interisano A, Basso L, et al. Management of perianal Crohn's disease. Results of a multicenter study in Italy. *Dis Colon Rectum.* 1995;38(2):121-124.
17. Gelbmann CM, Rogler G, Gross V, et al. Prior bowel resections, perianal disease, and a high initial Crohn's disease activity index are associated with corticosteroid resistance in active Crohn's disease. *Am J Gastroenterol.* 2002;97(6):1438-1445.
18. Tozer PJ, Burling D, Gupta A, Phillips RK, Hart AL. Review article: medical, surgical and radiological management of perianal Crohn's fistulas. *Aliment Pharmacol Ther.* 2011;33(1):5-22.
19. Khan KJ, Ullman TA, Ford AC, et al. Antibiotic therapy in inflammatory bowel disease: a systematic review and meta-analysis. *Am J Gastroenterol.* 2011;106(4):661-673.
20. Dejaco C, Harrer M, Waldhoer T, Miehslder W, Vogelsang H, Reinisch W. Antibiotics and azathioprine for the treatment of perianal fistulas in Crohn's disease. *Aliment Pharmacol Ther.* 2003;18(11-12):1113-1120.
21. Dewint P, Hansen BE, Verhey E, et al. Adalimumab combined with ciprofloxacin is superior to adalimumab monotherapy in perianal fistula closure in Crohn's disease: a randomised, double-blind, placebo controlled trial (ADAFI). *Gut.* 2014;63(2):292-299.
22. Maeda Y, Ng SC, Durdey P, et al. Randomized clinical trial of metronidazole ointment versus placebo in perianal Crohn's disease. Br J Surg. 2010;97(9):1340-1347.

23. Pearson DC, May GR, Fick GH, Sutherland LR. Azathioprine and 6-mercaptopurine in Crohn disease. A meta-analysis. *Ann Intern Med.* 1995;123(2):132-142.
24. Kotze PG, Shen B, Lightner A, et al. Modern management of perianal fistulas in Crohn's disease: future directions. *Gut.* 2018;67(6):1181-1194.
25. Yarur AJ, Kanagala V, Stein DJ, et al. Higher infliximab trough levels are associated with perianal fistula healing in patients with Crohn's disease. *Aliment Pharmacol Ther.* 2017;45(7):933-940.
26. Schwartz DA, White CM, Wise PE, Herline AJ. Use of endoscopic ultrasound to guide combination medical and surgical therapy for patients with Crohn's perianal fistulas. *Inflamm Bowel Dis.* 2005;11(8):727-732.
27. Park EJ, Song KH, Baik SH, et al. The efficacy of infliximab combined with surgical treatment of fistulizing perianal Crohn's disease: comparative analysis according to fistula subtypes. *Asian J Surg.* 2018;41(5):438-447.
28. Regueiro M, Mardini H. Treatment of perianal fistulizing Crohn's disease with infliximab alone or as an adjunct to exam under anesthesia with seton placement. *Inflamm Bowel Dis.* 2003;9(2):98-103.
29. Yang BL, Chen YG, Gu YF, et al. Long-term outcome of infliximab combined with surgery for perianal fistulizing Crohn's disease. *World J Gastroenterol.* 2015;21(8):2475-2482.
30. Lavy A, Weisz G, Adir Y, Ramon Y, Melamed Y, Eidelman S. Hyperbaric oxygen for perianal Crohn's disease. *J Clin Gastroenterol.* 1994;19(3):202-205.
31. Prosst RL, Joos AK. Short-term outcomes of a novel endoscopic clipping device for closure of the internal opening in 100 anorectal fistulas. *Tech Coloproctol.* 2016;20(11):753-758.
32. Chidi V, Shen B. Endoscopic needle knife fistulotomy technique for ileal pouch-to-pouch fistula. *Endoscopy.* 2015;47(suppl 1 UCTN):E261.
33. Paine E, Shen B. Endoscopic therapy in inflammatory bowel diseases (with videos). *Gastrointest Endosc.* 2013;78(6):819-835.
34. Senejoux A, Siproudhis L, Abramowitz L, et al. Fistula plug in fistulising ano-perineal Crohn's disease: a randomised controlled trial. *J Crohns Colitis.* 2016;10(2):141-148.
35. Kotze PG, Albuquerque IC, da Luz Moreira A, Tonini WB, Olandoski M, Coy CS. Perianal complete remission with combined therapy (seton placement and anti-TNF agents) in Crohn's disease: a Brazilian multicenter observational study. *Arq Gastroenterol.* 2014;51(4):284-289.
36. de Groof EJ, Sahami S, Lucas C, Ponsioen CY, Bemelman WA, Buskens CJ. Treatment of perianal fistula in Crohn's disease: a systematic review and meta-analysis comparing seton drainage and anti-tumour necrosis factor treatment. *Colorectal Dis.* 2016;18(7):667-675.
37. van Koperen PJ, Bemelman WA, Gerhards MF, et al. The anal fistula plug treatment compared with the mucosal advancement flap for cryptoglandular high transsphincteric perianal fistula: a double-blinded multicenter randomized trial. *Dis Colon Rectum.* 2011;54(4):387-393.
38. Dietz AB, Dozois EJ, Fletcher JG, et al. Autologous mesenchymal stem cells, applied in a bioabsorbable matrix, for treatment of perianal fistulas in patients with Crohn's disease. *Gastroenterology.* 2017;153(1):59-62.e2.
39. Uzzan M, Stefanescu C, Maggiori L, Panis Y, Bouhnik Y, Treton X. Case series: does a combination of anti-tnf antibodies and transient ileal fecal stream diversion in severe Crohn's colitis with perianal fistula prevent definitive stoma? *Am J Gastroenterol.* 2013;108(10):1666-1668.
40. Coscia M, Gentilini L, Laureti S, et al. Risk of permanent stoma in extensive Crohn's colitis: the impact of biological drugs. *Colorectal Dis.* 2013;15(9):1115-1122.
41. Shwaartz C, Munger JA, Deliz JR. Fistula-associated anorectal cancer in the setting of Crohn's disease. *Dis Colon Rectum.* 2016;59(12):1168-1173.
42. Maejima T, Kono T, Orii F, et al. Anal canal adenocarcinoma in a patient with longstanding Crohn's disease arising from rectal mucosa that migrated from a previously treated rectovaginal fistula. *Am J Case Rep.* 2016;17:448-453.
43. Thomas M, Bienkowski R, Vandermeer TJ, Trostle D, Cagir B. Malignant transformation in perianal fistulas of Crohn's disease: a systematic review of literature. *J Gastrointest Surg.* 2010.14(1):66-73.
44. Beaugerie L, Carrat F, Nahon S, et al. High risk of anal and rectal cancer in patients with anal and/or perianal Crohn's disease. *Clin Gastroenterol Hepatol.* 2018;16(6):892-899.e2.
45. Wisniewski A, Fléjou JF, Siproudhis L, Abramowitz L, Svrcek, Beaugerie L. Anal neoplasia in inflammatory bowel disease: classification proposal, epidemiology, carcinogenesis, and risk management perspectives. *J Crohns Colitis.* 2017;11(8):1011-1018.
46. Lightner AL, Moncrief SB, Smyrk TC, et al. Long-standing Crohn's disease and its implication on anal squamous cell cancer management. *Int J Colorectal Dis.* 2017;32(5):661-666.
47. Satsangi J, Silverberg MS, Vermeire S, Colombel JF. The Montreal classification of inflammatory bowel disease: controversies, consensus, and implications. *Gut.* 2006;55(6):749-753.

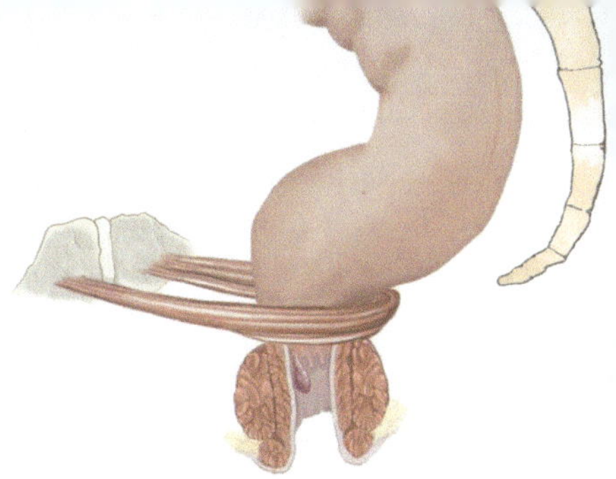

8

Rectal Prolapse

Bidhan Das, MD, FACS

KEY POINTS

- Rectal prolapse is a clinically diagnosed protrusion that is distinctly different from hemorrhoidal disease but often has the same functional etiologies.
- Rectal prolapse can be differentiated at the bedside based on texture, concentricity of the mucosal folding, degree of prolapsing tissue, and thickness of the protruding tissue.
- Diagnosis of rectal prolapse is based on clinical evaluation and physical examination, but endoscopic evaluation may be helpful to evaluate for underlying causes.
- It is critical to realize that rectal prolapse may concomitantly exist with other pelvic prolapses or pelvic floor diseases in order to offer the patient an appropriate, multidisciplinary approach to care.
- Rectal prolapse is fundamentally a surgically treated disease, but perineal operations offer less morbidity and higher recurrence rates; however, abdominal approaches to correction offer slightly higher morbidity and reduced recurrence rates.
- Recurrent rectal prolapse can be treated largely the same way as an initial prolapse, but it is crucial to understand what operative approach was chosen in the first operation in order to avoid creating colonic ischemia.
- SRUS has a wide array of presentations but fundamentally is a focal area of the rectum affected by trauma or inflammation and almost always associated with ongoing straining and the same mechanisms that relate to rectal prolapse.
- The vast majority of efficacious therapies for treating SRUS patients revolve around medical management rather than surgical management. This situation is notably in stark contrast to the management of rectal prolapse as an entity of its own; however, should rectal prolapse be causing SRUS, the prolapse should be corrected.

Qureshi W, ed. *Diagnosis and Management Guide for Anorectal Disease: A Clinical Reference* (pp 89-97).

Rectal prolapse has a long history in the medical literature, with its etiology based on 2 major theories. Moschcowitz[1] believed that rectal prolapse was effectively a hernia through the endopelvic fascia. Broden and Snellman[2] believed that prolapse started with intrarectal circumferential intussusception of the rectum. Current thoughts demonstrate that these processes are likely part of the same spectrum of disease, and, truly, invagination of the anterior aspect of the rectum could be considered a herniation that would effectively create an intussusception that has yet to become fully circumferential, leading to a classic prolapse. No matter the mechanism, procidentia is the protrusion of the rectum so that it is outside of the body. Its appearance is a erythematous, congested at times, large intestinal protuberance that is a true intussusception of the rectum through the sphincters.

More common in women, rectal prolapse traditionally has been thought of as a disease of elderly female patients with maximal incidence in the seventh decade of life, but there has been a rise in young male patients who have consistent defecatory straining resulting in rectal prolapse. Women are thought to have a higher incidence of prolapse due to anatomic differences, namely that they have a wider pelvic width and a deeper peritoneal reflection. Childbirth is thought to damage the pelvic fascia and pelvic floor with vaginal deliveries also affecting pudendal innervation, resulting in pelvic floor disorders, such as increased perineal descent and issues with incontinence. Men with prolapse tend to be younger (20 to 40 years of age) and usually have an associated prior disorder (ongoing issues of aggressive straining, psychiatric illness, or congenital anal atresia).

Additionally, there are several predisposing factors that may also typify patients with rectal prolapse. As noted previously, constipation and straining predominate the symptomatology of patients with rectal prolapse,[3] with a high percentage of patients having diarrhea as a predominant symptom. Pregnancy, neurologic disease, and psychiatric illness are all factors for prolapse. Pathologic anatomic issues associated with patients with rectal prolapse include pelvic floor diastasis/levator diastasis, deepening of the pouch of Douglas, and occasionally redundant rectosigmoid colons.

Rectal prolapse is also seen in infants, often associated with straining and congenital abnormalities of the sacrum, most commonly those whose sacral concavity is significantly less than normal.

Pathophysiology

The 2 theories mentioned earlier effectively work together to create rectal prolapse. The sliding hernia description can be translated as the anterior rectal wall invaginating to create a partial intussusception not yet involving the entire bowel circumference. In such a way, both theories describe rectal prolapse, but its etiology is somewhat elusive. While many patients share laxity of the pelvic floor and pelvic musculature, it has been well studied through cinedefecography that rectal prolapse starts its intussusception well above the pelvic floor. It has been suggested previously[4] that there is a common pathophysiology for full-thickness rectal prolapse, rectal prolapse, anterior mucosal prolapse, and solitary rectal ulcer. Anorectal pressures at rest, during contraction, during serial distention of the rectum, and during straining were measured in patients with rectal prolapse, and it was shown that both basal and squeeze pressures were significantly lower in these patients compared with the control groups.[4] Although abdominal pressure was increased, anal pressure was lower than the maximal rectal pressure when compared with the control groups. Serial distention testing would demonstrate that the vast majority of these affected patients would have repetitive rectal contractions. In the affected group, the highest anal pressure was lower than the rectal pressure, and the threshold volume needed to feel a need to defecate and the maximal tolerable volume were lower in the affected patient group. These findings would suggest that this group of patients, and thus rectal prolapse patients, have a rectum that is more hypersensitive and hyperreactive. With the relative weakness of the anal sphincter and the presence of this hyperreactivity, one can see how conditions are met that allow rectal prolapse to occur.

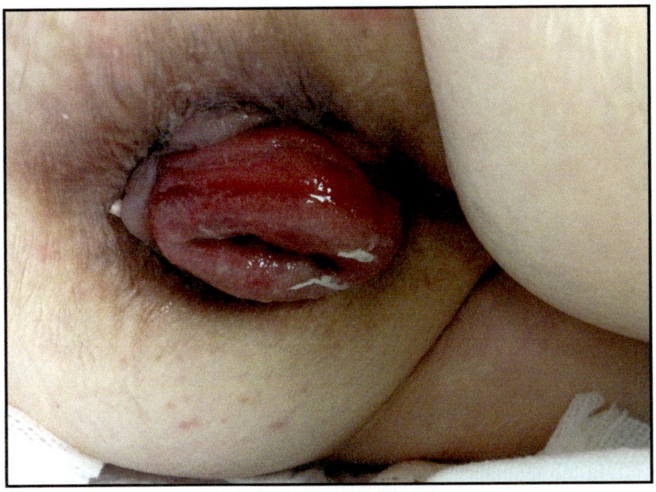

Figure 8-1. Reducible full-thickness circumferential rectal prolapse (circular mucosal folds visible) with viable mucosa. (Reprinted with permission from Marcus Aquino, MD, FACS.)

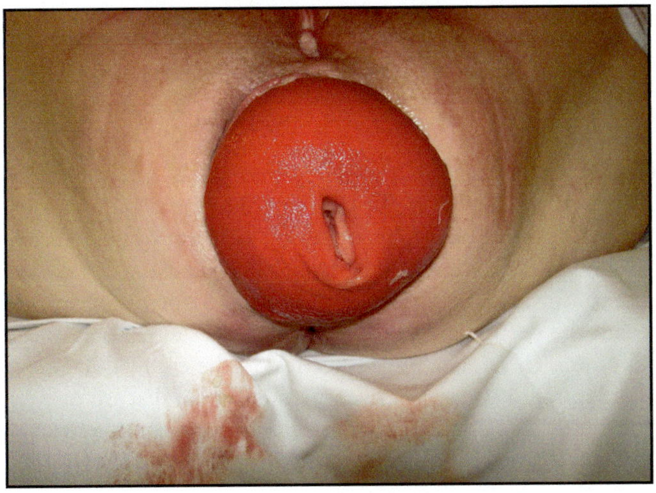

Figure 8-2. Reducible near full-thickness rectal prolapse seen during active straining (note the absence of mucosal folds). (Reprinted with permission from Marcus Aquino, MD, FACS.)

Signs and Symptoms

The presenting symptoms of rectal prolapse can vary wildly, from mucoid discharge that is minimally noticed to a dramatic, florid protrusion. The complaints can be related to the protrusion or issues with continence (from wet mucosa or frank stool that is brought with the rectum down beyond the sphincters) that may accompany it. In earlier stages, the protrusive mass may extrude only while defecating or immediately after (Figure 8-1), but as the procidentia gets more advanced, the protrusion may extrude even with virtually no exertion or at times of mild straining, such as coughing or sneezing (Figure 8-2). Sensations of tenesmus, incomplete evacuation, or the need for continued wiping after defecation may be part of early presentations of rectal prolapse. The fullness of an intussuscepting rectum or an ongoing protrusion/permanently extruded prolapsed rectum can cause ongoing excoriation, bleeding, and soiling of the clothing with stool. Worse yet, there can often be impairment of anorectal sensation from persistent dilation of the extruded mass as well as permanent reduction in the anal sphincter tone. It is worth noting that other pelvic organs may also be prolapsing, and in addition to fecal incontinence, there is often associated urinary incontinence; such a combination of presenting findings may warrant a multidisciplinary team involving urology, colorectal surgery, gynecology, and urogynecology to handle these issues concomitantly.

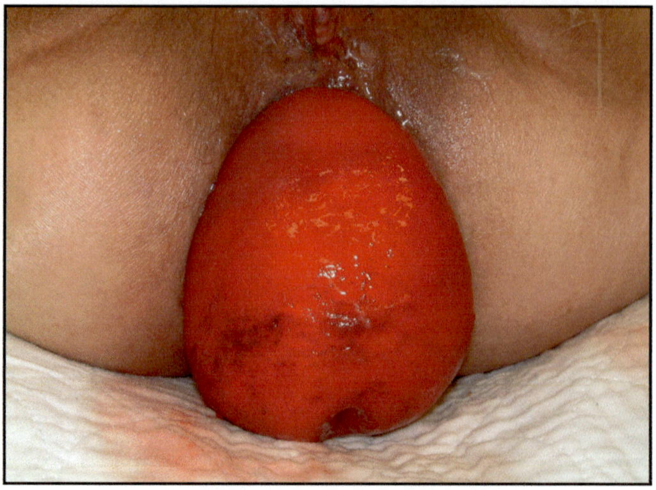

Figure 8-3. Incarcerated irreducible full-thickness rectal prolapse with lack of mucosal folds due to underlying edema. Early signs of mucosal hemorrhage/ischemia noted sparingly. (Reprinted with permission from Marcus Aquino, MD, FACS.)

Diagnosis

PHYSICAL EXAMINATION

When rectal prolapse is fully presented, it protrudes with a large red mass that, upon initial examination, may already be reduced and not evident. However, the anal sphincters may be very loose with the anus being quite patulous. Putting the patient on a toilet or sitting position while performing a prolonged Valsalva maneuver reveals the full thickness of the rectal wall prolapsing downward, with the concentric folds around the center of the anus being noted. Indirect anoscopy is performed this way with a small mirror placed beneath the perineum. Other abnormalities such as a cystocele and rectocele may be seen using this technique. This appearance is critical to the clinical diagnosis. Mucosal prolapse (extrusion of just the redundant mucosa) or even hemorrhoidal disease demonstrates radial folding pointing toward the center of the anus. In more critical phases, there can be ulceration and chronic oozing from the injected mucosa given the tension of the prolapse.

Notably, upon palpation of the prolapse, there will be a marked lack of pain when palpating the prolapse itself. Certainly, the patient may be in pain with an acutely extruded prolapse because the stretching of the anal canal suddenly may be uncomfortable, but the intussuscepted rectum itself is not painful. Furthermore, palpation of this tissue reveals it is the entire thickness of the rectum rather than simply just the mucosal lining. Additionally, it is worth noting that the sphincter tone and voluntary squeeze during digital examination may be diminished, with responses being nearly absent while the prolapse is extruded.

Flexible endoscopy or proctoscopy with the prolapse returned may reveal an anterior erythema and focal inflammation, which may be almost circumferential but very focal. Other causes will be seen as well, which may be occult lead points via mucosal abnormalities.

COMPLICATED PRESENTATIONS

Certain presentations of rectal prolapse warrant an aggressive or immediate consultation with a colorectal surgeon and are uncommon presentations of rectal prolapse; therefore, they may go unnoticed by the initial triaging providers. Uncommonly, a rectal prolapse may become incarcerated acutely (Figure 8-3). In almost every situation, a full-thickness rectal prolapse can be reduced manually once recognized. Tips for reduction include providing a local perianal anesthetic block and using an osmotic change agent (sugar in packets is often discussed) to apply liberally to the mucosal surface to reduce the edematous incarceration. When reducing a prolapse, gentle but continued and even pressure that reduces the most distal aspect first (recall that the intussusception leading edge would be returned to being the most proximal) is key to reduction success. However, there are times when bowel viability is clearly in question, and incarceration is truly strangulation. Such a situation requires emergency perineal rectosigmoidectomy. Much more extremely rare complicated presentations include a ruptured rectal prolapse. These situations are hallmarked by excessive straining and sudden prolapse leading to tearing of the anterior rectal wall, resulting in exposure of intraperitoneal contents and evisceration of the small bowel or omentum. Immediate consultation with a colorectal surgeon is warranted, and emergent operation through an abdominal approach would likely be necessary.

DIFFERENTIAL DIAGNOSIS

Understanding common mimickers of this pathology is critical to the clinical diagnosis and further therapy in rectal prolapse patients. Many times in the inpatient or even emergency room setting, the mucosa can appear just at the anal verge, and it is frankly quite difficult to determine whether or not the clinician is dealing with hemorrhoidal disease, rectal prolapse, or mucosal prolapse. Full-thickness rectal prolapse will have furrows of the prolapsed mucosa in a concentric ring around the center of the anus. Mucosal prolapse will have radial groves pointing to the center of the anus. Another clinical point is that in full-thickness rectal prolapse, there is a clear fold between the anus itself and the prolapsed rectum. In mucosal prolapse, there is no such sulcus, and the tissue is thinner.

FURTHER INVESTIGATION

Colonoscopy should be considered to rule out mucosal anomalies that may act as a lead point, but should the patient's endoscopic screening status be up to date, rigid proctoscopy or flexible sigmoidoscopy and/or a contrast study of the distal bowel are appropriate for further evaluation. The contrast study will demonstrate a redundant sigmoid colon that, if associated with significant constipation, could be resected as part of the rectopexy. Defecography and its variant modalities may be helpful when rectal prolapse is suspected but not readily demonstrable in the office setting. Furthermore, it may help delineate other functional pelvic floor disorders that may present concomitantly; however, it is often not warranted in the treatment of many patients because the main defecatory dysfunction would be treatable by treating the prolapse. Anorectal manometry can help assess sphincter function; however, it is widely argued that with full-thickness prolapse patients, the sphincter pressures will be lower in any case due to chronic dilation and the pathophysiologic nature of these patients (discussed previously). However, it is worth discussing with the patients what their pre-prolapse continence was using a fecal incontinence scoring system in order to determine the appropriate choice for future operations. Colonic transit times combined with defecography may be warranted in the patient with a long history of prolonged constipation, again so that the appropriate corrective operation may be performed in the future.

TREATMENT AND FOLLOW-UP

Correction of rectal prolapse is primarily an operative intervention; nonoperative techniques such as limiting straining, dealing with underlying defecatory disorders, and dealing with longstanding constipation are essential in the "pre-prolapse" or intra-anal intussusception phase before those conditions have progressed to the rectal prolapse state, should there even be a true progression. The decision in the treatment of rectal prolapse correction is whether to pursue an abdominal approach for correction or a perineal approach. There are many approaches, variations, and modifications that are beyond the scope of this text; as such, only the most common and most salient to the treatment of prolapse will be discussed.

PERINEAL PROCEDURES

Thiersch Procedure

Thiersch first described anal encirclement in 1891, and it represents the simplest of methods to treat rectal prolapse. The procedure is not to correct the prolapse but truly to narrow the anus enough that the prolapse is confined to the rectum, with a success rate reported at 54% to 100%.[5,6] Two centimeters distal from the anal verge, a curved instrument is used to tunnel around the external anal sphincter in such a way as to allow an encircling material to be drawn around the entirety of the external anal sphincter as a reinforcing buttress. The material is then secured and tightened with a finger in the anus as a judge of tightness. Notably, there are some impressive complications; namely, there can be breakage of the material, fecal impaction from the tightness, erosion, and infection. Its failure to correct prolapse as well as the morbidity make it reserved for only the most seriously ill patients who are unable to undergo other perineal procedures. This procedure is rarely performed today.

Perineal Rectosigmoidectomy

Perineal rectosigmoidectomy was popularized by Altemeier and is now called the *Altemeier procedure*. This type of procedure can be performed under general, spinal, or local anesthetic with sedation. In this procedure, a circumferential incision is made in the rectal wall just above the dentate line. In essence, the prolapsed rectum is amputated along with the redundant sigmoid colon, and the proximal end of the colon is sutured to the dentate line. Dissection is undertaken until the intussusceptum is separated from the intussuscipiens. Once the prolapse is completely unfolded, the peritoneum is entered, and the rectum and its associated redundant sigmoid (or even more proximally) colon are continually pulled down and out of the perineal approach, advancing more proximally while the blood supply is taken sequentially in such a way as to not devascularize the more proximal bowel. This process continues until there is no more redundant bowel to bring down. The bowel and associated mesentery are divided and reanastomosed to the anus for coloanal anastomosis. While the pelvic floor is exposed with the perineal extrusion, the patient can also undergo levator plication before the anastomosis, which can assist in continence.[7,8] The mortality rate is quite low for the procedure, but morbidity can range from 5% to 24%. It is worth noting that most issues stem from preexisting problems, and the recurrence rates in follow-up to 5 years are up to 10%. Given the higher recurrence rate but the reduced risk to patients, perineal rectosigmoidectomy can be optimal for high-risk patients. Furthermore, there is often value for the procedure in the male patient who is at higher risk for impotency issues because the dissection avoids working near structures that convey potency.

Delorme Procedure

Described by Delorme,[9] the premise of the procedure is to strip the mucosa and submucosa away from the prolapsed bowel and then plicate the residual muscular wall, which is reanastomosed to the mucosal ring. Such a procedure is ideally suited for patients with full-thickness prolapse that is fairly minimal or partial circumferential full-thickness prolapse (the anterior wall, as we have described previously). This perineal procedure can also be performed under general, spinal, or local anesthesia. Once the bowel is maximally extruded, a partial-thickness incision is made just proximal to the dentate line to expose the submucosa of the outer cylinder. The mucosa and submucosa of the outer cylinder are dissected from the underlying muscular coat, effectively revealing more and more of the proximal muscular coat, which is then plicated with gathering sutures and tied to the mucosal ring left behind from the initial incision to complete the anastomosis. Due to the extensive nature of the mucosectomy, it is understandable why the Delorme procedure may be best suited for full-thickness, short-segment prolapse. The recurrence rates are higher than in the Altemeier procedure at 7% to 22% at 1 to 13 years, with incontinence improving in 40% to 50% of patients.[10]

ABDOMINAL PROCEDURES

Abdominal Rectopexy With or Without Sigmoid Colectomy

Simple suture rectopexy without sigmoid colectomy has been reported as an effective surgical treatment for rectal prolapse. The recurrence rate is markedly minimal, and in many studies with prolonged follow-up, it is less than 10%. Notably, the fundamental steps are (1) complete mobilization of the rectum to the pelvic floor while keeping the lateral stalks intact, (2) suture fixation of the lateral rectal stalks to the presacral fascia below the sacral promontory in the midline, and (3) obliteration of the cul-de-sac. Most modern surgeons do not perform the third step of closing the cul-de-sac because it does not seem to contribute to the correction of rectal prolapse. Sigmoid colectomy is often performed by certain colorectal surgeons who believe that resection of all excess sigmoid colon/left colon is key to reducing the risk of recurrence. Such people think that given the process of straightening the left colon such that it is only held by the proximal phrenicocolic ligament creates a lack of mobility that prevents the colon and rectum from further sliding, and controlling the length of the bowel is one of the few absolutes that can be surgically remedied. The cul-de-sac may deepen with age or pelvic floor changes, but the length of the bowel cannot change. With a newly reanastomosed colon to the rectum, even if the fixated rectum loses fixation as time goes on, the tethering of the anastomosis to a colon without any redundancy does not allow the rectum to descend to create rectal prolapse. However, surgeons must often weigh the pros and cons of such an approach because the recurrence rates with additional resection are not substantially improved relative to simple rectopexy. Furthermore, the additional bowel resection subjects a patient to additional morbidity of a large bowel resection. Many colon rectal surgeons feel that sigmoid resection is an ineffective and pointless addition to rectopexy because there are no studies to show that sigmoid colectomy in any way impacts slow transit constipation or future recurrence of the prolapse. Sigmoid colectomy adds to the length and complexity of the surgery and carries its own list of complications.

Mesh Rectopexy

In 1963, Drs. Ripstein and Lanter[11] created a mesh-based rectopexy, with the thought being that if they could fixate and straighten the rectum itself to the fascia, there would be a markedly decreased risk of prolapse. In such a way, rectal mobilization is undertaken as described previously only with some resection of the lateral stalks. After mobilization, prosthetic mesh is wrapped around the rectum and sutured to the rectum, and then the edges are sutured to the sacral fascia. Such a procedure has fallen out of favor in recent times due to the placement of mesh around the bowel and the possibility of injuring the rectum or even creating an obstruction from fibrotic stenosis, particularly in light of other therapies that do not involve the use of mesh.

Another prosthetic rectopexy method is that of the Ivalon sponge (FABCO), which has been popular in the United Kingdom since the late 1950s. Described by Wells in 1959,[12] the operation is performed by mobilizing the rectum as described previously and then wrapping a piece of Ivalon sponge that is sutured three-quarters of the way around the rectum, leaving the anterior aspect free of sponge. The peritoneum is then closed over the sponge to exclude it from the peritoneal cavity and into the true pelvis.

Again, adhering to the principle of keeping to a simple and effective procedure, the addition of mesh to proctopexy adds morbidity and contributes nothing to the outcome. Modern colorectal surgeons are moving away from implanting permanent prosthetics directly against the rectal wall.

Follow-up

After a perineal approach for correction of rectal prolapse, the patient is maintained on an enhanced recovery after surgery approach overnight and discharged home the next day. Traditionally, these patients are seen postoperatively in a few weeks, and they are sequentially evaluated.

Table 8-1

SURGICAL MANAGEMENT OPTIONS FOR RECURRENT RECTAL PROLAPSE

INITIAL OPERATION	OPTIONS FOR MANAGEMENT OF RECURRENCE
Perineal rectosigmoidectomy	Redo perineal rectosigmoidectomy Abdominal rectopexy (avoid resection)
Abdominal rectopexy	Redo abdominal rectopexy (+/− sigmoid colectomy) Perineal rectosigmoidectomy
Abdominal rectopexy + resection	Redo abdominal rectopexy (+/− re-resection) Avoid perineal rectosigmoidectomy

RECURRENT RECTAL PROLAPSE

Unfortunately, despite many procedures and procedure types, there is still a substantial recurrence rate associated with the treatment of rectal prolapse, with the preponderance of the surgical literature noting that perineal procedures are associated with a higher rate of recurrence when compared with an abdominal approach. When a recurrence is deemed to be full thickness, it is recommended to reassess the patient according to the guidelines presented earlier, in particular paying attention to defecatory behaviors that may not have been able to be assessed in the initial presentation or workup. Comorbid conditions that have accumulated since the prior operation also need to be assessed.

One of the most important decisions in handling full-thickness rectal prolapse recurrence is the operation that is most appropriate for the patient, and the crux of this issue relies on appreciating the residual blood supply that is available for the final operation. The management options in this situation are summarized in Table 8-1.

Of note, it is encouraging that treatment of recurrent full-thickness rectal prolapse can be appropriately managed using the same operative options, and the successful treatment of recurrence ranges from 85% to 100%.[13,14] Interestingly, most literature discussing recurrent prolapse fails to note the secondary operative technique in order to guide future clinicians on choosing an appropriate course for most patients based on a purely evidentiary basis.

RELATED PATHOLOGY

SOLITARY RECTAL ULCER SYNDROME

While stressing the importance of avoiding straining in the setting of rectal prolapse, one entity readily associated with straining and often thought to be related to rectal prolapse (often erroneously) is that of solitary rectal ulcer syndrome (SRUS). This entity is often a misnomer because the entity may not be solitary, may not be ulcerative, or may be associated with multiple ulcerations.

SRUS is considered to be a clinical condition that is characterized by the presence of rectal bleeding and deep-seated anorectal pain, which is usually not intense. Tenesmus and obstructive defecation may also be associated symptoms. It is worth noting that straining is almost always the cause for SRUS, with the common feature producing the pathology being chronic inflammation or chronic trauma. To mirror the causes discussed previously, the inflammation/trauma causing SRUS may be ischemic, pressure related, internal intussusception, rectal prolapse, direct digital trauma, direct trauma from the insertion of objects, or ongoing straining to evacuate stool.

Physical examination of the lesions will result in an area of induration that can be felt, with ulcerations seen on the anterior rectal wall between 4 and 10 cm from the anal verge. The ulcerations are shallow and gray-white with an irregular shape and raised edges. The mucosa leading to the ulcerated areas is hyperemic and may appear nodular. Rectal prolapse may well be demonstrated during straining in patients with SRUS.

Confirming the diagnosis of SRUS usually requires endoscopic evaluation of the distal colon and rectum to reveal lesions, with the differential diagnosis of lesions being resolved with adequate endoscopic biopsy. The pathology demonstrates a characteristic appearance with superficial mucosal ulceration, hyperplastic epithelium, and, particularly, obliteration of the lamina propria by fibrosis and growth of the muscularis mucosae toward the bowel lumen. Defecography can also be very helpful for understanding the underlying disorder causing SRUS, often demonstrating issues with failure to relax the pelvic floor or internal intussusception.

Treating SRUS is focused on reducing symptoms or preventing the proposed causes. Eating a high-fiber diet, increasing water intake, and avoiding straining are the usual hallmarks of therapy. Medications such as 5-aminosalicylic acid–derivative enemas have been tried with some success.[15] Persistent symptoms with failure of medical management may warrant localized resection (ranging from transanal excision to coloanal pull through), while those with prolapse as the cause of SRUS warrant the operations discussed previously.

References

1. Moschcowitz AV. The pathogenesis, anatomy and cure of prolapse of the rectum. *Surg Gynecol Obstet.* 1912;15:7-21.
2. Broden B, Snellen B. Procidentia of the rectum studied with cineradiography: a contribution of the discussion of causative mechanism. *Dis Colon Rectum.* 1968;2013:330-347.
3. Zbar AP, Takashima S, Hasegawa T, Kitabayashi K. Perinal rectosigmoidectomy (Altemeier's procedure): a review of physiology, technique and outcome. *Tech Coloproctol.* 2002;6(2):109-116.
4. Sun WM, Read NW, Donnelly TC, Bannister JJ, Shorthouse AJ. A common pathophysiology for full thickness rectal prolapse, anterior mucosal prolapse and solitary rectal ulcer. *Br J Surg.* 1989;76(3):290-295.
5. Goldman J. Concerning prolapse of the rectum with special emphasis on the operation by Thiersch. *Dis Colon Rectum.* 1988;31(2):154-155.
6. Williams JG. Perineal approaches to repair of rectal prolapse. *Semin Colon Rectal Surg.* 1991;2:198-204.
7. Prasad ML, Pearl RK, Abcarian H, Orsay CP, Nelson RL. Perineal proctectomy, posterior rectopexy, and postanal levator repair for the treatment of rectal prolapse. *Dis Colon Rectum.* 1986;29(9):547-552.
8. Ramanujam PS, Venkateh KS. Perineal excision of rectal prolapse with posterior levator ani repair in elderly high-risk patients. *Dis Colon Rectum.* 1988;31(9):704-706.
9. Delorme E. Sur le traitement des prolapsus du rectum totaux pour l'excision de la muqueuse rectale ou rectocolique. *Bull Mem Soc Chir Paris.* 1900;26:499-578.
10. Whitlow CB, Beck DE, Opelka FG, Gathright JB Jr, Timmcke AE, Hicks TC. Perineal repair of rectal prolapse. *J La State Med Soc.* 1997;149(1):22-26.
11. Ripstein CB, Lanter B. Etiology and surgical therapy of massive prolapse of the rectum. *Ann Surg.* 1963;157:259-264.
12. Wells C. New operation for rectal prolapse. *Proc R Soc Med.* 1959;52:602-603.
13. Fengler SA, Pearl RK, Prasad ML, et al. Management of recurrent rectal prolapse. *Dis Colon Rectum.* 1997;40(7):832-834.
14. Pikarsky AJ, Joo JS, Wexner SD, et al. Recurrent rectal prolapse: what is the next good option? *Dis Colon Rectum.* 2000;43(9):1273-1276.
15. Malatjalian DA, Williams CN. 5-ASA therapy in solitary rectal ulcer syndrome. Report of three patients. *Can J Gastroenterol.* 1988;2:18-21.

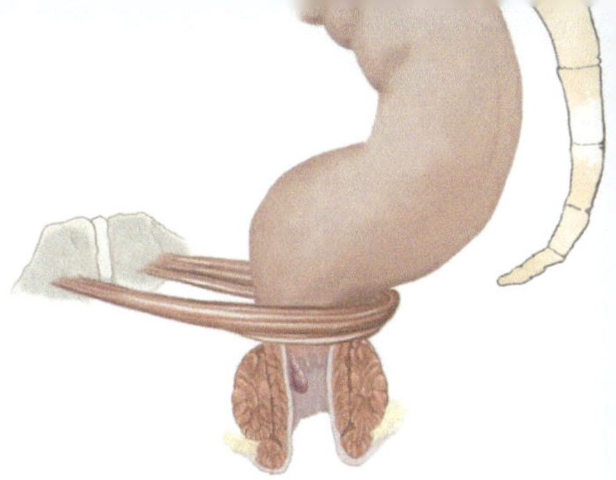

9

Solitary Rectal Ulcer Syndrome

Vineet S. Gudsoorkar, MD and Gulchin A. Ergun, MD, AGAF, FACG

Key Points

- Solitary rectal ulcer syndrome (SRUS) is a challenging disorder, often with a delayed or missed diagnosis. A high index of clinical suspicion should be maintained to avoid misdiagnosis.
- The term *solitary rectal ulcer syndrome* is a misnomer because lesions may not be solitary, confined to the rectum, or always ulcerated.
- A multidisciplinary approach involving gastroenterology, radiology, and pathology is required to make an accurate diagnosis.
- Management begins with improving the bowel regimen, avoiding constipation, and assessing and correcting abnormal behavioral aspects of dyssynergic defecation. This is coupled with an evaluation of anatomic abnormalities of the pelvic floor.

SRUS is a rare, benign disease entity that is defined by a combination of symptoms and endoscopic and histologic findings. It would be prudent to recognize at the outset that the term *solitary rectal ulcer* is a misnomer because the syndrome may have mucosal involvement ranging from mild erythema to multiple, full-blown ulcers.[1,2]

Epidemiology

Almost all epidemiologic data have been derived from smaller, typically retrospective studies and, therefore, are quite heterogeneous. Additionally, the lack of awareness and nonuniform disease presentations have led to underdiagnosis and misdiagnosis of this condition; thus, the available data

Qureshi W, ed. *Diagnosis and Management Guide for Anorectal Disease: A Clinical Reference* (pp 99-108).

may not be representative of the true epidemiologic picture.[1] Based on some of the larger data sets, the incidence of SRUS appears to be anywhere from 1 to 3.6 per 100,000 patients per year.[1,2] Among the adult population, the median age of diagnosis of SRUS is typically in the third to fourth decades of life; however, it has been well documented in pediatric and geriatric populations. Sex distribution is perhaps equal between males and females because some case series suggest a female predominance, whereas others indicate a male predominance.[3,4] Of note, the average time from the onset of symptoms to diagnosis is 5 years, ranging from 3 months to 30 years in adults,[4] which reflects the previously mentioned diagnostic challenges. Although the earliest description of this disease entity was reported almost 200 years ago,[5] its pathogenesis still remains poorly defined, thus compounding the clinical complexity of the disease. With advanced understanding of the neuromuscular physiology of the anorectum, some light has been shed on the putative mechanisms at play leading to the development of this unique disease process.

Pathophysiology

Clues to the pathogenesis and subsequent management of SRUS lie in understanding the normal anatomy and physiology of the rectum and anal canal and their relationship with the pelvic floor. For the purpose of this chapter, it is helpful to consider the distal rectum, anorectal ring, and anal canal as a single unit (ie, the anorectum) and to review the pertinent structural and functional characteristics. Filling of the rectal ampulla, either by mass movements or by emptying of the sigmoid into the ampulla, results in a complex interaction of rectoanal reflexes, which, coupled with voluntary controls, results either in the process of defecation or delaying of it.

The rectum is attached to the mesorectum within the curve of the sacrum with limited mobility. Continence is maintained by several anatomic structures working in concert including the circular muscle tone of the rectal wall; superior, middle, and inferior rectal valves of Houston; internal anal sphincter; hemorrhoidal venous plexus; and external anal sphincter including the puborectalis muscle. A large portion of the resting anal tone has been attributed to the internal anal sphincter.[6]

The anorectum receives sympathetic nerve supply from the thoracolumbar spinal segment and parasympathetic input via the S2, S3, and S4 roots (ie, the nervi erigentes). The cortical area for anorectal motor control is represented bilaterally in the superior motor cortex. Somatic innervation of the external anal sphincter is derived from the inferior rectal nerve, a branch of the pudendal nerve. The inferior rectal nerves also carry the cutaneous sensation from below the dentate line. The rectum and proximal anal canal respond primarily to distension and mechanical shearing stimuli. However, the exact mechanism of visceral sensation remains obscure, and theories exist whether the visceral pain is caused by incremental activation of the visceral nociceptors (eg, increasing volumes of mechanical distension) or a result of impulse generation in certain spatiotemporal patterns.[7] A combination of anatomic factors, vascular insufficiency, and neural dysfunction has been implicated in the final pathogenesis of SRUS.

Broadly, 2 factors, namely rectal prolapse and dyssynergic defecation, are thought to play a central role in the pathogenesis of SRUS. Earlier studies suggested that an abnormal descent of the pelvic floor was an important theme in defecatory disorders including rectal prolapse and, therefore, a predisposition to SRUS.[8] Indeed, a study evaluating the incidence of radiographic abnormalities associated with SRUS suggested that 68% of patients with SRUS had internal or external rectal prolapse.[9] However, a conclusive cause-effect relationship has not been established between the 2 because not all patients with rectal prolapse develop SRUS. Moreover, when the anorectal physiology of patients with SRUS was compared with those with rectal prolapse (with or without mucosal changes), the SRUS group had increased anal squeeze pressures and paradoxical contraction of the puborectalis muscle,[10] suggesting that the pathophysiology of SRUS extends beyond the rectal prolapse and raises the question as to whether rectal prolapse is a cause of SRUS or an effect of the mechanisms that may play a role in the development of SRUS.

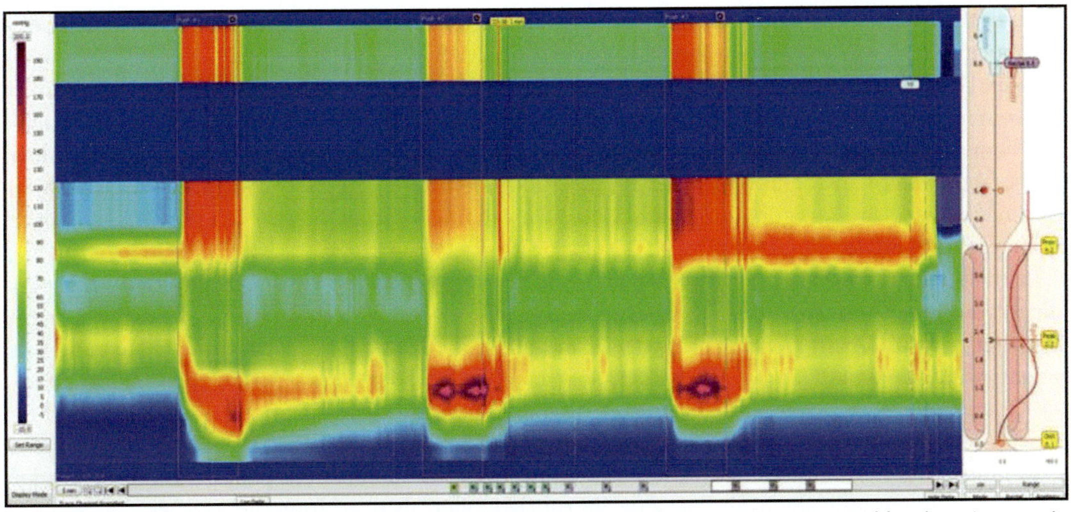

Figure 9-1. Anorectal manometry in dyssynergic defecation. In type I dyssynergia (represented here), an increase in intrarectal pressure is observed along with a paradoxical increase in anal sphincter pressure.

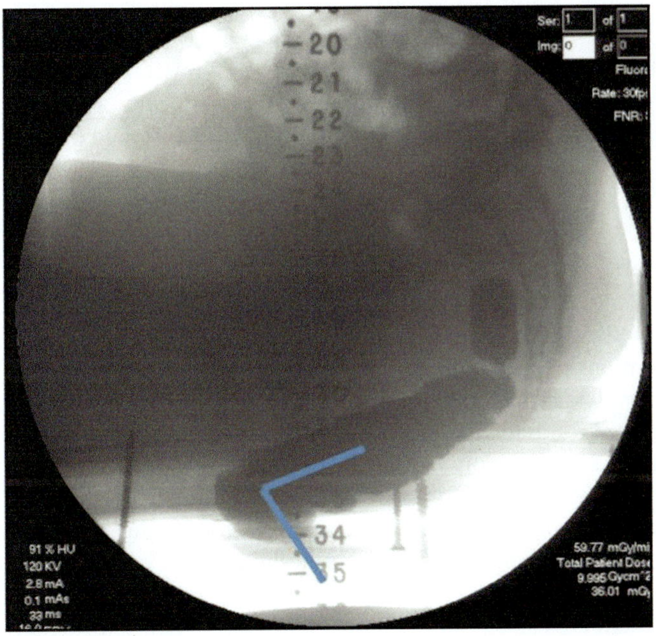

Figure 9-2. A defecogram demonstrating paradoxical contraction of the puborectalis muscle. During straining and defecation, the anorectal angle should become more obtuse to allow for opening of the anal canal and rectal evacuation. With puborectalis dyskinesia, the anorectal angle fails to widen; therefore, it becomes difficult to empty the rectal vault of stool.

Anorectal physiologic abnormalities have been reported more consistently with SRUS. When compared with case-matched groups of patients without SRUS and patients with overt rectal prolapse, patients with SRUS were noted to have significantly elevated anal squeeze pressures on anorectal manometry (Figure 9-1), whereas defecography showed paradoxical contraction of the puborectalis muscle (Figure 9-2), failure to completely empty the rectum, and a longer mean straining duration.

This suggested that despite similar symptoms, a cause-effect relationship between SRUS and rectal prolapse cannot be established.[10] Two other studies comparing anorectal manometry and the balloon expulsion test between patients with SRUS and healthy controls showed statistically significant abnormal balloon expulsion tests and impaired anal relaxation in the SRUS group. Both of these studies confirmed the presence of a higher anal squeeze pressure in the SRUS group, with one of them reaching statistical significance.[3,11] Thus, dyssynergic defecation, an acquired behavioral disorder, appears to play a large role in the pathogenesis of SRUS.

Pelvic floor weakness resulting in excessive perineal descent and rectal prolapse was thought to lead to stretch neuropathy of the pudendal nerve.[12] Although subsequent studies refuted this theory,[13,14] emerging work did show evidence of autonomic dysfunction using gut mucosal blood flow as a surrogate marker of autonomic innervation in patients with SRUS.[15] Thus, mucosal ischemia, from neurovascular dysregulation in addition to mechanical forces, appears to play a part in the pathogenesis of SRUS.

Interestingly, the psychological state has been shown to affect the gut mucosal blood flow, presumably via autonomic neural activity.[16] This finding aligns well with the concept of a psychological contribution to the pathogenesis of SRUS. A unique study evaluating biopsychological profiles of patients with proven SRUS showed that 82% of the patients had an underlying psychological disorder. Obsessive-compulsive disorder (or trait) was the most prevalent diagnosis at 62% followed by anxiety disorder (50%). A multitude of other psychological comorbidities including physical and sexual abuse were also noted.[17] Thus, a gastroenterologist caring for these patients should consider these not-so-apparent triggers and provide appropriate referrals to address these issues.

Direct trauma from repetitive digitation has been discussed as a contributing factor in the pathogenesis of SRUS, although most ulcers are located as much as 10 cm proximal to the anal verge, an area where digitation is unlikely to inflict direct trauma, making this explanation unlikely.

Finally, one prospective study of SRUS patients speculated that SRUS is a regional presentation of a systemic process.[18] In a cohort of 22 biopsy-proven SRUS patients, 20% had HLA-B27 positivity, 18% had recurrent oral ulcers, 31% had sacroiliitis, and 1 patient had erythema nodosum. Although not conclusive, these findings might suggest that an underlying immune-mediated systemic disease process may exist in SRUS patients.

Clinical Features

Patients with SRUS typically present with a constellation of symptoms that include rectal bleeding, mucus discharge, perineal or abdominal pain, straining, constipation, or diarrhea, although this may be reflective of the sense of incomplete evacuation and resultant frequent passage of small-volume stools. Some patients report the need for manual digital fecal evacuation. One retrospective study reported as many as 26% of patients did not have any symptoms associated with SRUS and that ulcers were detected on colonoscopy performed for other indications; however, upon detailed direct questioning, more than half of these patients reported mild abdominal symptoms including rectal bleeding.[19] Table 9-1 shows predominant symptoms found in some studies in patients with SRUS.

Endoscopically, the majority of ulcers are located on the anterior rectal wall anywhere from 3 to 18 cm from the anal verge, but most of them are clustered between 6 and 10 cm.[3,20] The endoscopic appearance ranged from erythematous ulcerated lesions to polypoid lesions.[3,19,21] The heterogeneous appearance of SRUS has resulted in cases of misdiagnosis, most commonly as inflammatory bowel disease (for the ulcerated variant) or rectal neoplasia (for the polypoid variant).[4]

Diagnosis

Diagnosing SRUS with accuracy involves a clinical suspicion, anorectal physiologic studies including defecation proctography (x-ray or magnetic resonance aided), anorectal manometry and balloon expulsion testing, endoscopy, and histology. The characteristic findings of the anorectal physiologic studies and endoscopy have been discussed previously in this chapter.

Table 9-1

A Summary of the Common Clinical Symptoms Reported in Some of the Larger Studies Across the World

FIRST STUDY AUTHOR (YEAR)	STUDY DESIGN	REGION	PATIENTS	PREDOMINANT SYMPTOMS	BOWEL HABITS
Tjandra (1992)[19]	Retrospective	United States	80	Rectal bleeding (56%) Straining (28%) Pelvic fullness (23%) Mucous discharge (18%) Incontinence (10%)	Constipation (35%) Diarrhea (20%) Variable (19%) Normal (26%) Digital evacuation (8%)
Ford (1982)[22]	Retrospective	United Kingdom	40	Rectal bleeding with mucus (97.5%) Straining (70%) Incomplete evacuation (62.5%) Anorectal/left lower abdominal pain (70%)	Constipation (22.5%) Diarrhea (45%) Variable (22.5%) Normal (~12%) Digital evacuation (73%) (19/26)
Derakhshani (2009)[23]	Retrospective	Middle East (Iran)	112	Rectal bleeding (67%) Mucous discharge (58%) Anorectal pain (48.2%) Straining (9.8%) Tenesmus (27.7%) Incomplete evacuation (23.2%) Incontinence (6.2%)	Constipation (46.4%) Diarrhea (14.3%) Digital evacuation (56.2%)
Behera (2015)[3]	Prospective	India	92	Rectal bleeding (83.7%) Straining at stool (31.5%) Mucus per rectum (28.8%) Abdominal/perianal pain (48%) Tenesmus (22.8%) Incomplete evacuation (18.4%)	Constipation (46.7%) Diarrhea (25%) Digital evacuation (36.9%)

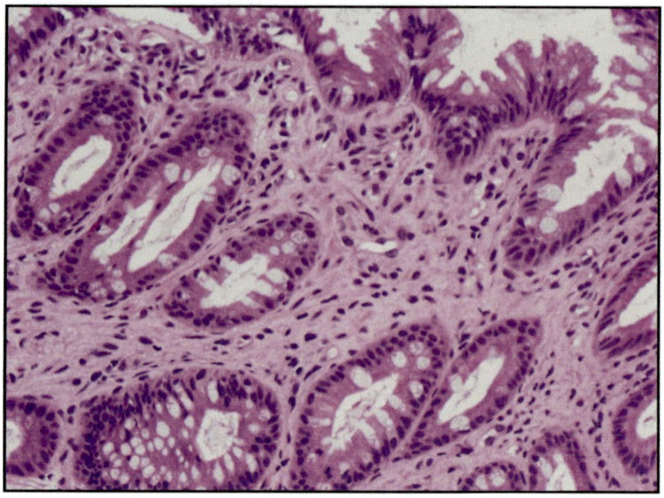

Figure 9-3. The histology of SRUS. A biopsy of SRUS showing proliferation of fine smooth muscle fibers in the lamina propria, mild mucosal fibrosis, mild hyperplastic change of surface epithelium, and absence of significant inflammation (hematoxylin and eosin staining, magnified ×20).

The histologic findings of SRUS have been well characterized and should be used as the most definite diagnostic criterion. The key histologic findings include fibromuscular obliteration of the lamina propria and superficial ulceration (Figure 9-3). Fibromuscular hyperplasia of the lamina propria appears to be the most consistent histologic feature. Also seen are thickening and upward splaying of the muscularis propria, resulting in crypt distortion and dilation. Typically, biopsies are characterized by a lack of significant inflammation.[3,20,21] The characteristic appearance of distorted crypts in rectal prolapse, which has sometimes been referred to as *diamond crypts*, can be suggestive of but *not* pathognomonic of SRUS.[24,25]

Despite extensive workup, occasionally it is still difficult to reliably differentiate between SRUS and rectal malignancy. Reports exist of SRUS mimicking malignancy[26] and vice versa[27] as well as the 2 conditions coexisting.[28,29] Rectal magnetic resonance imaging (MRI) and endoscopic rectal ultrasound (ErUS) have been used as anecdotally adjunct imaging modalities, attempting to further differentiate the 2 conditions. A case report describing the use of MRI reported the appearance of SRUS as an area of focal thickening in the anterior rectal wall with a central ulceration confined to the mucosa; the muscularis propria was intact with no enlarged regional lymph nodes or fatty stranding. The authors concluded that the magnetic resonance appearance of SRUS was nonspecific and indistinguishable from malignancy.[30] ErUS has also been studied in the evaluation of SRUS as part of a small case series. This series described a marked thickening of the third layer (the upper portion of the muscularis propria) of the rectal wall without any destruction of the 5-layer structure in all 5 of the patients.[31] Van Outryve et al[32] also reported thickening of the muscularis propria but, importantly, found the echostructure to be disturbed in 9 of 15 patients with fading of the borders between the mucosa and the muscularis propria. More recently, a retrospective case series evaluated patients with a final histologic diagnosis of SRUS who were initially diagnosed with rectal cancer. Among the 6 patients who had undergone ErUS, the diagnosis of cancer was excluded in only 1 patient. Similarly, of the 4 patients who underwent MRI, it was nondiagnostic in 1 patient, whereas the other 3 suggested cancer. A final diagnosis of SRUS was made in all patients with deep macrobiopsies. Therefore, the authors concluded that even with the use of MRI and ErUS, misdiagnosis between these 2 conditions is common unless an intact 5-layer structure of the rectal wall is clearly maintained.[33] Thus, these 2 modalities currently do not hold a place in the routine diagnostic algorithm of suspected SRUS.

Management

The management of SRUS is complex because its pathogenesis is poorly understood. Ideally, it should consist of a multipronged approach including pharmacologic management for constipation, behavioral management for dyssynergic defecation, and surgical management of overt anatomic abnormalities of the pelvic floor.

PHARMACOLOGIC MANAGEMENT

This strategy is often the first step because it is easy to administer, noninvasive, and generally well tolerated. It aims at producing stools that are soft and easy to expel without straining and achieving regulation of bowel habits. Pharmacologic management is perhaps more appropriate for patients with mild disease without evidence of obvious anatomic abnormalities. In a study published in 1984 that included 21 patients followed longitudinally on a high-fiber diet (30 to 40 g fiber daily), the authors reported complete healing of the ulcer in 15 patients at the average follow-up period of 10.5 months.[34] Anecdotal reports exist of adding sucralfate or 5-aminosalicylic acid derivatives topically[35,36]; one study with 6 patients who received sucralfate enemas reported that all patients had endoscopic but not histologic healing of the ulcer at the mean follow-up of 8 months. However, the other study did not replicate this success when patients were treated with a high-fiber diet, stool softeners, and bulking laxatives, resulting in only 20% endoscopic healing. The addition of sulfasalazine enemas led to overall improvement in 28% of patients. Thus, pharmacotherapy alone has a variable success rate and is probably best reserved for patients without underlying rectal prolapse.

BIOFEEDBACK

The main purpose of biofeedback therapy is to train or retrain a patient to achieve a coordinated effort of adequate expulsion synchronized with complete anal relaxation. This is typically used in conjunction with dietary and pharmacologic modifications to avoid constipation and straining. Additionally, biofeedback may also be used as an adjunct to surgery. Vaizey et al[37] studied 13 consecutive patients in 1997 who underwent biofeedback therapy and reported, after a median follow-up of 9 months, that symptom improvement or elimination occurred in the need to strain (7/13 patients), digitation (7/11 patients), laxative use (5/9 patients), the time in the toilet (median of 10 minutes, down from 30 minutes), and the number of visits to the toilet. Of note, none of the patients had complete healing of the ulcer. The presence of paradoxical contraction of the pelvic floor did not influence the outcome.[37] In another study of 16 patients without overt rectal prolapse, 12 (75%) had symptomatic improvement, and 5 (31%) had endoscopic resolution of the ulcer. Additionally, mucosal blood flow, which was lower in the SRUS group, also showed improvement with biofeedback.[38] Rao et al[39] reported a series of 11 patients with refractory SRUS who underwent biofeedback therapy for a median duration of 3 months. After biofeedback, straining effort and stool frequency decreased, and bowel satisfaction scores improved. There was complete ulcer healing in 4 (36%) patients and ≥50% healing in 2 (18%) patients. Moreover, follow-up anorectal function studies demonstrated a decrease in rectal pressure as well as reduced balloon expulsion time.[39] Although all of these studies were limited by a relatively short-term follow-up, a questionnaire-based study by Malouf et al[40] noted that, at a median follow-up of 36 months, approximately 50% of the patients who have early clinical benefit from biofeedback will experience deterioration across variable parameters such as laxative use, the need to strain, visits to the toilet, and the time spent in the toilet.

Thus, to summarize, biofeedback appears to be helpful in mitigating various symptoms associated with SRUS, but the resolution of ulcers is achieved only in approximately one-third of patients. Similarly, the effects may not be durable, and patients may need repeat sessions. The utility of biofeedback appears to be higher if associated dyssynergic defecation is present because biofeedback may improve dyssynergia. It is critical to recognize that the current evidence for biofeedback in SRUS management is of limited quality because of the small number of patients, relatively short follow-up, and open-label design.

ENDOSCOPIC AND SURGICAL MANAGEMENT

Topical therapies delivered endoscopically have been anecdotally reported. In a case series of 12 patients, human fibrin, a stimulator of angiogenesis, was endoscopically applied in 6 patients in addition to diet and behavioral modifications. The comparator group received only diet and behavioral modifications. At 14 days posttreatment, all 6 patients who received human fibrin application had ulcer healing; in the other group, none of the patients had ulcer healing at 14 days, but 3 of the 6 patients had ulcer healing at the 1-year follow-up.[41] Botulinum toxin injections were used in 4 patients with paradoxical rectal spasm, which resulted in symptom improvement in all patients, but ulcer healing was noted only in 2 of the 4 patients.[36]

Surgery is reserved for patients refractory to nonoperative management as outlined previously or for those with associated rectal prolapse. Several surgical approaches have been described in the literature, ranging from proximal colostomy creation, low anterior resection, mucosal resection (Delorme procedure), and rectopexy to local resection. It is important to address the underlying behavioral issues such as pelvic floor dyssynergia and colonic transit abnormalities before subjecting a patient to surgery. A quick review of the surgical literature would suggest that rectopexy is favored among the other techniques. In 1998, Sitzler et al[42] reported that, of 49 patients undergoing rectopexy, the rectopexy failed in 22 patients (45%) at the 7.5-year follow-up. The Delorme procedure was performed in 9 patients, with 4 failures at the 3-year follow-up. Similarly, 4 of 7 patients undergoing anterior resection eventually required ostomy.[42] Similar outcomes were reported by Marchal et al,[43] who reported a 60% success rate (measured as symptom improvement or ulcer healing). Another retrospective study by Torres and colleagues[44] reported a better success rate, with ulcer healing achieved in 13 of 16 patients undergoing surgery. In this cohort, low anterior resection was the most common procedure because of the presence of large ulcerations. Of the 16 patients, 4 had persistent symptoms, 3 had sexual dysfunction, and 2 had rectal bleeding requiring surgery, yielding an overall complication rate of approximately 44%.

A retrospective European study analyzing outcomes of the laparoscopic approach indicated a 100% ulcer healing rate at the 1-year follow-up in 11 patients. Of the 7 patients available for long-term follow-up, none had ulcer recurrence, and 6 had symptom resolution.[45] Although this study did not directly compare outcomes with conventional open laparoscopy, it would appear that a laparoscopic approach may have favorable outcomes compared with an open procedure.

Thus, in summary, a surgical approach should be reserved for a select group of patients who are refractory to noninvasive management strategies. The success rate is variable, with larger studies indicating approximately 60% success, although newer studies seem to have improved outcomes. Rectopexy, particularly laparoscopic, may have better outcomes. Local resection may be favored when there is no overt or complete prolapse.

REFERENCES

1. Haray PN, Morris-Stiff GJ, Foster ME. Solitary rectal ulcer syndrome—an underdiagnosed condition. *Int J Colorectal Dis.* 1997;12(5):313-315.
2. Martin CJ, Parks TG, Biggart JD. Solitary rectal ulcer syndrome in Northern Ireland. 1971-1980. *Br J Surg.* 1981;68(10):744-747.
3. Behera MK, Dixit VK, Shukla SK, et al. Solitary rectal ulcer syndrome: clinical, endoscopic, histological and anorectal manometry findings in north Indian patients. *Trop Gastroenterol.* 2015;36(4):244-250.

4. Tjandra JJ, Fazio VW, Petras RE, et al. Clinical and pathologic factors associated with delayed diagnosis in solitary rectal ulcer syndrome. *Dis Colon Rectum*. 1993;36(2):146-153.
5. Cruveilhier J. *Ulcere Chronique du Rectum. Anatomie Pathologique du Corps Humain*. Paris, France: JB Bailliere; 1829.
6. Barleben A, Mills S. Anorectal anatomy and physiology. *Surg Clin North Am*. 2010;90(1):1-15, Table of Contents.
7. Bharucha AE. Pelvic floor: anatomy and function. *Neurogastroenterol Motil*. 2006;18(7):507-519.
8. Levine DS. "Solitary" rectal ulcer syndrome. Are "solitary" rectal ulcer syndrome and "localized" colitis cystica profunda analogous syndromes caused by rectal prolapse? *Gastroenterology*. 1987;92(1):243-253.
9. Halligan S, Nicholls RJ, Bartram CI. Evacuation proctography in patients with solitary rectal ulcer syndrome: anatomic abnormalities and frequency of impaired emptying and prolapse. *AJR Am J Roentgenol*. 1995;164(1):91-95.
10. Morio O, Meurette G, Desfourneaux V, D'Halluin PN, Bretagne JF, Siproudhis L. Anorectal physiology in solitary ulcer syndrome: a case-matched series. *Dis Colon Rectum*. 2005;48(10):1917-1922.
11. Sharma A, Misra A, Ghoshal UC. Fecal evacuation disorder among patients with solitary rectal ulcer syndrome: a case-control study. *J Neurogastroenterol Motil*. 2014;20(4):531-538.
12. Henry MM, Parks AG, Swash M. The pelvic floor musculature in the descending perineum syndrome. *Br J Surg*. 1982;69(8):470-472.
13. Jorge JM, Wexner SD, Ehrenpreis ED, Nogueras JJ, Jagelman DG. Does perineal descent correlate with pudendal neuropathy? *Dis Colon Rectum*. 1993;36(5):475-483.
14. Ryhammer AM, Laurberg S, Hermann AP. No correlation between perineal position and pudendal nerve terminal motor latency in healthy perimenopausal women. *Dis Colon Rectum*. 1998;41(3):350-353.
15. Emmanuel AV, Kamm MA. Laser Doppler measurement of rectal mucosal blood flow. *Gut*. 1999;45(1):64-69.
16. Emmanuel AV, Mason HJ, Kamm MA. Relationship between psychological state and level of activity of extrinsic gut innervation in patients with a functional gut disorder. *Gut*. 2001;49(2):209-213.
17. Daghaghzadeh H, Mohammadi N, Afshar H, Mazaheri M, Tavakoli H. Solitary rectal ulcer syndrome: a biopsychosocial assessment. *Int J Body Mind Culture*. 2016;3(1):55-63.
18. Tandon RK, Atmakuri SP, Mehra NK, Malaviya AN, Tandon HD, Chopra P. Is solitary rectal ulcer a manifestation of a systemic disease? *J Clin Gastroenterol*. 1990;12(3):286-290.
19. Tjandra JJ, Fazio VW, Church JM, Lavery IC, Oakley JR, Milsom JW. Clinical conundrum of solitary rectal ulcer. *Dis Colon Rectum*. 1992;35(3):227-234.
20. Madigan MR, Morson BC. Solitary ulcer of the rectum. *Gut*. 1969;10(11):871-881.
21. Abid S, Khawaja A, Bhimani SA, Ahmad Z, Hamid S, Jafri W. The clinical, endoscopic and histological spectrum of the solitary rectal ulcer syndrome: a single-center experience of 116 cases. *BMC Gastroenterol*. 2012;12:72.
22. Ford MJ, Anderson JR, Gilmour HM, Holt S, Sircus W, Heading RC. Clinical spectrum of "solitary ulcer" of the rectum. *Gastroenterology*. 1983;84(6):1533-1540.
23. Derakhshani S, Pakzad M, Vafaie M, Tehrani-Tarighat S, Abdollahi M. A report of 112 cases of solitary rectal ulcer syndrome from Iran. *Cent Eur J Med*. 2009;4(1):49-53.
24. Al-Brahim N, Al-Awadhi N, Al-Enezi S, Alsurayei S, Ahmad M. Solitary rectal ulcer syndrome: a clinicopathological study of 13 cases. *Saudi J Gastroenterol*. 2009;15(3):188-192.
25. Warren BF, Dankwa EK, Davies JD. 'Diamond-shaped' crypts and mucosal elastin: helpful diagnostic features in biopsies of rectal prolapse. *Histopathology*. 1990;17(2):129-134.
26. Delgado J, Delgado B, Sztarkier I, Sperber AD, Walfisch S. A solitary rectal ulcer mimicking rectal cancer. *Gastrointest Endosc*. 2005;62(2):309; discussion 309.
27. Li SC, Hamilton SR. Malignant tumors in the rectum simulating solitary rectal ulcer syndrome in endoscopic biopsy specimens. *Am J Surg Pathol*. 1998;22(1):106-112.
28. Monkemuller KE. Solitary rectal ulcer syndrome and rectal cancer. *Am J Gastroenterol*. 1999;94(5):1417.
29. Tsuchida K, Okayama N, Miyata M, et al. Solitary rectal ulcer syndrome accompanied by submucosal invasive carcinoma. *Am J Gastroenterol*. 1998;93(11):2235-2238.
30. Amaechi I, Papagrigoriadis S, Hizbullah S, Ryan SM. Solitary rectal ulcer syndrome mimicking rectal neoplasm on MRI. *Br J Radiol*. 2010;83(995):e221-224.
31. Hizawa K, Iida M, Suekane H, et al. Mucosal prolapse syndrome: diagnosis with endoscopic US. *Radiology*. 1994;191(2):527-530.
32. Van Outryve MJ, Pelckmans PA, Fierens H, Van Maercke YM. Transrectal ultrasound study of the pathogenesis of solitary rectal ulcer syndrome. *Gut*. 1993;34(10):1422-1426.
33. Blanco F, Frasson M, Flor-Lorente B, Minguez M, Esclapez P, Garcia-Granero E. Solitary rectal ulcer: ultrasonographic and magnetic resonance imaging patterns mimicking rectal cancer. *Eur J Gastroenterol Hepatol*. 2011;23(12):1262-1266.
34. van den Brandt-Gradel V, Huibregtse K, Tytgat GN. Treatment of solitary rectal ulcer syndrome with high-fiber diet and abstention of straining at defecation. *Dig Dis Sci*. 1984;29(11):1005-1008.

35. Zargar SA, Khuroo MS, Mahajan R. Sucralfate retention enemas in solitary rectal ulcer. *Dis Colon Rectum*. 1991;34(6):455-457.
36. Bulut T, Canbay E, Yamaner S, Gulluoglu M, Bugra D. Solitary rectal ulcer syndrome: exploring possible management options. *Int Surg*. 2011;96:45-50.
37. Vaizey CJ, Roy AJ, Kamm MA. Prospective evaluation of the treatment of solitary rectal ulcer syndrome with biofeedback. *Gut*. 1997;41(6):817-820.
38. Jarrett ME, Emmanuel AV, Vaizey CJ, Kamm MA. Behavioural therapy (biofeedback) for solitary rectal ulcer syndrome improves symptoms and mucosal blood flow. *Gut*. 2004;53(3):368-370.
39. Rao SS, Ozturk R, De Ocampo S, Stessman M. Pathophysiology and role of biofeedback therapy in solitary rectal ulcer syndrome. *Am J Gastroenterol*. 2006;101(3):613-618.
40. Malouf AJ, Vaizey CJ, Kamm MA. Results of behavioral treatment (biofeedback) for solitary rectal ulcer syndrome. *Dis Colon Rectum*. 2001;44(1):72-76.
41. Ederle A, Bulighin G, Orlandi PG, Pilati S. Endoscopic application of human fibrin sealant in the treatment of solitary rectal ulcer syndrome. *Endoscopy*. 1992;24(8):736-737.
42. Sitzler PJ, Kamm MA, Nicholls RJ, McKee RF. Long-term clinical outcome of surgery for solitary rectal ulcer syndrome. *Br J Surg*. 1998;85(9):1246-1250.
43. Marchal F, Bresler L, Brunaud L, et al. Solitary rectal ulcer syndrome: a series of 13 patients operated with a mean follow-up of 4.5 years. *Int J Colorectal Dis*. 2001;16(4):228-233.
44. Torres C, Khaikin M, Bracho J, et al. Solitary rectal ulcer syndrome: clinical findings, surgical treatment, and outcomes. *Int J Colorectal Dis*. 2007;22(11):1389-1393.
45. Tweedie DJ, Varma JS. Long-term outcome of laparoscopic mesh rectopexy for solitary rectal ulcer syndrome. *Colorectal Dis*. 2005;7(2):151-155.

10

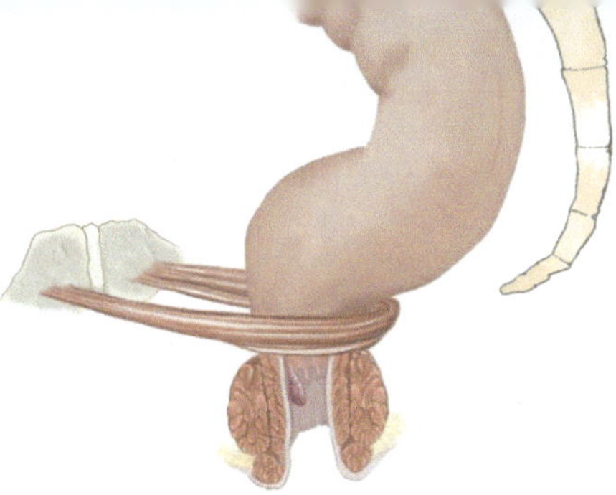

Chronic Constipation

Assessment and Treatment

Mehnaz A. Shafi, MD

Key Points

- Chronic constipation is a highly prevalent disorder that affects 20% of the US population. It impairs quality of life and imposes an enormous economic burden on society.
- Three broad subsets of chronic constipation have been identified: slow transit constipation, rectal outlet disorders, and normal transit constipation, which is the largest subgroup. There is considerable overlap among the subgroups. Irritable bowel syndrome (IBS) with constipation, a common etiology of chronic constipation, often has associated symptoms of abdominal bloating and pain. Chronic constipation may present with upper abdominal symptoms such as nausea.
- A detailed history, physical examination, and digital rectal examination are important in identifying primary and secondary constipation.
- Several advances have been made in the diagnosis and management of constipation.
- The prevalence and diagnosis of dyssynergic constipation are better understood, leading to improved management and use of biofeedback therapy. Physiologic tests such as colon transit studies and anorectal manometry can help diagnose the subtype of chronic constipation.
- Several treatment options are available including intestinal secretagogues, peripherally acting mu receptor antagonists for opioid-induced constipation (OIC), and biofeedback therapy. Surgery is rarely indicated and is considered in refractory slow transit constipation.

Qureshi W, ed. *Diagnosis and Management Guide for Anorectal Disease: A Clinical Reference* (pp 109-119).

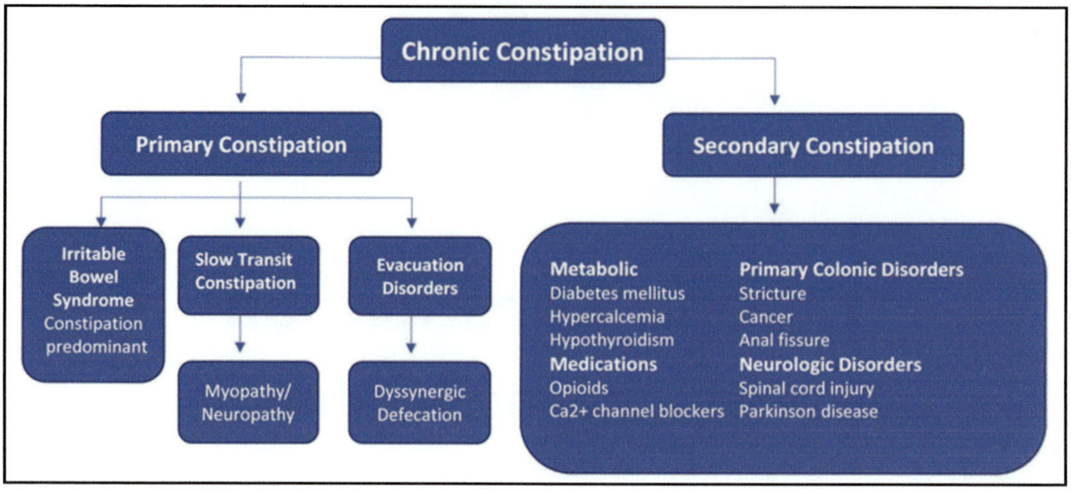

Figure 10-1. Etiologies of primary and secondary constipation.

Constipation is used to describe altered bowel habits. It involves a range of symptoms including infrequent bowel movements, hard stools, straining, small-volume evacuation, abdominal bloating, and pain. It is one of the commonest gastrointestinal (GI) conditions seen in primary care and GI practices. It can cause physical and psychological stress and adversely affect the quality of life of the patient. The prevalence of constipation is 14% to 16% in the United States.[1] This increases with age and can be up to 33% in the elderly.[2] Women, non-White race, and a lower socioeconomic status are associated with chronic constipation. Symptoms of constipation often overlap with other GI conditions, such as IBS and dyspepsia. Anxiety and depression are seen more often in patients with chronic constipation than in the general population. Constipation alone in the absence of alarm symptoms suggestive of organic disease is not associated with a higher risk of colorectal cancer. The American Society of Gastrointestinal Endoscopy recommends average-risk screening in patients with constipation in the absence of alarm symptoms.

Subtypes and Pathophysiology

Chronic constipation can be a primary disorder or a secondary condition due to metabolic conditions or drugs. Primary constipation is more frequent than secondary causes and results from factors such as insufficient dietary fiber, a sedentary lifestyle, or neuromuscular dysregulation of the colon and the rectum that involves disturbances in the brain-gut axis, resulting in disordered colonic propulsion or rectal evacuation.[3,4]

Secondary constipation is due to metabolic conditions such as diabetes, hypercalcemia, hypothyroidism, or pregnancy; various drugs including opioids and calcium channel blockers; neurologic conditions such as Parkinson disease and multiple sclerosis; or an intrinsic pathology of the colon such as colon cancer, an anal stricture, or an anal fissure[5] (Figure 10-1).

Primary constipation can be subcategorized into 3 groups that overlap considerably[6,7]: slow transit constipation, normal transit constipation, and rectal outlet disorder. Colonic propulsion depends on mass movements associated with contraction of the colon wall. Contractions of the large bowel wall lead to increased intraluminal pressure and result in high-amplitude propagating contractions. These are associated with mass movement of colonic contents from the cecum to the rectum.[8]

Slow transit constipation, or colonic inertia, results from dysfunction of the colonic smooth muscle of the colocolonic reflexes or neuropathy and results in delayed passage of stool through the colon. Patients have decreased colonic motor activity, diminished gastrocolic reflexes, and blunted or

Table 10-1

Rome IV Diagnostic Criteria for Functional Constipation

Must include 2 or more of the following: • Straining during more than 25% of defecations • Lumpy or hard stools (Bristol stool types 1 or 2) more than 25% of defecations • Sensation of incomplete evacuation more than 25% of defecations • Manual maneuvers to facilitate more than 25% of defecations (eg, digital evacuation and support of the pelvic floor)
Loose stools are rarely present without the use of laxatives
Insufficient criteria for IBS
Criteria fulfilled for the last 3 months with symptom onset at least 6 months prior to diagnosis.

absent high-amplitude propagated contractions. The loss of interstitial cells of Cajal has been demonstrated. Alterations in the colonic microbiota may also contribute to colonic inertia. A small fraction of these patients may develop chronic megacolon associated with decreased colonic compliance.

Rectal outlet dysfunction results from the discoordination of abdominal and pelvic floor muscles to effectively expel stool.[9-11] Dyssynergic defecation, an example of this, results from functional impairment of the pelvic floor and the anal sphincter muscles. This is seen in two-thirds of patients with expulsion difficulties. Often, this is a behavioral disorder.[12,13] Discoordination of the abdominal and anal muscles leads to paradoxical anal contractions or impaired anal relaxation while attempting to evacuate. Other causes of outlet dysfunction include a rectocele, solitary rectal ulcer syndrome, or a weak pelvic floor.

The largest group of patients with primary chronic constipation do not have slow transit constipation or rectal outlet dysfunction. This subset is called *functional constipation* or *normal transit constipation*. IBS with constipation predominant (IBS-C) is an example of this subgroup[9] (Table 10-1). The pathophysiology of IBS is multifactorial and incompletely understood. IBS-C is a functional disorder that manifests with recurrent abdominal pain. Visceral hyperalgesia is a distinct feature of IBS.

The Rome IV diagnostic criteria for IBS-C include recurrent pain on average at least 1 day/week in the last 6 months associated with at least 2 of the following symptoms: related to defecation, associated with a change in the frequency of stools, and associated with a change in the form of stool (with > 25% Bristol stool type 1 or 2; Table 10-2).

About 10% of patients have postinfectious IBS after an acute illness with *Escherichia coli* O157:H7, *Campylobacter jejuni*, or *Giardia*. Small bowel bacterial overgrowth may contribute to the development of IBS-C.[10]

A new category of constipation is OIC, which is a change in bowel habits associated with opioid use.[9] It can result in a decrease in bowel frequency, development or worsening of straining, and a sense of incomplete evacuation. OIC develops due to the actions of opioids on the GI tract and the central nervous system. As opiate use has increased, so has the recognition that these drugs can cause adverse effects on the GI tract. This is not categorized as a distinct functional disorder but rather a result of the adverse effects of opioids. Frequently, the symptoms of OIC overlap with those of functional constipation.

Table 10-2

Rome IV Diagnostic Criteria for Irritable Bowel Syndrome With Predominant Constipation

Recurrent abdominal pain on average at least 1 day/week in the last 3 months associated with 2 or more of the following criteria: • Related to defecation • Associated with a change in frequency of stool • Associated with a change in form (appearance) of stool (> 25%, Bristol stool types 1 or 2)
Criteria fulfilled for the last 3 months with symptom onset at least 6 months prior to diagnosis.

Clinical Evaluation

An important initial step in diagnosis should be to rule out alarm symptoms suggestive of an organic disorder, such as colon cancer. These include blood in the stool, new onset of constipation or a change in bowel habits after 50 years of age, anemia, weight loss, and a family history of colon cancer. The timing of symptom onset and its association with a trigger event, such as a new medication, poor oral intake, or surgery, should be reviewed. Symptoms associated with chronic constipation are similar among the different subtypes and overlap considerably. These include excessive straining, hard stools, infrequent bowel movements, a sense of incomplete evacuation, abdominal bloating, and pain. Patients should be asked which symptom is predominant, what laxatives or suppositories have been used, and if any maneuvers are used to assist with defecation such as straining and digital maneuvers. The presence of bloating, distention, and pain along with constipation is suggestive of IBS-C.

The history should include an assessment of stool consistency using the validated Bristol stool form scale.[14] The Bristol stool form scale is a visual chart showing 7 different stool consistencies from liquid to hard lumps. Bowel diaries are a reliable method to assess stool colonic transit time. Self-reported stool frequency is often unreliable, and decreased stool frequency alone is not a good predictor of slow transit constipation.[14,15]

Digital Rectal Examination

Digital rectal examination is a key component in the evaluation of constipation. External perianal inspection may show a prolapsed hemorrhoid or anal fissure. Digital rectal examination can reveal a stricture, mass, or impacted stool. The external anal sphincter should be assessed for the resting tone. By asking the patient to squeeze the puborectalis, anterior lift is elicited. When asked to bear down, corresponding relaxation of the puborectalis and perianal descent are felt.[16] In dyssynergia, this response is often impaired with paradoxical contraction of the anal sphincter during attempted evacuation. Digital rectal examination can also reveal a fissure, rectocele, and stool or mass in the rectum.

Rectal Balloon Expulsion Test

This is a noninvasive test to screen for evacuation disorders. It evaluates a patient's ability to expel a water-filled balloon.[17] The deflated balloon is placed in the rectum and inflated to 50 mL. The time taken to expel the rectal balloon while in the seated position should be less than 1 minute. Patients with pelvic floor dysfunction require a longer time to expel the balloon. In a study of 106 patients with constipation and 24 patients with defecatory disorders, rectal balloon expulsion was 87.5% sensitive and 89% specific, with positive and negative predictive values of 64% and 97% for diagnosing defecatory disorders, respectively.[18] However, this test does not distinguish between functional and anatomic causes, and an abnormal result requires further testing.

ANORECTAL MANOMETRY

Conventional and high-resolution anorectal manometry are physiologic tests that assess the external anal sphincter tone, rectoanal reflexes, and rectal pressure changes during defecation and at rest. These tests are useful in diagnosing anorectal disorders such as dyssynergic defecation and its subtypes. Four subtypes of dyssynergia can be identified by anorectal manometry.[19,20] A high anal resting pressure, typically ≥ 90 mm Hg with relatively little voluntary effort, is suggestive of nonrelaxing pelvic floor/sphincter dysfunction. Biofeedback therapy can be tailored to the type of dyssynergia diagnosed with anorectal manometry such as the pushing effort in dyssynergic defecation type 2, improved relaxation in dyssynergic defecation type 3, or both in dyssynergic defecation type 4. This test also detects rectal hyposensitivity.[21]

COLON TRANSIT TESTS

Colonic transit time can be evaluated by radiopaque markers or a wireless motility capsule. The capsule test can detect dysmotility in proximal segments of the gut as well.

Radiopaque Markers

This is a simple, noninvasive test to assess colonic transit time. It involves oral intake of tiny radiopaque markers in a capsule followed by an abdominal x-ray after a defined period of time. Many testing variations exist, but a commonly used method is the Hinton method.[22] A capsule with 20 to 24 small ringlike radiopaque markers is given to the patient to swallow on day 1. An abdominal plain film is obtained on day 5. Retention of more than 20% of the rings is suggestive of slow transit constipation.

Wireless Motility Capsule Test

A pH- and temperature-sensitive capsule can be used to determine segmental and whole-gut transit times based on changes in pH in different parts of the gut.[23] The patient is asked to stop all acid-suppressing medications 5 to 7 days before the test. On ingestion, a prompt decrease in the intraluminal pH below 4 is consistent with the low gastric pH, a rise in the pH by 3 units is indicative of entry into the small bowel, and a decrease by 1 unit occurs when the capsule enters the cecum. The capsule can also detect the amplitude of contractions. A physiologic increase in activity can be seen after meals. There is a good correlation between the wireless motility capsule and radiopaque markers in measuring colon transit time in patients with chronic constipation.

Whole-gut transit studies have shown that more than one-third of patients with constipation have additional transit abnormalities beyond the colon.[24] Thus, the capsule can provide added information for patients with overlapping symptoms of the upper and lower GI tract.

DEFECOGRAPHY

This test is used to determine the function and anatomy of the anorectum. Images can be obtained with contrast such as barium or with functional magnetic resonance imaging. These can diagnose rectal intussusception, rectal prolapse, or a rectocele. Findings include inadequate (spastic) or excessive (flaccid or descending perineum syndrome) widening of the anorectal angle and perineal descent during defecation.[7] However, most defecography is performed in the supine position, which is not physiologic.

DIAGNOSTIC SUMMARY

This diagnostic evaluation of patients with constipation should lead to an assessment of 1 or more of the following categories[8]:

1. Normal colonic transit and defecation (some patients in this group have symptoms of IBS [eg, abdominal pain, bloating, and incomplete defecation])
2. Slow transit constipation when pelvic floor function is normal and there is evidence of slow colon transit time
3. Defecatory disorders (dyssynergia or descending perineal syndrome and other flaccid disorder)
4. Combination of 2 and 3 (some patients also have features of IBS)
5. Organic constipation
6. Opioid-induced constipation

TREATMENT

LIFESTYLE MODIFICATIONS

Fluid Intake

Although an increase in fluid intake is widely advised to improve symptoms of constipation, no convincing data or randomized controlled trials have shown that constipation can be treated by increasing fluid intake.

Increased physical activity is associated with less constipation. Mild physical activity increases intestinal gas clearance and reduces bloating, and moderate to vigorous physical activity (20 to 60 minutes 3 to 5 days/week) has been shown to improve symptoms of life and quality of life in patients with IBS.[25]

High-Fiber Diet

Fiber is a complex carbohydrate that is poorly digested and can bulk stools and draw water into the gut. Fiber accelerates colon transit, and most guidelines recommend a high-fiber diet for patients with constipation with an intake of 25 to 30 g or more per day.[26] Oral intake of soluble fiber such as pectins, gums, and polysaccharides, which are present in oat bran, nuts, beans, barley, and lentils, is recommended, as are psyllium fiber supplements.[27] Data on insoluble fibers, which are present in wheat bran and whole grain, are conflicting and may worsen symptoms in patients with IBS-C. Worsening of bloating and distention limits fiber intake. Diets low in fermentable oligosaccharides, disaccharides, monosaccharides, and polyols may be helpful in chronic constipation, but the evidence for IBS-C is poor.

PHARMACOLOGIC AGENTS

The major classes of drugs used in chronic constipation include laxatives (stimulant and osmotic), prosecretory agents, and serotonergic 5-hydroxytryptamine 4 (5-HT4) agonists. Peripherally acting mu-opioid receptor antagonists are used to treat OIC (Table 10-3). In patients who do not respond to lifestyle modifications, a systematic approach to treatment with laxatives, intestinal secretagogues, and, where applicable, the use of biofeedback therapy is indicated (Figure 10-2).

Table 10-3

Pharmacological Treatment of Constipation

DRUG	MECHANISM OF ACTION	ADVERSE EVENTS
Osmotic Laxatives		
Polyethylene glycol	Creation of an osmotic gradient draws water into the small intestine	Diarrhea and abdominal distention
Lactulose		Abdominal gas, bloating and cramping can occur and are dose-dependent
Poorly absorbed salts		Excessive use, particularly in patients with renal insufficiency or elderly patients, may lead to electrolyte disturbances
Stimulant Laxatives		
Anthraquinones	Stimulation of water and electrolyte secretion, intestinal motility and prostaglandin release by acting on the enteric nervous system	Diarrhea and abdominal pain are common
Bisacodyl		
Sodium picosulfate		
Prosecretory Agents		
Lubiprostone	Chloride channel protein 2 agonist	Nausea
Linaclotide	Guanylate cyclase-C receptor agonists, which increase intracellular cyclic guanosine monophosphate levels and promote chloride secretion through cystic fibrosis transmembrane conductance regulator	Diarrhea
Plecanatide		
Serotonergic Agents		
Prucalopride	5-hydroxytryptamine 4 receptor agonist	Headache, nausea, abdominal pain and diarrhea

Osmotic Laxatives

In patients who do not respond to lifestyle modifications, the first line of treatment is osmotic laxatives. These laxatives create an intraluminal osmotic gradient causing water and electrolyte secretion into the lumen, which leads to increased stool volume. Polyethylene glycol has shown improvement in chronic constipation compared with placebo in randomized controlled trials; it has also been shown to be superior to lactulose in head-to-head trials.[28]

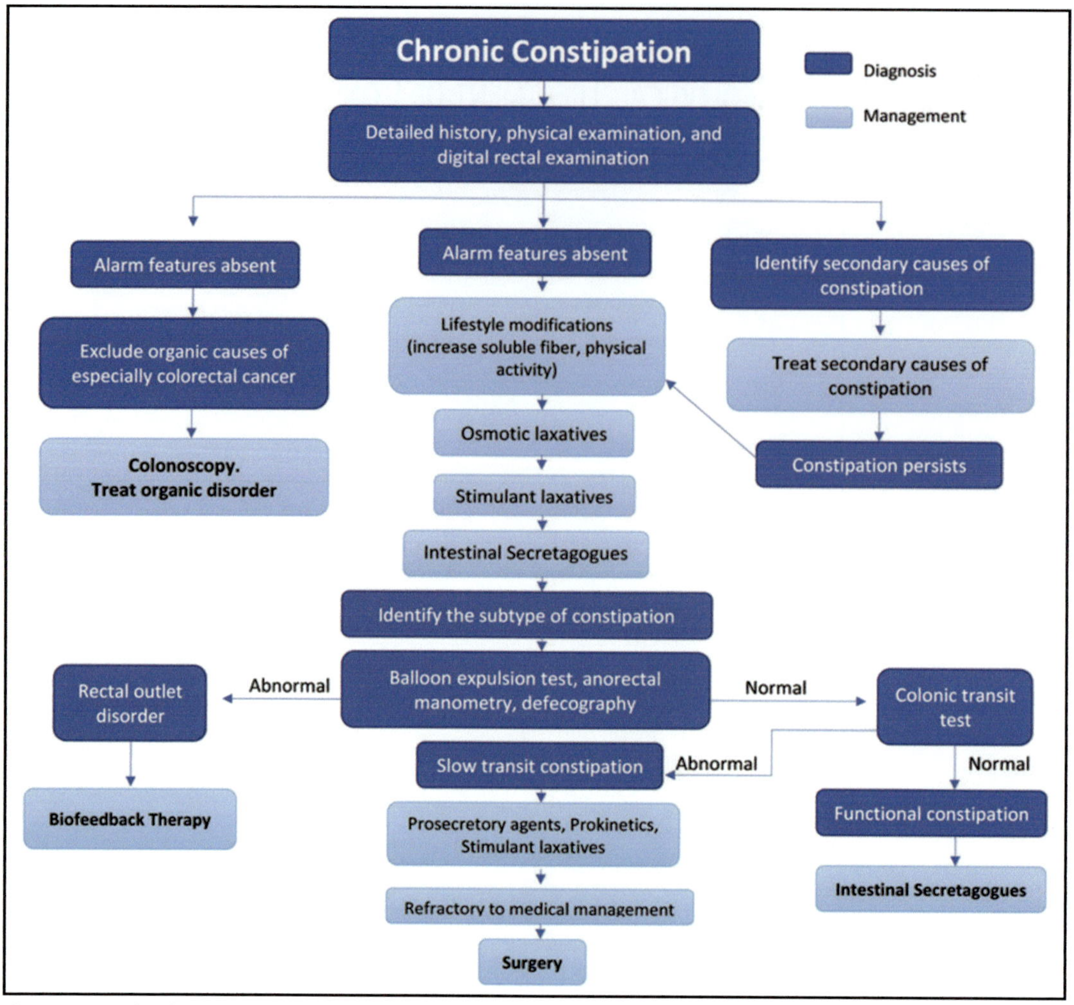

Figure 10-2. The diagnosis and management algorithm for chronic constipation. The algorithm is adapted based on data from studies by Rao et al[6] and Camilleri et al.[12]

Stimulant Laxatives

These laxatives are recommended when osmotic laxatives have not been effective in relieving symptoms of chronic constipation. Stimulant laxatives induce water and electrolyte secretion and stimulate intestinal motility, causing an increase in colonic transit time. Chronic use of stimulant laxatives does not lead to drug tolerance or rebound constipation on stopping the drug.

Prosecretory Agents

These are intestinal secretagogues that create a net efflux of ions and water into the intestinal lumen, which accelerates colon transit and also facilitates ease of defecation. These drugs (lubiprostone, linaclotide, and plecanatide) promote fluid secretion by direct action on the intestinal epithelial cells. Lubiprostone increases chloride secretion into the lumen of the gut, which is followed by sodium and water to maintain electrical neutrality. In a randomized controlled trial, 4-week treatment with lubiprostone increased stool frequency, reduced straining and bloating, and improved overall constipation symptoms compared with placebo.[29] The most common side effect is nausea.

Linaclotide and plecanatide are guanylate cyclase-C receptor agonists that increase cyclic guanosine monophosphate in the intestinal epithelial cells resulting in chloride and bicarbonate secretion into the intestinal lumen and acceleration of GI transit. In 2 randomized controlled trials, 12 weeks of linaclotide was better than placebo in increasing stool frequency and improving stool consistency and straining.[30] The efficacy of plecanatide is similar to that of linaclotide. The most common side effect for both is diarrhea, reported in 16% with linaclotide and 5.9% with plecanatide.

Serotonin Agonist

Prucalopride is a highly selective 5-HT4 receptor agonist that facilitates intestinal motility. It has been shown to accelerate GI and colonic transit in constipation.[31] Serotonin 5-HT4 receptors are extensively present on enteric neurons; 5-HT4 receptor agonists induce the release of neurotransmitters such as acetylcholine and induce mucosal secretion by activating submucosal neurons.

Several clinical trials have shown an improvement in stool frequency and straining with prucalopride compared with placebo.[32] The most common side effect is diarrhea. This drug is now available in the United States.

Opioid Receptor Antagonists

OIC is increasing in prevalence due to the increase in prescriptions for opioids. The Food and Drug Administration has approved peripherally acting mu-opioid receptor antagonists that can reverse the opioid effects peripherally without affecting the central analgesic effect. The initial step in treatment is discontinuing opioids if possible and then the use of peripherally acting mu-opioid receptor antagonists. Naloxegol is an oral agent that is effective in OIC in doses of 12.5 and 25 mg.[33,34] Methylnaltrexone is a naltrexone derivative available in oral and subcutaneous forms. Several trials have shown that oral and subcutaneous methylnaltrexone is effective in inducing the first bowel movement and improving stool frequency.

Anorectal Biofeedback Therapy

Pelvic floor retraining by biofeedback therapy is a valuable tool in the management of constipation due to defecatory disorders. Biofeedback is a behavioral training technique in which anorectal physiology is shown to the patient using visual clues of anorectal and pelvic floor muscle activity. The muscle activity is recorded by surface electromyographic sensors or manometry. Patients learn to coordinate abdominal and pelvic floor muscles during simulated defecation. They are taught to appropriately increase intra-abdominal pressure and relax the pelvic floor muscles during defecation. They practice by expelling an air-filled balloon. In patients with reduced rectal sensation, sensory retraining, in which patients learn to recognize weaker sensations of rectal filling, can also be taught. Controlled studies have shown that biofeedback is more effective than sham feedback or diazepam treatment. Most biofeedback sessions are 30 to 60 minutes every 2 weeks.[34-37] The length of training is variable and may involve 5 to 6 sessions. Overall, 70% of patients will respond to biofeedback therapy.

Surgery

Surgery for chronic constipation is rarely indicated. Only patients with intractable slow transit constipation who have failed medical therapy may be appropriate candidates. Secondary causes of constipation should be treated or excluded. Surgery is not recommended for patients with pelvic floor dysfunction or IBS-C.[38] For combined dyssynergic disorders and slow transit constipation, pelvic floor dysfunction should be corrected before consideration of surgery.[8] Delayed transit in both the small and large bowel may occur as a consequence of a primary delayed transit in the colon or diffuse GI dysmotility. Patients with diffuse GI dysmotility disorders have poorer outcomes than those with isolated slow transit constipation.

Patients with slow transit constipation may benefit from total colectomy. The recommended surgery is total colectomy with iliorectal anastomosis.[39-41] This can almost always be performed laparoscopically. In patients with severe uncorrected pelvic floor dysfunction, the only surgery that may relieve symptoms is an ileostomy. Surgery may also be done to repair a rectocele or rectal intussusception. The selection of surgical candidates by strict criteria results in good surgical outcomes. In a study of 74 patients who underwent colectomy with iliorectal anastomosis, 97% reported improved quality of life.[40]

References

1. Suares NC, Ford AC. Prevalence of and risk factors for, chronic idiopathic constipation in the community: systematic review and meta-analysis. *Am J Gastroenterol.* 2011;106(9):1582-1591.
2. Mugie SM, Benninga MA, Di Lorenzo C. Epidemiology of constipation in children and adults: a systemic review. *Bet Pract Res Clin Gastroenterol.* 2011;25(1):3-18.
3. Rao SS. Constipation: evaluation and treatment of colonic and anorectal motility disorders. *Gastrointest Endosc Clin N Am.* 2009;19(1):117-139.
4. Rao SS, Seaton K, Miller MJ, et al. Psychological profiles and quantity of life differ between patients with dyssynergia and those with slow transit constipation. *J Psychom Res.* 2007;63(4):441-449.
5. Burgell RE, Lelic D, Carrington EV, et al. Assessment of rectal afferent neuronal function and brain activity in patients with constipation and rectal hypersensitivity. *Neurogastroenterol Motil.* 2013;25(3):260-267.
6. Rao SS, Rattanakovit K, Patcharatatrakul T. Diagnosis and management of chronic constipation in adults. *Nat Rev Gastroenterol Hepatol.* 2016;13(5):295-305.
7. Bharucha AE, Wald A, Enck P, et al. Functional anorectal disorders. *Gastroenterology.* 2006;130(5):1510-1518.
8. Bharucha AE, Pemberton JH, Locke GR III. American Gastroenterology Association technical review on constipation. *Gastroenterology.* 2013;144(1):218-238.
9. Drossman DA. Functional gastrointestinal disorders: history, pathophysiology, clinical features of Rome IV. *Gastroenterology.* 2016;150(12):1262-1279.
10. Spiller R, Lam C. An update on post-infectious irritable bowel syndrome: role of genetics, immune activation, serotonin and altered microbiome. *J Neurogastroenterol Motil.* 2012;18(3):258-268.
11. Ravi K, Bharucha AE, Camilleri M, et al. Phenotypic variation of colonic motor functions in chronic constipation. *Gastroenterology.* 2010;138(1):89-97.
12. Camilleri M, Ford AC, Mawe GM, et al. Chronic constipation. *Nat Rev Dis Primers.* 2017;3:17095.
13. Rao SS, Leelasinjaroan P, Amieva-Aalmori M, et al. Characterization of dyssenergia phenotypes with high resolution anorectal manometry (HRAM). *Gastroenterology.* 2016;150(4):S158-S159.
14. Saad RJ, Rao SSC, Koch KL, et al. Do stool form and frequency correlate with whole-gut and colonic transit? Results from a multicenter study in constipated individuals and healthy controls. *Am J Gastroenterol.* 2010;105(2):403-411.
15. Ashraf W, Park F, Lof J, et al. An examination of the reliability of reported stool frequency in the diagnosis of idiopathic constipation. *Am J Gastroenterol.* 1996;91(1):26-32.
16. Tantiphlachiva K, Rao P, Attaluri A, et al. Digital rectal examination is a useful tool for identifying patients with dyssynergia. *Clin Gastroenterol Hepatol.* 2010;8(11):955-960.
17. Rao SS, Hatfield R, Soffer E, et al. Manometric tests of anorectal function in healthy adults. *Am J Gastroenterol.* 1999;94(3):773-783.
18. Minguez M, Herreros B, Sanchiz V, et al. Predictive value of the balloon expulsion test for excluding the diagnosis of pelvic floor dyssynergia in constipation. *Gastroenterology.* 2004;126(1):57-62.
19. Faubion SS, Shuster LT, Bharucha AE. Recognition and management of nonrelaxing pelvic floor dysfunction. *Mayo Clin Proc.* 2012;87(2):187-193.
20. Jones MP, Post J, Crowell MD. High-resolution manometry in the evaluation of anorectal disorders: a simultaneous comparison with water-perfused manometry. *Am J Gastroenterol.* 2007;102(4):850-855.
21. Camilleri M, Bharucha AE, di Lorenzo C, et al. American Neurogastroenterology and Motility Society Consensus statement on intraluminal measurement of gastrointestinal and colonic motility in clinical practice. *Neurogastroenterol Motil.* 2008;20(12):1269-1282.
22. Hinton JM, Lennard-Jones JE, Young AC. A new method for studying gut transit times using radiopaque markers. *Gut.* 1969;10(10):842-847.
23. Rao SS, Kuo B, McCallum RW, et al. Investigation of colonic and whole gut transit with wireless motility capsule and radiopaque markers in constipation. *Clin Gastroenterol Hepatol.* 2009;7(5):537-544.

24. Kao B, Maneerattanaporn M, Lee AA, et al. Generalized transit delay on wireless motility capsule testing in patients with clinical suspicion of gastroparesis, small intestinal dysmotility or STC. *Dig Dis Sci.* 2011;56(10):2928-2938.
25. Johannesson E, Simren M, Strid H, Bajor A, Sadik R. Physical activity improves symptoms in irritable bowel syndrome: a randomized controlled trial. *Am J Gastroenterol.* 2011;106(5):915-922.
26. Suares NC, Ford AC. Systematic review: the effects of fibre in the management of chronic idiopathic constipation. *Aliment Pharmacol Ther.* 2011;33(8):895-901.
27. Ford AC, Moyyedi P, Lacy BE, et al. American College of Gastroenterology monograph on the management of IBS and chronic idiopathic constipation. *Am J Gastroenterol.* 2014;109(suppl 1):S2-S26.
28. Dipalma J, Cleveland MV, McGowan J, Herrera JL. A randomized multicenter placebo controlled trial of polyethylene glycol laxative for chronic treatment of chronic constipation. *Am J Gastroenterol.* 2007;102:1436-1441.
29. Johnson JF, Morton D, Geenen J, Ueno R. Multicenter 4 week double blind randomized placebo controlled trial of lubiprostone, a locally acting type 2 chloride channel activator, in patients with chronic constipation. *Am J Gastroenterol.* 2008;103(1):170-177.
30. Lembo AJ, Schneier HA, Shiff SJ, et al. Two randomized trials of linaclotide for chronic constipation. *N Engl J Med.* 2011;365(6):527-536.
31. Ford A, Suares N. Effect of laxatives and pharmacological therapies in chronic idiopathic constipation: systematic review and meta-analysis. *Gut.* 2011(2);60:209-218.
32. Quigley EM, Vandeplassche L, Kerstens R, Ausma J. Clinical trial: the efficacy, impact on quality of life, and safety and tolerability of prucalopride in severe chronic constipation—a 12-week, randomized, double-blind, placebo-controlled study. *Aliment Pharmacol Ther.* 2009;29(3):315-328.
33. Chey WD, Webster L, Sostek M, Lappalainen J, Barker PN, Tack J. Naloxegol for opioid-induced constipation in patients with non-cancer pain. *N Engl J Med.* 2014;370(25):2387-2396.
34. Chiarioni G, Salandini L, Whitehead WE. Biofeedback benefits only patients with outlet dysfunction, not patients with isolated slow transit constipation. *Gastroenterology.* 2005;129(1):86-97.
35. Chiarioni G, Whitehead WE, Pezza V, Morelli A, Bassotti G. Biofeedback is superior to laxatives for normal transit constipation due to pelvic floor dyssynergia. *Gastroenterology.* 2006;130(3):657-664.
36. Rao SS, Seaton K, Miller M, et al. Randomized controlled trial of biofeedback, sham feedback, and standard therapy for dyssynergic defecation. *Clin Gastroenterol Hepatol.* 2007;5(3):331-338.
37. Heymen S, Scarlett Y, Jones K, Ringel Y, Drossman D, Whitehead WE. Randomized, controlled trial shows biofeedback to be superior to alternative treatments for patients with pelvic floor dyssynergia-type constipation. *Dis Colon Rectum.* 2007;50(4):428-441.
38. Pemberton JH, Rath DM, Ilstrup DM. Evaluation and surgical treatment of severe chronic constipation. *Ann Surg.* 1991;214(4):403-411.
39. Pinedo G, Zarate AJ, Garcia E, Molina ME, Lopez F, Zúñiga A. Laparoscopic total colectomy for colonic inertia: surgical and functional results. *Surg Endosc.* 2009;23(1):62-65.
40. Nyam DC, Pemberton JH, Ilstrup DM, Rath DM. Long-term results of surgery for chronic constipation. *Dis Colon Rectum.* 1997;40(3):273-279.
41. Hassan I, Pemberton JH, Young-Fadok TM, et al. Ileorectal anastomosis for slow transit constipation: long-term functional and quality of life results. *J Gastrointest Surg.* 2006;10(10):1330-1336.

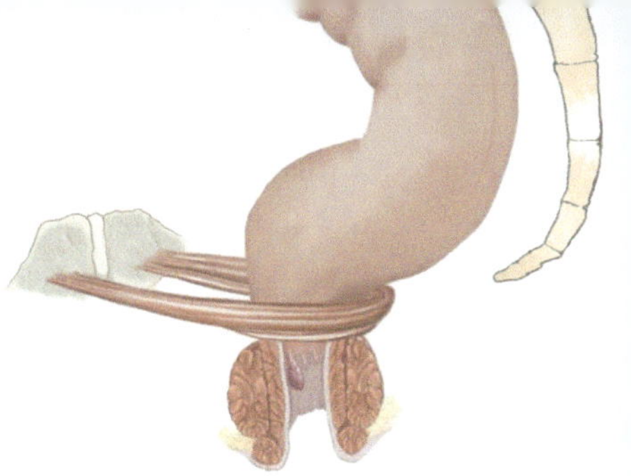

Section 3

Benign Soft Tissue, Perianal, Perineal, and Complicated Conditions

11

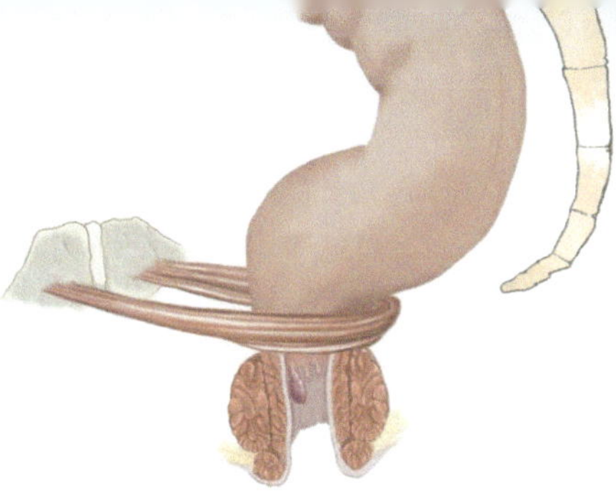

Pruritus Ani

Andy Tau, MD and Waqar Qureshi, MD, FRCP, FACP, FACG, FASGE

Key Points

- Ask about diabetes, corticosteroids, and sexually transmitted disease risk factors (anal sex). Perform a careful perianal examination with anoscopy and a perianal swab. Perform a "tape test" if the patient has symptomatic kids in the household.
- Ask about the consistency and frequency of stool and incontinence. Ask about the sensation of prolapse.
- Soaps, perfumes, and moisturizers can often exacerbate symptoms. Instruct the patient to stop using them.
- Careful physical examination, digital rectal examination, and anoscopy are invaluable. If a prolapsing rectal mass is suspected, flexible sigmoidoscopy or colonoscopy is mandatory.
- Psoriasis is the most common dermatologic cause of pruritus ani. Dermatology consultation and biopsy are invaluable.
- Paget's and Bowen's disease are very rare, whereas squamous cell carcinoma, melanoma, and rectal neoplasia are rarely going to present as pruritus ani alone. However, these diagnoses can never be missed and must be ruled out first. They should be found on examination.
- Ask about food associations, in particular coffee intake. Keep in mind that triggers will differ from one patient to another.
- Take a careful history of both oral and topical anal medications. Remember colchicine and quinidine are particularly notable. In those recently or currently hospitalized, high-dose intravenous steroids can produce a rebound itch phenomenon.

Qureshi W, ed. *Diagnosis and Management Guide for Anorectal Disease: A Clinical Reference* (pp 123-133).

- Just before one makes a diagnosis of the exclusion of idiopathic pruritus ani, screen for systemic illnesses, which can rarely cause anal itching.
- You will most likely secure the diagnosis on history alone. A systemic query using the "ITCHeS" mnemonic is easiest.
- Pay particular attention for hemorrhoids, fissures, skin lesions around the anus, and palpable masses during digital rectal examination. If hemorrhoids are present and suspected to be the cause, treat them in the same visit using office-based therapy if available.
- Topical therapies can be started empirically at the initial visit with 1% hydrocortisone 3 times/day. Avoid prolonged therapy or higher potency steroids.
- Office-based injectable therapy with methylene blue is effective for chronic refractory cases.

Pruritus ani is defined as unpleasant perianal itching or a burning sensation.[1] The prevalence in the general population is up to 5%[2] and is commonly encountered by general practitioners and specialists alike. Despite this, pruritus ani is arguably a neglected anorectal disease given its perception as a benign condition of poor hygiene. However, pruritus ani can seriously affect the quality of life of patients and can be caused by serious underlying etiologies like infection, systemic diseases, or neoplasia. Determining the etiology of pruritus ani demands systematic history taking, careful physical examination, and a broader differential diagnosis than most other anorectal pathologies.

Pathophysiology

The sensation of itching is mediated by superficial pain fibers, which are stimulated at a lower threshold than pain fibers (tickling and fibers of wool). Histamine, kallikrein, papain, bradykinin, and trypsin can produce itching in experimental models.[3] A cutaneous injury from scratching produces a transient but inadequate negative feedback to the pain fibers that mediate itching. However, the itching soon returns, and the enlarging area of the cutaneous injury triggers more pruritus. Further scratching enlarges the area of the cutaneous injury without durable relief, and an itch-scratch cycle maddeningly continues. Other stimuli like heat, cold, and pain/stinging (eg, alcohol or pepper extract) can produce more durable inhibitory feedback of itching relative to scratching.[4] To break the itch-scratch cycle requires identifying and eliminating the underlying etiology or severing a critical mediator from the itch-scratch cycle. Perianal skin appears to be more sensitive to itching than other parts of the body.[5]

Etiology

Pruritus ani is classified as either primary (idiopathic) or secondary to an underlying disease process. After a thorough history and physical examination, if no other etiologies can be found, this condition is classified as idiopathic pruritus ani. Idiopathic pruritus ani accounts for 50% to 90% of all cases of pruritus.[6] The differential diagnosis of pruritus ani is quite daunting (Table 11-1).[7,8] In the following sections, etiologies that were specifically reviewed based on both prevalence and clinical pertinence are discussed. At the end of each subsection, a note is made about what questions to ask during history taking, physical examination findings, and practical tests to order during the evaluation.

Table 11-1

Causes of Pruritis Ani: ITCHeS

INFECTION	
Fungal	Candidiasis, dermatophytes (*Tinea cruris*)
Parasitic	Oxyuris (pinworm), amebiasis cutis, cimicosis (bed bugs), trichomoniasis, schistosomiasis cutis, scabies, pediculosis (lice), larva currens, larva migrans
Viral	Molluscum contagiosum, herpes zoster, cytomegalovirus
Bacterial	*Staphylococcus aureus*, beta-hemolytic *Streptococcus*, pilonidal disease/abscess, tuberculosis
Sexually Transmitted Infections	Gonorrhea, syphilis, chancroid, granuloma inguinale, lymphogranuloma venereum, molluscum contagiosum, herpes simplex virus, condyloma acuminatum
TOPICAL IRRITANTS	Fecal contamination (poor hygiene, diarrhea, incontinence) Contact dermatitis—chemical in toilet paper, perfumes, wet wipes, alcohol, witch hazel, topical anesthetics
CONCOMITANT ANORECTAL DISEASE	Hemorrhoids, fistula, fissure, tags, prolapsing anal papilla, surgical scars, radiation dermatitis/proctitis
CUTANEOUS DISEASE (DERMATOSES)	Psoriasis, seborrheic dermatitis, atopic dermatitis, lichen sclerosis, lichen planus, lichen simplex
CANCER/ NEOPLASIA	Bowen's disease (anal intraepithelial neoplasia), Paget's disease, squamous call carcinoma variants, villous adenomas (diarrhea), prolapsing rectal neoplasia
HYPER-SENSITIVITY	Food—coffee, chocolate, cola, milk, peanuts, tomato, and citrus Medications—colchicine, quinidine, high dose steroids (IV)
SYSTEMIC ILLNESS	Cholestatic liver disease, diabetes, chronic renal failure (uremia), iron deficiency, thyroid disease, leukemia/lymphoma, polycythemia vera

The "ITCHeS" mnemonic can be used to remember the most common causes of pruritus ani.[9]

- I: Infection
- T: Topical irritants (fecal, soaps, wipes, ointments, and perfumes)
- C: Concomitant anorectal pathology, Cutaneous disorders, Cancer
- H: Hypersensitivity (food/medications)
- S: Systemic illnesses

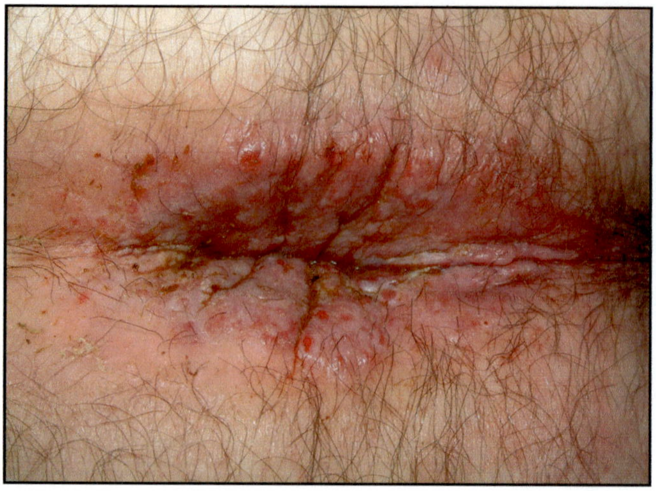

Figure 11-1. Fungal infection with *Candida* as cause of the pruritus. (Reprinted with permission from Marcus Aquino, MD, FACS, FASCRS.)

INFECTION

Although perianal infections (fungal, bacterial, and viral) in children are the first to be considered, infections account for a minority of pruritus ani in adults. Nevertheless, they are often the simplest to cure.

Fungal infections are attributable to pruritus ani in up to 15% of cases in 2 large series of 47 and 200 patients.[10,11] Figure 11-1 shows a case of perianal candidiasis. In contrast, in the series by Smith et al., none of the 75 patients, all of whom had scrapings and fungal culture, were found to have fungal infection as the cause of their perianal itching.[12] Specifically, *Candida albicans* appears to have no association with pruritus ani, being cultured equally in those with and without pruritus ani.[13] In this study, 35% of patients were culture positive for *C. albicans*, which was equally prevalent in those with pruritus ani (26%) and in those without (28%). In populations who are taking steroids or who have diabetes, *C. albicans* can be pathogenic secondary to an attenuated immune response. Dermatophytes, while accounting for only 1% to 2% of anal pruritus cases, are consistently pruritic when culture positive, suggesting reliable pathogenicity. In a series of 200 patients with pruritus ani, 28 (14%) had a fungal infection, 1 was diabetic, 14 were on corticosteroids, and 6 were on antibiotics.[14]

Viral infections appear to have no role in pruritus ani directly. Indirectly, condylomata acuminata and anal intraepithelial neoplasia, which are caused by human papillomavirus, can present with pruritus. Likewise, molluscum contagiosum (poxvirus) can cause itching in the perianal area, identifiable as small clusters of papillary lesions with central umbilication. All of these perianal lesions are likely causing pruritus indirectly by contributing to fecal seepage and hindering proper hygiene. Herpes simplex virus infections typically are painful with vesicular eruptions and do not itch.

Bacterial infections can also be a form of pruritus ani. In particular, sexually transmitted diseases (chlamydia and gonorrhea), when symptomatic, tend to occur acutely at the onset of the infection and are reliably diagnosed on perianal swab samples. Non–sexually transmitted bacterial infections like staphylococcus, beta-hemolytic streptococcus, and erythrasma (*Corynebacterium minutissimum*) can cause chronic itching. In particular, erythrasma was found by Wood's light fluorescence in 15 of 81 patients (18%) who failed routine therapy[14] and in 32 of 200 patients (16%) in a larger series.[11] In the latter series, over one-quarter of the patients infected were symptomatic for over 5 years. Intertriginous areas (skinfolds) of the thighs, toes, and groin were commonly involved, and erythromycin rapidly resolved all *C. minutissimum* infections.

Pinworm infections (*Enterobius vermicularis*) are the most common cause of pruritus in children[15] and must be at the top of the differential diagnosis in adults with symptomatic children because pinworms can rapidly spread to infect whole families. Adult pinworms emerge from the anus at night to lay eggs, which causes an inflammatory process, triggering an itch-scratch cycle. Scratching colonizes the space under the fingernails and mobilizes the infection to other hosts. The "tape test" of the perianal area is administered 3 times consecutively at night and remains the most reliable method of diagnosis.

FECAL CONTAMINATION

Fecal contamination is a well-described cause of perianal itching and can routinely be treated at home by the patient before seeking medical consultation. Caplan[5] studied 27 patients with and without prior pruritus ani using autologous stool patch testing on the inner arm and in the perianal area. In total, 12 of the 27 (44%) developed pruritus ani, whereas 0 of the 10 control patients who received sham patches developed itching. In the subgroup analysis, one-third of those with prior pruritus ani developed recurrent itching, whereas over one-half of those without prior pruritus developed incident itching. Only 4% of patients had itching on their forearm patch. Rapid onset (within 6 hours) and the relief of symptoms with washing suggest an irritant rather than an allergic effect.[5]

In a study of 75 patients with pruritus ani, 50% had reported loose stools and at least daily soiling in 41%.[12] Other studies have demonstrated that stool leakage (as tested by saline infusion) occurs sooner in patients with pruritus ani[16] and that patients with pruritus ani have a more pronounced anal inhibitory reflex (ie, more prominent reduction in the anal sphincter tone with rectal distention).[17,18]

If the history suggests soiling or seepage, then the next step is to immediately refocus the differential diagnosis to fecal incontinence, which includes postsurgical incontinence, diarrheal illness, or anorectal pathology like prolapsing hemorrhoids or mass lesions.

Moisture and heat exacerbate underlying itching. Although no clothing is specifically known to cause pruritus ani, cotton or other moisture-wicking fabrics are routinely recommended, in particular for those with seasonal or warm weather symptoms.

ALLERGIC CONTACT DERMATITIS

Allergic contact dermatitis may be distinguished from irritant dermatitis (moisture/stool) by the presence of eczematous inflammation with redness, scaling, and erupting vesicles. Given the location of pruritus ani, rarely are the typical culprits like latex or nickel involved. More commonly, they are iatrogenic and include topical anesthetics, antibiotics, soaps, detergents, perfumes, and dyes. In a large study using patch testing, 55 of 80 patients (69%) tested positive. Among these, 38 of 55 tested positive to medications or the fragrance mixed into the ointments.[19] Common chemicals found in cleansers, wet wipes, or moisturizing creams, such as lanolin, neomycin, anesthetics (procaine), and parabens, have all been described as causing a sensitization reaction. Many of these agents are combined in steroid preparations, which may initially mask the inflammation (steroid effect) but, subsequently and paradoxically, with more broad use, increase the affected area. Ointments have fewer preservatives than creams and are less likely to sensitize.

CONCOMITANT ANORECTAL PATHOLOGY

Coexisting anal conditions commonly produce itch or worsen itching. Nearly one-half of the pruritus ani cases are attributable to concomitant anorectal pathology,[20,21] including hemorrhoids (most common), fissure, fistula, abscess, condyloma, and ulcerative proctitis. All of these causes can be visualized, underscoring the importance of a careful perianal examination. Hemorrhoids slide in and out of the anus, shuttling stool onto the anoderm, whereas fissures and fistulas leak stool. All 3 perianal entities produce pruritus by chronic fecal soiling. Hemorrhoids were found to be the sole cause or attributable to pruritus ani in one-quarter (43/200) of patients with pruritus ani.[14] In a study of 82 patients with hemorrhoids, pruritus was more common in age- and sex-matched cohorts with

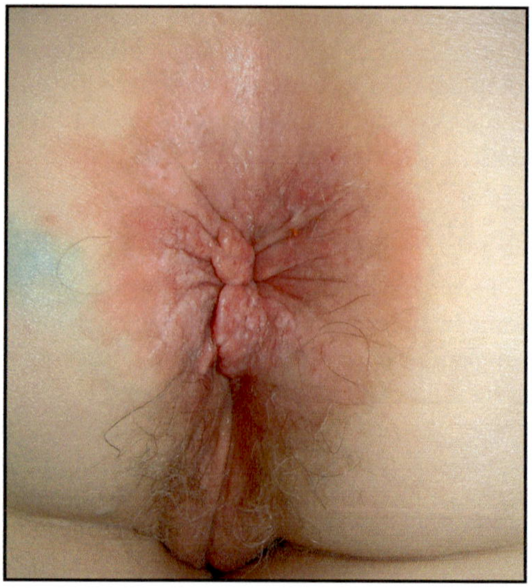

Figure 11-2. Paget's disease diagnosed following complaints of anal pruritus. (Reprinted with permission from Marcus Aquino, MD, FACS, FASCRS.)

hemorrhoids than without, and the correction of hemorrhoids using rubber band ligation improved or eliminated itching.[22] Indirect evidence has suggested that correcting anorectal pathology reduces fecal soiling by eliminating the presence (culture) of *Candida* and dermatophytes in over 85% of cases in a surgical series.[23] Unfortunately, anorectal surgery itself via postsurgical scarring can cause persistent pruritus. However, more immediate postsurgical wound healing produces an itch that responds well to antihistamine creams and is overall short lived.[4]

CUTANEOUS CONDITIONS (DERMATOSES)

Psoriasis is the most common dermatologic etiology of pruritus ani. It can be found as an isolated entity on perianal skin[24] and is a significant etiology of pruritus ani in several series. In a prospective series of 40 patients referred to a colorectal dermatology clinic, 22 (45%) were found to have psoriasis.[25] In larger series in nonspecialty clinics, 5.5% to 8% of patients were found to have psoriasis as a cause of itching.[12,14] In 82 patients diagnosed with psoriatic perianal lesions, treatment with fluocinolone acetonide 0.025% successfully resolved all the of lesions and the itching.[26] The typical appearance of psoriasis is often not present due to maceration/moisture. Concomitant psoriasis should be sought elsewhere, particularly in the extensor surfaces of the forearms, elbows, knees, base of scalp, ear canals, eyelids, navel, and external genitalia.

Lichen sclerosis, while most commonly involving the vulva in women and the penis in men, can also affect the perianal area. The lesion appears pale, wrinkled, and atrophic. Diagnosis is easily confirmed on biopsy, and high-dose topical corticosteroids are effective. Importantly, refractory cases must be biopsied because concomitant squamous cell carcinoma is found in 5% of cases.[27]

CANCER/NEOPLASIA

Perianal Paget's disease can present with chronic anal itching.[28] Figure 11-2 is a case of Paget's disease. Likewise, perianal Bowen's disease (intraepithelial squamous cell carcinoma in situ), while rare, presented with pruritus ani in 60% of patients in one series.[29] Squamous cell carcinoma (Figures 11-3 and 11-4) and melanoma most commonly present with bleeding and pain rather than pruritus.[30-32] However, any tumor that prolapses out of the anus, like a distal rectal neoplasia, can produce chronic fecal soiling and itching.[21] In one series, one-quarter of the local causes of pruritus ani were due to anal or rectal neoplasm.[2] As such, in any adult over 50 years of age with chronic idiopathic pruritus, colonoscopy is recommended.

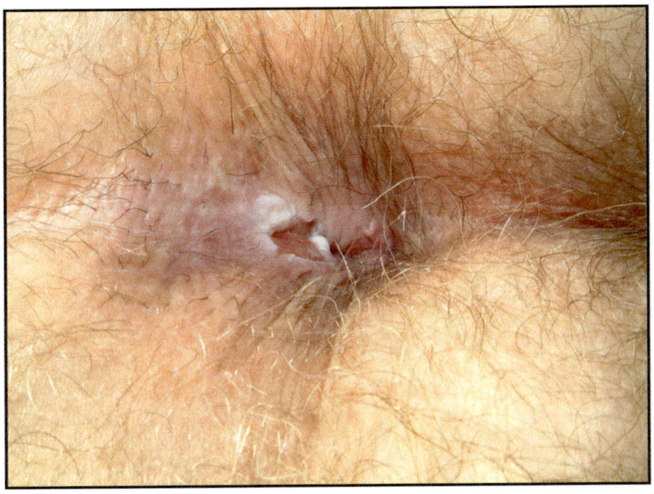

Figure 11-3. Case of squamous cell anal cancer presenting with pruritus. (Reprinted with permission from Marcus Aquino, MD, FACS, FASCRS.)

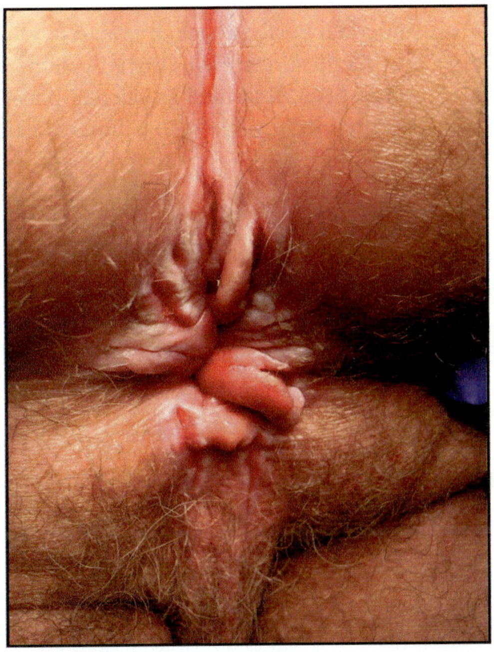

Figure 11-4. Case of squamous cell anal cancer presenting with pruritus. (Reprinted with permission from Marcus Aquino, MD, FACS, FASCRS.)

FOODS

Although no controlled trials have proven any food factors to be directly related to pruritus ani, certain foods have been reported to trigger or exacerbate pruritus ani. These dietary triggers include coffee, chocolate, cola, milk, peanuts, tomatoes, and citrus, which have been implicated in studies using an elimination diet.[4,5,7,10,21] The pathophysiology of each food implicated is not known. Notably, coffee intake was demonstrated to lower anal pressures and to be associated with poorly formed stools.[12] In one study, the average coffee intake in those with idiopathic pruritus ani appeared to be around 6 cups/day vs 3.5 cups/day in patients with secondary pruritus ani.[21]

MEDICATIONS

Prolonged topical steroid use can thin the perianal skin and contact dermatitis from sensitization. In addition to topical steroids, well-described itching occurs as a rebound phenomenon upon

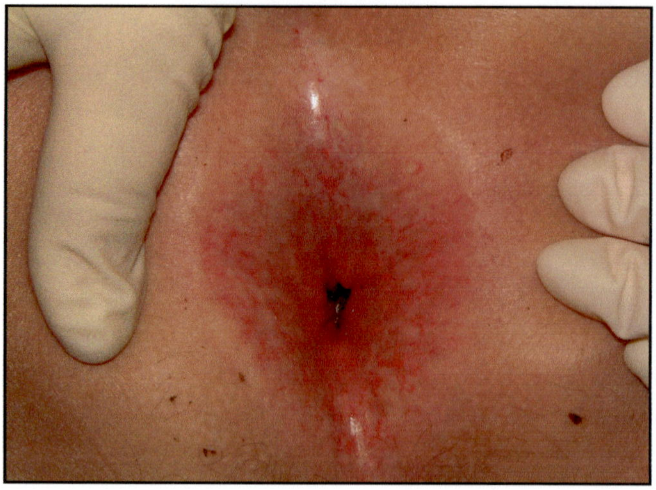

Figure 11-5. Severe radiation proctitis causing anal pruritus. (Reprinted with permission from Marcus Aquino, MD, FACS, FASCRS.)

discontinuing systemic (intravenous) corticosteroids. This is remedied by a gradual taper and complete discontinuation of steroids over several weeks. Other oral medications including colchicine, quinidine, peppermint oil, and other laxatives and antibiotics have been described as causing perianal itch.[33,34] The mechanism is either a combination of contact irritation or simply loosening stools.

SYSTEMIC DISEASE

Systemic diseases like hepatobiliary disease (particularly cholestatic jaundice), leukemia, myeloma, uremia, and iron deficiency can cause generalized itching, including perianal itching. If none of these obvious causes are clearly identified, screening with an iron profile, ferritin, liver function tests, creatinine, and a complete blood count is a reasonable next step to identify a systemic cause of anal itching.[35]

History and Physical Examination

HISTORY

A detailed history is the most important first step in diagnosing the cause of pruritus ani. The majority of causes can be detected on history itself, including infection, topical irritants, hypersensitivity, and many systemic illnesses ("I-T-H-S" from the ITCHeS mnemonic). The "C's" and a few infections require a physical examination and further testing (see Table 11-1).

First, it is important to query patients about anal seepage, diarrhea (frequency and consistency), and incontinence. Ask about hygiene habits (wipes, perfumes, creams/ointments, and soaps) and trauma. Then ask about oral and topical medications, risk factors for sexually transmitted infections (anal sex), diabetes/immunosuppressed (candidiasis), and other systemic illnesses. In some cases, radiation proctitis may be responsible for the pruritus (Figure 11-5).

PHYSICAL EXAMINATION

The physical examination during the initial visit should focus carefully on concomitant anorectal pathology (prolapsing internal hemorrhoids) and cancerous and cutaneous lesions of the anoderm. The examination should include 3 components: inspection, digital rectal examination (palpation and tone), and, ideally, anoscopy. If an infection or dermatosis is seen and suspected (especially if risk factors are present), a culture, biopsy, and consultation with a dermatologist are recommended. Patients over 50 years of age or those with diarrhea, bleeding, or any palpable mass are all indications for a full colonoscopy.

Treatment

Perianal Hygiene

All patients regardless of etiology should be counseled on proper hygiene and avoidance of potential food/fluid triggers. Both potential topical irritants and foods/fluids that cause loose stools should be avoided. Proper hygiene involves minimizing moisture and excessive trauma and avoiding perfumes, soaps, and excessive traumatic cleansing. Patients should wear breathable cotton undergarments and use a thin piece of cotton tissue left in place during the day. After cleansing, the patient can air-dry with a hair dryer on a cool setting to avoid trauma. During the initial visit, one should begin increasing fiber intake (balanced with fluid intake) to achieve regular-formed bowel movements.

If no obvious secondary cause of pruritus ani is found and proper hygiene is undertaken, then idiopathic pruritus is the diagnosis of exclusion, and empiric treatment should begin for idiopathic pruritus ani beginning with topical and then injectable therapies.

Topical Therapies

The use of a weak topical steroid like 1% hydrocortisone cream 3 times/day for 14 days is reasonable during the first visit to break the itch-scratch cycle. In a randomized, placebo-controlled trial, 1% hydrocortisone for 2 weeks showed a 68% reduction in the visual analog scale and a 75% reduction in Dermatology Life Quality Index scores favoring 1% hydrocortisone therapy.[36] However, prolonged or potent steroid use can thin the anoderm and worsen pruritus paradoxically.[20]

Topical capsaicin is theorized to reduce pruritus by inhibiting the release or effects of substance P, a neuropeptide that triggers burning and itching.[37] Capsaicin (0.006%) has also been studied in a randomized, placebo-controlled trial in patients with chronic pruritus ani (>3 months). Among 44 patients, 31 (70%) had relief of their itching, with 4 patients withdrawing because of the side effects. At least a once daily application appeared to be required in order to provide durable symptom relief.[37]

Anorectal Injection/Tattoo

Intradermal injection or tattoo with methylene blue has demonstrated effectiveness for the treatment of intractable pruritus ani. The mechanism is theorized to be the destruction of subcutaneous nerve endings.[20]

In one series,[38] under intravenous sedation, 30 to 40 mL 0.025% bupivacaine and 1:200,000 epinephrine plus an equal volume of lidocaine were injected into the subcutaneous anoderm and intracutaneous perianal tissue (total = 60 to 80 mL). They then injected 30 mL 0.05% methylene blue with a 22- to 25-gauge needle. The majority of the patients (21/23) in the series had either short- or long-term relief; however, 3 patients developed skin necrosis related to large volumes in the subcutaneous tissue.[38]

In another series,[39] office-based injections were performed without sedation using 7 to 8 mL 2% methylene blue mixed with equal volumes of 0.5% lidocaine via a 22-gauge needle (total = 10 to 15 mL). The needle targeted the dermoepidermal junction. Among 30 patients, 80% were symptom-free by 1 month. The total response rate was 93.3% if a rescue injection was allowed at 1 month if only a partial response was achieved. No major complications (including necrosis) were reported. The outcome was durable, with 77% of patients maintaining a complete response at the 1-year follow-up.[39] The improved results and better safety profile relative to the first study are attributed to less volume and less superficial injection. This is the preferred modality in current practice.

Conclusion

Pruritus ani is easily the most ignored component of perianal disease. One author described anal itching as the "least researched everyday symptom from which humans suffer".[40] However, rational diagnosis and treatment of pruritus ani demand a notably larger fund of knowledge than other anorectal conditions. The differential diagnosis is broad for these "ITCHeS." Proper hygiene and avoiding topical and dietary irritants are key followed by a systematic search for secondary causes, including infection, concomitant anorectal pathology, cutaneous cancer, and systemic diseases. Effective topical and injectable modalities are available for the remaining idiopathic cases.

References

1. Billingham RP, Isler JT, Kimmins MH, et al. The diagnosis and management of common anorectal disorders. *Curr Probl Surg.* 2004;33(7):586-645.
2. Zuccati G, Lotti T, Mastrolorenzo A, et al. Pruritus ani. *Dermatol Ther.* 2005;18(4): 355-362.
3. Davidson S, Zhang X, Yoon CH, Khasabov SG, Simone DA, Giesler Jr GJ. The itch-producing agents histamine and cowhage activate separate populations of primate spinothalamic tract neurons. *J Neurosci.* 2007;27:10007-10014.
4. Bernhard JD. *Itch: Mechanisms and Management of Pruritus.* New York: McGraw-Hill; 1994.
5. Caplan RM. The irritant role of feces in the genesis of perianal itch. *Gastroenterology.* 1966;50:19-23.
6. Metcalf A. Anorectal disorders. Five common causes of pain, itching and bleeding. *Postgrad Med.* 1995;98(5):81-84, 87-89, 92-94.
7. Corman ML. *Colon and rectal surgery.* 2nd ed. Philadelphia, PA: Lippincott; 1989:287.
8. Stamos MJ, Hicks TC. Pruritus ani: diagnosis and treatment. In: *Perspectives in Colon and Rectal Surgery.* 1998;11(1):1-20. Thieme Medical Publishers.
9. Henderson PK, Cash BD. Common anorectal conditions: evaluation and treatment. *Curr Gastroenterol Rep.* 2014;16:408.
10. Verbov J. Pruritus ani and its management—a study and reappraisal. *Clinical and Experimental Dermatology.* 1984;9:46-52.
11. Weismann K, Sand Petersen C, Roder B. Pruritus ani caused by beta-haemolytic streptococci. *Acta Derm Venereol.* 1996;76:415.
12. Smith LE, Henrichs D, McCullah RD. Prospective studies on the etiology and treatment of pruritus ani. *Dis Colon Rectum.* 1982;25:358-363.
13. Dodi G, Pirone E, Bettin A, Veller C, Infantino A, Pianon P, et al. The mycotic flora in proctological patients with and without pruritus ani. *Br J Surg.* 1985;72:967-969.
14. Bowyer A, McColl I. A study of 200 patients with pruritus ani. *Proc R Soc Med.* 1970;63(Suppl):96-98.
15. Stermer E, Sukhotnic I, Shaoul R. Pruritus ani: an approach to an itching condition. *J Pediatr Gastroenterol Nutr.* 2009 May;48(5):513-516.
16. Allan A, Ambrose NS, Silverman S, Keighley MR. Physiological study of pruritus ani. *Br J Surg.* 1987;74:576-579.
17. Farouk R, Duthie GS, Pryde A, Bartolo DC. Abnormal transient internal sphincter relaxation in idiopathic pruritus ani: physiological evidence from ambulatory monitoring. *Br J Surg.* 1994;81:603-606.
18. Eyers AA, Thomson JP. Pruritus ani: is anal sphincter dysfunction important in aetiology? *BMJ.* 1979;2:1549-1551.
19. Harrington CI, Lewis FM, McDonagh AJ, Gawkrodger DJ. Dermatological causes of pruritus ani. *BMJ.* 1992;305:955.
20. Siddiqi S, Vijay V, Ward M, et al. Pruritus ani. *Ann R Coll Surg Engl.* 2008;90(6):457-463.
21. Daniel GL, Longo WE, Vernava AM. III Pruritus ani. Causes and concerns. *Dis Colon Rectum.* 1994;37:670-674.
22. Murie JA, Sim AJ, Mackenzie I. The importance of pain, pruritus and soiling as symptoms of haemorrhoids and their response to haemorrhoidectomy or rubber band ligation. *Br J Surg.* 1981;68:247-249.
23. Pirone E, Infantino A, Masin A, et al. Can proctological procedures resolve perianal pruritus and mycosis? A prospective study of 23 cases. *Int J Colorectal Dis.* 1992;7:18-20.
24. Alexander-Williams J. Pruritus ani. *Br Med J (Clin Res Ed).* 1983;287:159-160.

25. Dasan S, Neill SM, Donaldson DR, Scott HJ. Treatment of persistent pruritus ani in a combined colorectal and dermatological clinic. *Br J Surg.* 1999;86:1337-1340.
26. Lochridge Jr E. Pruritus ani-perianal psoriasis. *South Med J.* 1969;62:450-452.
27. Carli P, Cattaneo A, De Magnis A, Biggeri A, Taddei G, Giannotti B. Squamous cell carcinoma arising in vulval lichen sclerosus: a longitudinal cohort study. *Eur J Cancer Prev.* 1995;4:491-495.
28. Sarmiento JM, Wolff BG, Burgart LJ, Frizelle FA, Ilstrup DM. Paget's disease of the perianal region—an aggressive disease? *Dis Colon Rectum.* 1997;40:1187-1194.
29. Marchesa P, Fazio VW, Oliart S, Goldblum JR, Lavery IC. Perianal Bowen's disease: a clinicopathologic study of 47 patients. *Dis Colon Rectum.* 1997;40:1286-1293.
30. Goldman S, Glimelius B, Pahlman L. Anorectal malignant melanoma in Sweden. Report of 49 patients. *Dis Colon Rectum.* 1990;33:874-877.
31. Brady MS, Kavolius JP, Quan SH. Anorectal melanoma. A 64-year experience at Memorial Sloan-Kettering Cancer Center. *Dis Colon Rectum.* 1995;38:146-151.
32. Enker WE, Heilwell M, Janov AJ, et al. Improved survival in epidermoid carcinoma of the anus in association with preoperative multidisciplinary therapy. *Arch Surg.* 1986;121:1386-1390.
33. Chaudhry V, Bastawrous A. Idiopathic pruritus ani. *Semin Colon Rectal Surg.* 2003;14:196-202.
34. Hanno R, Murphy P. Pruritus ani. Classification and management. *Dermatol Clin.* 1987;5:811-816.
35. Etter L, Myers SA. Pruritus in systemic disease: mechanisms and management. *Dermatol Clin.* 2002;20(3):459-472, vi-vii.
36. Al-Ghnaniem R, Short K, Pullen A, et al. 1% Hydrocortisone ointment is an effective treatment of pruritus ani: a pilot randomized controlled crossover trial. *Int J Colorectal Dis.* 2007;22(12):1463-1467.
37. Lysy J, Sistiery-Ittah M, Israelit Y, et al. Topical capsaicin—a novel and effective treatment for idiopathic intractable pruritus ani: a randomized, placebo controlled, crossover study. *Gut.* 2003;52(9):1323-1326.
38. Eusebio EB, Graham J, Mody N. Treatment of intractable pruritus ani. *Dis Colon Rectum.* 1990;33(9):770-772.
39. Mentes BB, Akin M, Leventoglu S, et al. Intradermal methylene blue injection for the treatment of intractable idiopathic pruritus ani: results of 30 cases. *Tech Coloproctol.* 2004;8(1):11-14.
40. Heard S. Pruritis ani. *Aust Fam Physician.* 2004;33(7):511-513.

12

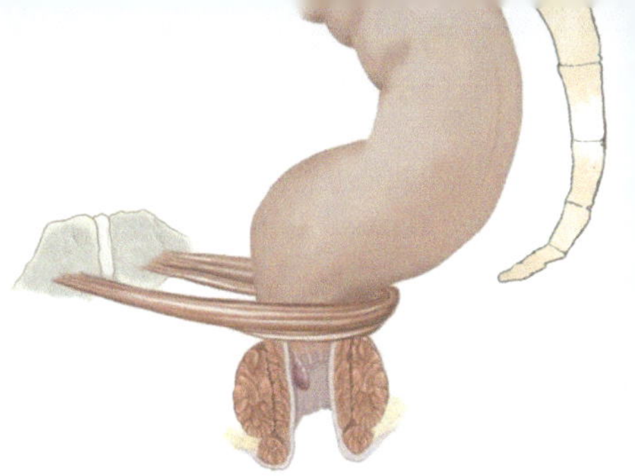

Pilonidal Disease

Roman Sargsyan, MD, PhD and Avo Artinyan, MD, MS

Key Points

- The etiology of pilonidal disease is most likely acquired in nature secondary to obstruction and infection of hair follicles in the natal cleft.
- Nonoperative treatment methods may be effective in selected cases but should not be considered definitive treatment.
- In the setting of acute pilonidal abscess, the treatment of choice is incision and drainage.
- The definitive management of chronic pilonidal disease requires surgical excision.
- Open excisional techniques (without primary wound closure) are associated with significantly delayed wound healing and patient discomfort.
- Primary wound closure is an effective alternative to open excisional techniques and is associated with significantly reduced healing times.
- Off-midline closure results in significantly fewer postoperative infections and recurrences compared with midline closure methods.

Background/Epidemiology

Pilonidal disease is a subcutaneous infectious and inflammatory process that generally occurs in the gluteal cleft and sacrococcygeal region. The original description of the disease itself has been attributed to Mayo,[1] who described a hair-containing cyst located just below the coccyx, with the term *pilonidal*, or "nest of hair," coined later in 1880 by Hodges.[2] Many terms have since been used interchangeably and somewhat indiscriminately to describe pilonidal disease, including *pilonidal sinus* and *pilonidal cyst*, although *cyst* is not an accurate term given that a surrounding epithelial wall is not present.

Qureshi W, ed. *Diagnosis and Management Guide for Anorectal Disease: A Clinical Reference* (pp 135-140).

Pilonidal disease is a common condition. The incidence and prevalence in the United States are unknown but were estimated at 26 per 100,000 individuals in a European study.[3] It is generally a condition of the young, affecting mostly teenagers and young adults in the second and third decades of life, and is at least twice as more common in males than females. Although not necessarily directly causative, hirsutism, a sedentary occupation, a positive family history, obesity, poor hygiene, and deep natal cleft anatomy have all been identified as risk factors for the development of pilonidal disease.[3]

Etiology/Pathophysiology

The etiology and pathophysiology of pilonidal disease have been the subject of considerable debate. Although initially thought to be congenital in origin, more recent evidence and experience favor an acquired etiology secondary to obstruction of hair follicles in the natal cleft.

The mechanism of the acquired theory has not been clearly elucidated. It has been postulated that affected hair follicles become distended with keratin, leading to infection, folliculitis, and the formation of an abscess that extends down into subcutaneous fat.[4] It has also been theorized that the disease is caused by loose hair ingrown into the skin, which causes chronic inflammation and infection, with secondary pits resulting from subcutaneous burrowing and additional hair entry.[5] Isolated reports of pilonidal sinuses occurring in unusual locations, such as the umbilicus, a healed amputation stump, and interdigital clefts, as well as the recurrence of disease in adequately excised areas support the acquired theory of disease.

Clinical Presentation and Diagnosis

Pilonidal disease can present in a variety of ways. In order to guide treatment, it is useful to categorize the disease as asymptomatic pilonidal disease, acute pilonidal abscess, or chronic pilonidal disease.

Asymptomatic disease may be discovered incidentally on examination, often in the process of evaluating and treating unrelated anorectal pathology. An acute pilonidal abscess generally presents with pain, induration, surrounding erythema, and occasionally spontaneous drainage. The hallmark of chronic pilonidal disease is the presence of chronically draining sinus tracts extending from the midline that are resistant to spontaneous healing. Chronic disease may also present with frequent recurrent episodes of painful induration and drainage consistent with recurrent acute abscesses with intervening asymptomatic intervals.

The diagnosis of pilonidal disease is clinical in nature and is normally made by a thorough history and physical examination. In the acute setting, physical examination reveals induration, erythema, and tenderness at or adjacent to the gluteal cleft. In an early, developing acute abscess, examination may be less conspicuous, showing only slight bulging of the skin in the cleft. Spontaneous drainage may relieve the patient's symptoms and improve physical findings. Fever and leukocytosis may also be present but are less common.

Chronic pilonidal disease is typified by the finding of midline pilonidal pits and indurated sinus tracts extending laterally from the midline natal cleft. These sinus tracts may cause secondary openings and sites of drainage off the midline, usually cephalad to the primary infected pit.

In the great majority of cases, imaging is unnecessary because a thorough history and physical examination are sufficient to both confirm the diagnosis and determine the extent of disease. In more complicated cases, magnetic resonance imaging may be helpful in determining the extent and location of multiple complex sinus tracts. In this setting, magnetic resonance imaging findings may assist surgical planning and can help rule out other potential diagnoses. The differential diagnosis of pilonidal disease includes perianal abscess, fistula-in-ano, perianal Crohn's disease, hidradenitis, and, less commonly, tubercular and actinomycotic infections. If the diagnosis is uncertain, additional studies such as anoscopy and proctosigmoidoscopy may help rule out other potential sources of perianal pathology.

Treatment

The treatment of pilonidal disease depends on the acuity and extent of disease at presentation. A variety of nonoperative, operative, and combined methods have been described, all with variable success rates. The main goals of treatment regardless of approach are to treat the acute infection; to eliminate the underlying disease with techniques that minimize the rate of recurrence; to minimize wound complications, patient discomfort, and disability; and, lastly, to affect good cosmesis.

NONOPERATIVE AND OTHER ADJUNCTIVE THERAPIES

Control of Hair Growth

Given the current understanding of the acquired nature of pilonidal disease, there has been significant interest in the control of hair growth as a means of both treating pilonidal disease and preventing its recurrence. Shaving and depilation via a number of methods have been investigated.[6-8] Because of its generally benign nature, shaving along the gluteal cleft and the surrounding region can be used as first-line treatment in cases without abscesses or as a standard component of postoperative treatment. The disease site and surrounding 5 cm should be shaved weekly until complete healing has occurred. Using this approach, a military study demonstrated complete resolution of symptoms in 101 consecutive patients at an average of 3 to 4 weeks from the beginning of shaving.[7]

Complete healing of recurrent pilonidal disease with laser depilation in a small series of patients has also been reported.[8] In addition to its potential role in symptom prevention and treatment of minimally symptomatic disease, the control of hair growth in the sinus region can play an important role in the prevention of recurrence after radical surgery. A recent systematic review that included multiple studies of small sample sizes demonstrated a lower rate of disease recurrence in surgically treated patients who underwent adjunctive laser depilation compared with patients who had razor or cream depilation or no hair removal at all.[9]

Although these studies are promising, hair control is not considered definitive therapy for pilonidal disease by most practicing physicians, as recurrences tend to occur with the cessation of hair control measures. Although these measures are benign, treatments may be tedious for the patient and, in the case of laser depilation, painful and financially burdensome as well.

Sclerosing Agents and Sealants

Ablation/sclerotherapy is another approach that has been attempted as a nonexcisional treatment measure for pilonidal disease. The most commonly used sclerosing agent is phenol, which can be used in many forms including liquid phenol solution (25% to 80%), crystalline phenol, and phenol cream/gel. It is unclear which preparation is most effective and, in the case of liquid phenol, which specific concentration is the most ideal for clinical treatment.

A common approach is to inject a phenol solution of up to 80% into a sinus tract after initial curettage and removal of hair and debris. The phenol solution is usually kept in the curetted sinus tract for 1 to 2 minutes, then flushed out. Care must be taken to avoid injury to the surrounding skin. Given that the procedure involves curettage, and phenol injection itself is painful, it is generally performed under local or general anesthesia. The success rates of phenol treatment vary from 60% to 95%.[10-12] The main problem with phenol therapy is its local toxicity and significant pain and discomfort, which may require inpatient admission.

Fibrin glue injection has also been explored as either monotherapy and/or as an adjunct to surgical excision. While small series demonstrate promising results, a recent *Cochrane Review*[13] did not demonstrate a clear benefit to this approach.

Antibiotic Use

Antibiotics have a limited role in the management of both acute and chronic disease. Primary, preoperative, or postoperative use does not improve wound infection rates, cure rates, or recurrence rates.[12] However, antibiotic use is advisable in patients who are immunosuppressed, have severe cellulitis, or have severe concomitant systemic disease.[14]

OPERATIVE TREATMENT

Acute Pilonidal Abscess

Simple incision and drainage under local anesthesia is the treatment of choice in most cases of acute pilonidal abscess, whereas larger abscesses or patient discomfort may necessitate a general anesthetic. The incision is generally placed over the area of greatest fluctuance, preferably off midline in longitudinal fashion to facilitate wound healing. The excision of midline pits and/or curettage of the abscess cavity at the time of drainage may be performed, but these additional maneuvers have not been definitively shown to improve healing rates or decrease recurrence.

Simple incision and drainage is effective at treating the acute infectious process, and the resulting wound will heal in a significant proportion of patients. However, simple incision and drainage may not adequately address the chronic underlying disease. As a result, approximately 50% of patients will eventually have recurrence of their disease either in the form of a recurrent acute pilonidal abscess or chronic pilonidal sinus tract formation.[15] Therefore, definitive surgical excision should be considered after resolution of the acute inflammatory process and wound healing, usually after a period of several months.

Chronic Pilonidal Disease

The definitive management of chronic pilonidal disease is surgical excision with or without some form of reconstruction. The goal of excision is to remove all diseased tissue, including all pilonidal pits, sinus tracts, and chronic abscess cavities. Many excisional techniques have been described through a variety of incisions, both midline and off-midline. After excision has been completed, the surgeon must decide on whether wound closure should be performed. If wound closure is elected, the surgeon must decide on which of the many techniques for wound reconstruction to use.

Over the course of the last several decades, the surgical management of pilonidal disease has evolved from the utilization of predominantly open techniques to a greater emphasis on wound closure. With wound closure, midline closure has fallen out of favor, whereas off-midline closure and more complex flap and plasty procedures have become the relative norm.

Excision With Secondary Wound Closure: "The Open Technique"

The open technique involves wide excision or simple unroofing of the pilonidal pits and the surrounding sinus tracts, with the resultant wound left open for secondary closure. While very simple and straightforward for the surgeon, this technique can be onerous for the patient because local wound care may be necessary for several weeks after treatment. Delays in healing can lead to significant patient discomfort, incapacity, and inability to return to normal activities. The application of a vacuum dressing may facilitate wound closure and minimize the difficulty of wound care. Because of its technical simplicity, the open technique remains commonly used worldwide. It is effective at treating chronic disease with acceptable recurrence rates. The major disadvantage of this procedure, as addressed earlier, is the morbidity associated with delayed wound closure and the burden of prolonged wound care for the patient.

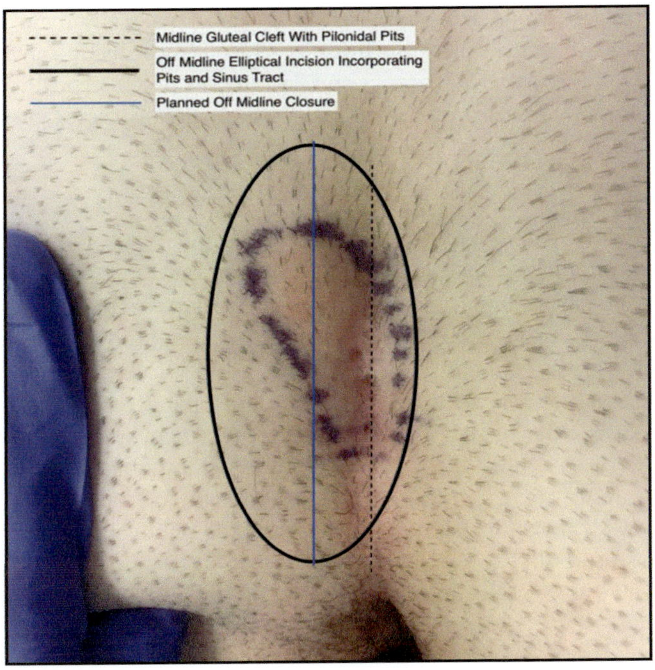

Figure 12-1. Planned incision and closure for a Karydakis flap procedure in a patient with chronic pilonidal sinus.

Excision With Wound Closure: "The Closed Technique"

Compared with open management, primary closure of pilonidal wounds after excision significantly reduces healing time.[16] Simple midline closure is associated with high rates of wound dehiscence and potentially higher recurrence rates; therefore, it has generally fallen out of favor.[17]

As a result, numerous off-midline, closed excision techniques have been described; the 3 most commonly used are the Karydakis flap,[5] Bascom cleft lift,[4] and Limberg flap. These techniques are associated with significantly fewer postoperative infections and recurrences compared with midline closure methods. A recent large meta-analysis comparing outcomes of multiple excision techniques in more than 80,000 patients demonstrated a recurrence rate of 0.6% at 24 months for the Karydakis and Bascom techniques and 1.8% for the Limberg flap technique, whereas primary midline closures were associated with a recurrence rate of 67.9%.[7]

Our preferred approach is the Karydakis off-midline excision technique (Figure 12-1). The technique involves the complete excision of all pilonidal pits and associated sinus tracts with a vertical elliptical incision that is oriented off the midline gluteal cleft. After complete excision down to the postsacral fascia, a thick subcutaneous flap is created medially, advanced laterally, and closed in layers over the midline postsacral fascia. In a review of over 6000 patients, Karydakis[18] identified a recurrence rate of less than 1% and a wound complication rate of 8.5%.

The Bascom technique, which we do not commonly perform, involves a lateral longitudinal incision to drain the sinus/abscess cavity with separate excision of each individual midline pit. After curettage of the abscess cavity, a fibrofatty flap consisting of the wall of the sinus cavity and subcutaneous fat is advanced over the midline postsacral fascia and secured with a suture to the bridge of skin between the midline cleft and the lateral incision. The pit excision sites are traditionally closed and the lateral incision is kept open, though tension-free closure is our preference. As discussed previously, this technique has satisfactory healing and recurrence rates, although it is less commonly used in practice today.

In addition to these procedures, multiple plasty operations have been adapted from experience with reconstruction of other disease sites. These include the Limberg rhomboid flap and other local forms of tissue transfer and advancement including V-Y advancement flaps and Z-plasties. These techniques are effective at treating chronic disease and preventing recurrence. The major disadvantage of these procedures is related to the need for significant tissue transfer, which is more technically demanding and may require prolonged hospitalization. Dehiscence and flap failures may also be difficult to manage. Additionally, the non–anatomic-appearing scar may not be cosmetically acceptable for some patients.

POSTOPERATIVE CARE

Both in the acute and chronic setting, pilonidal sinus incision or excision procedures are performed almost exclusively in the outpatient or short-stay setting. With incision and drainage, wound care is performed in the outpatient setting with either daily dressing changes or a vacuum dressing until closure of the wound.

With excision of chronic pilonidal disease, we generally see the patient postoperatively 1 week after surgery. If the wound has been closed, as is our most common practice, the patient is evaluated at this time for wound infection. If infection is evident, we treat the patient with antibiotics, and we consider the removal of 1 or 2 of the inferior-most sutures to allow for drainage. We have found that even in the setting of an infected wound, closed incisions managed with the removal of 1 to 2 sutures result in minimal discomfort and morbidity to the patient and still result in good wound healing. The sutures are generally removed 2 to 3 weeks after surgery. The patient is thereafter followed expectantly.

REFERENCES

1. Mayo OH. *Observations on Injuries and Diseases of the Rectum*. London, UK: Burgess and Hill; 1833.
2. Hodges RM. Pilonidal sinus. *Boston Med Surg J*. 1880;103:485-486.
3. Søndenaa K, Andersen E, Nesvik I, Søreide JA. Patient characteristics and symptoms in chronic pilonidal sinus disease. *Int J Colorectal Dis*. 1995;10(1):39-42.
4. Bascom JU. Repeat pilonidal operations. *Am J Surg*. 1987;154(1):118-122.
5. Karydakis GE. New approach to the problem of pilonidal sinus. *Lancet*. 1973;2(7843):1414-1415.
6. Khanna A, Rombeau JL. Pilonidal disease. *Clin Colon Rectal Surg*. 2011;24(1):46-53.
7. Armstrong JH, Barcia PJ. Pilonidal sinus disease. The conservative approach. *Arch Surg*. 1994;129(9):914-917, discussion 917-919.
8. Odili J, Gault D. Laser depilation of the natal cleft—an aid to healing the pilonidal sinus. *Ann R Coll Surg Engl*. 2002;84(1):29-32.
9. Pronk AA, Eppink L, Smakman N, Furnee EJB. The effect of hair removal after surgery for sacrococcygeal pilonidal sinus disease: a systematic review of the literature. *Tech Coloproctol*. 2018;22(1):7-14.
10. Hegge HG, Vos GA, Patka P, Hoitsma HF. Treatment of complicated or infected pilonidal sinus disease by local application of phenol. *Surgery*. 1987;102(1):52-54.
11. Dogru O, Camci C, Aygen E, et al. Pilonidal sinus treated with crystallized phenol: an eight-year experience. *Dis Colon Rectum*. 2004;47(11):1934-1938.
12. Humphries AE, Duncan JE. Evaluation and management of pilonidal disease. *Surg Clin North Am*. 2010;90(1):113-124.
13. Lund J, Tou S, Doleman B, Williams JP. Fibrin glue for pilonidal sinus disease. *Cochrane Database Syst Rev*. 2017;1:CD011923.
14. Segre D, Pozzo M, Perinotti R, Roche B; Italian Society of Colorectal Surgery. The treatment of pilonidal disease: guidelines of the Italian Society of Colorectal Surgery (SICCR). *Tech Coloproctol*. 2015;19(10):607-613.
15. Velasco AL, Dunlap WW. Pilonidal disease and hidradenitis. *Surg Clin North Am*. 2009;89(3):689-701.
16. Al-Hassan HK, Francis IM, Neglen P. Primary closure or secondary granulation after excision of pilonidal sinus? *Acta Chir Scand*. 1990;156(10):695-699.
17. Stauffer VK, Luedi MM, Kauf P, et al. Common surgical procedures in pilonidal sinus disease: a meta-analysis, merged data analysis, and comprehensive study on recurrence. *Sci Rep*. 2018;8(1):3058.
18. Karydakis GE. Easy and successful treatment of pilonidal sinus after explanation of its causative process. *Aust N Z J Surg*. 1992;62(5):385-389.

13

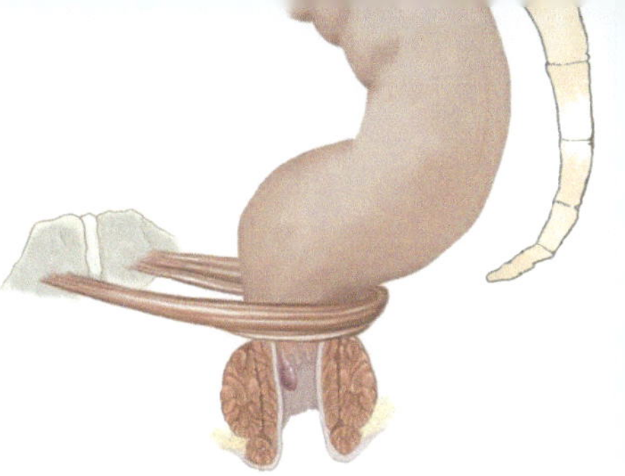

Trauma and Foreign Body Extraction From the Rectum

Rishi D. Naik, MD, MSCI and
Keith L. Obstein, MD, MPH, FASGE, FACG, AGAF

Key Points

- Patients can present with vague symptoms such as rectal bleeding, constipation, or abdominal pain without mention of a foreign object. Often, there is a delayed presentation due to embarrassment of the act or fear of repercussion.
- Physical examination can exhibit abdominal pain, sometimes with a palpable mass; rectal examination may reveal damage to the anal sphincter or even visualization of the retained object. Pay careful attention to evaluate for signs of peritonitis to rule out a perforation.
- Laboratory tests are limited in use but should involve a complete metabolic profile and in the case of perforation or need to proceed to the operating room, a type and screen, coagulation profile, and basic metabolic profile (for anesthesia purposes).
- Radiographic imaging is of higher yield because it can visualize the retained object and evaluate for free air (ie, concern for perforation). A flat and upright plain film (x-ray) or computed tomographic (CT) scan can be checked.
- Removal at bedside can be attempted (if not a drug packet, which should be monitored with x-rays and physical examination because it passes through the gastrointestinal tract and out of the patient without mechanical intervention), but when this fails, the patient needs anesthesia to help relax the anal sphincter and facilitate removal. Spinal anesthesia or a pudendal nerve block can often help, in which case the operating room is the next step for removal.
- Careful consideration should be placed when the provider encounters sharp objects, lumen-occluding blunt objects, or body packers with retained drug packets.

Qureshi W, ed. *Diagnosis and Management Guide for Anorectal Disease: A Clinical Reference* (pp 141-150).

- If there is a perforation or the object cannot be removed transanally, the patient needs to be moved to the operating room.
- Once the object is removed, evaluation of the mucosa after object extraction should be completed (sigmoidoscopy).
- The patient will need psychiatric and emotional support postextraction to help address the underlying causes and potentially prevent future episodes.

While rectal foreign bodies are uncommon findings with rising incidence, their clinical impact is important given the possibility of rectal bleeding and perforation. The first report of a rectal foreign body dates back to the 16th century and, unfortunately since this time, the literature only has case reports and case series with no prospective trials, randomized clinical trials, or higher level of evidence to help guide management.[1] Several review articles have opinions on management, which have served as the background for management of these patients but also explains the variability in approach. Highlighting some of these disparities is the lack of adequate epidemiologic data on the true incidence or prevalence of this condition. The incidence of rectal foreign bodies varies based on location; one large teaching hospital reported an incidence of 1 rectal foreign body/year, whereas small community-based settings have reported much lower incidence rates of 0.15 per 100,000 population.[2,3] Two-thirds of patients with retained rectal foreign bodies are males in their 30s to 40s, although the range has been reported to include patients 90 years of age.[4,5]

Patients often present with vague symptoms of rectal pain or bright red blood per rectum without giving information of a swallowed or anally inserted rectal object, which leads to a delay in diagnostics and a need for heightened suspicion from the treating provider. Retained rectal foreign bodies range from orally swallowed drug packets and batteries to anally inserted fruits, vegetables, light bulbs, deodorant bottles and cans, and cigar cases[3] (Figure 13-1). The rationale for insertion ranges from self-insertion for sexual pleasure to forced external insertion (ie, individuals who are incarcerated, raped, or forced into drug trafficking).

There can be a delay in presentation for those with a retained rectal foreign object due to embarrassment of the situation/object or the illegal nature of the act. This poses great pressure on the provider to take an accurate history and perform a careful physical examination to gain the patient's trust and expedite diagnosis. The delay in diagnosis can increase the risk of mucosal trauma, such as mucosal bleeding or even colonic perforation. Identifying patients with peritoneal signs on physical examination can help triage patients toward surgery more expeditiously. Extraction techniques are varied in case reports, ranging from manual bedside extraction to utilization of devices, such as obstetric suction, uterine clamps, or transanal use of a surgical port (SILS Port, Medtronic).[6-8] Unfortunately, even after extraction, there can be delayed perforation, bleeding, and delayed motility.

Pathophysiology

Rectal foreign bodies are typically placed voluntarily for sexual gratification. Foreign bodies can also be seen in cases of rape, assault, or body packing by drug traffickers. The literature details case reports of several objects, including apples, cucumbers, bottles, utensils, vibrators, dildos, knives, deodorant bottles, and drug packets. Injury from these objects includes direct trauma to the rectal mucosa, which can cause hematomas, lacerations, bleeding, and perforations. Although no formal rectal foreign body scale has been created, adaptation of the American Association for the Surgery of Trauma rectal organ injury scale (Table 13-1) can be applied to blunt and penetrating trauma to the rectum.[9] In this manner, the distinctions of injury include hematoma, degree of laceration, and a devascularized segment. Knowing the etiology of the foreign body can help understand the severity of the trauma; sharp objects or lumen-occluding objects can cause direct injury to the mucosa, which may necessitate surgical repair.

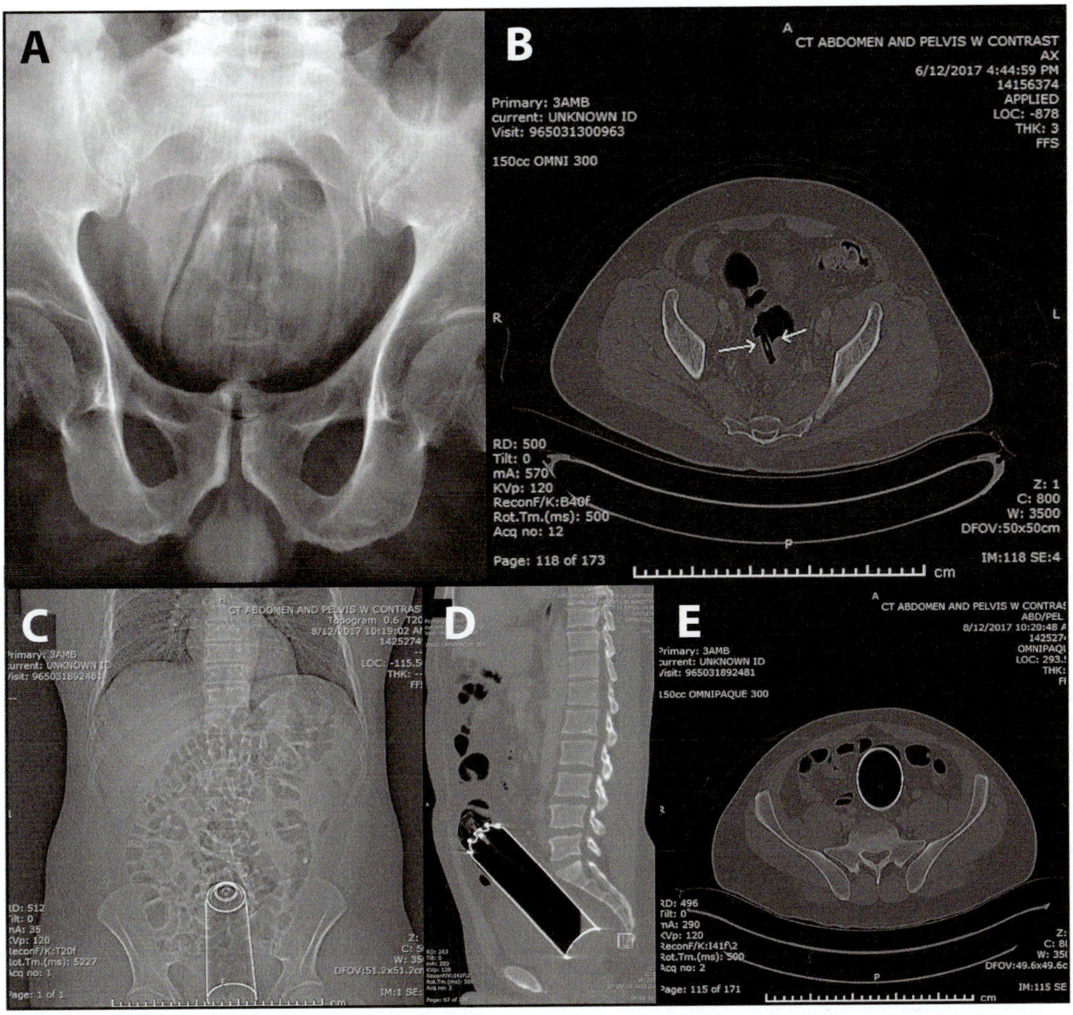

Figure 13-1. (A) Mango fruit in the rectum. (B) An ink pen in the rectum. (C-E) A potpourri spray can in the rectum. (Reprinted with permission from Collin Bray, MD.)

Table 13-1

American Association for the Surgery of Trauma Rectal Organ Injury Scale

GRADE	TYPE OF INJURY	DESCRIPTION OF INJURY
I	Hematoma	Contusion or hematoma with devascularization
	Laceration	Partial-thickness laceration
II	Laceration	Laceration <50% of circumference
III	Laceration	Laceration ≥50% of circumference
IV	Laceration	Full-thickness laceration with extension into the perineum
V	Vascular	Devascularized segment

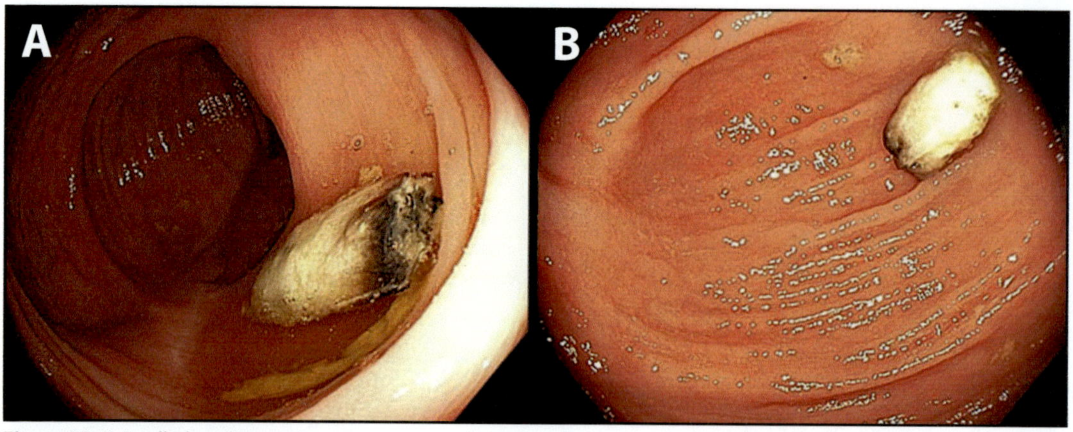

Figure 13-2. A rolled marijuana cigarette seen on colonoscopy.

Beyond immediate injury to the colon, body packing of illicit drugs can pose significant challenges; despite the outside packing not being inherently dangerous, rupture of the packet can lead to life-threatening toxicity due to the drug itself (ie, heroin or cocaine). Body packing, first described in 1973, is the transportation of drugs by internal concealment (ie, smuggling of cocaine, heroin, 3,4-methylenedioxymethamphetamine ["ecstasy"], or marijuana as means of transportation).[10-14] Often there are multiple drugs swallowed; 1 kg of a drug can be divided into as many as 50 to 100 packets, and a single packet of cocaine, heroin, or amphetamine may contain a life-threatening dose.[10] Body stuffing is the swallowing of relatively small amounts of loosely wrapped drugs due to the fear of arrest. Figure 13-2 shows a marijuana cigarette found in the rectum during colonoscopy. In this non–life-threatening case, the marijuana cigarette was removed using a standard foreign body removal technique (a retrieval basket) with little risk of damage to the mucosa or systemic drug toxicity.

Involuntary nonsexual foreign rectal objects are usually found in the elderly, children, or those with intellectual disability who have swallowed objects unintentionally, such as toothpicks, chicken bones, plastic objects, toys, or coins. Regardless of the rectal foreign body, all objects should be treated as potentially hazardous with a risk of severe injury. Fortunately, most rectal foreign objects cause grade I or II injuries, although perforation has been reported, and, therefore, a high degree of suspicion is required for prompt evaluation and management.

Signs and Symptoms

Due to the nature of the foreign body (whether placed involuntarily or voluntarily), there is often a lack of overt facts from patients on the circumstances leading to their presentation. Instead, they can present with a chief complaint of rectal bleeding, constipation, abdominal pain, or rectal mucus discharge. Due to the nature of the foreign body and embarrassment or illegal nature of the act, there is often a delay with attempts at home to try to expulse the object. Sometimes, this is successful, but patients can have subsequent bleeding or pain that prompts their visit. In these cases, high suspicion for a rectal foreign body should be maintained to help prevent overlooking a complication from the foreign body. If the foreign body is lumen occluding, then obstructive symptoms can occur with nausea, vomiting, and the inability to pass flatus or bowel movements. In these cases, patients may have signs of dehydration and are at increased risk for aspiration if obstructed.

When suspected, the provider should establish a therapeutic relationship with the patient to allow for an honest and open history on the events leading to the presentation without perceived embarrassment of the act. Approaching these symptoms in a nonconfrontational way helps build the therapeutic alliance and leads to more expeditious management. As stated earlier, some of these rectal foreign bodies are placed involuntarily, whether by rape or assault, and, hence, emotional support should also be provided given the trauma of the act.

When these symptoms are encountered, a thorough physical examination should be performed. An abdominal examination can reveal rebound tenderness as a sign of perforation, and focal pain can sometimes localize the area of the retained object. A detailed visual perianal and rectal examination for signs of trauma, bleeding, or a retained object should be performed. Prior to digital rectal insertion, we recommend evaluating the rectum under good lighting to evaluate for any sharp objects that can cause harm to the provider with digital insertion and to avoid digital examination if drug packets are suspected to prevent inadvertent packet puncture. Particular attention should be placed on the anal sphincter because involuntary insertion can cause damage to this area. If there is sphincter injury, there may be increased tone secondary to muscular spasms due to the upstream retained foreign body.[15] If the retained object is in the distal rectum, this can often be palpated on digital rectal examination.

Diagnosis

The physical examination can often lead to diagnosis, whether by palpating an object on abdominal examination or via a thorough rectal examination. If there is rebounding or guarding, then a laboratory examination can help confirm this diagnosis because an elevated white blood cell count, low bicarbonate, or elevated lactate leading to anion gap metabolic acidosis can be seen. In case surgery is needed, a basic metabolic profile and type and screen should be obtained to help with anesthesia planning and potential complications of bleeding during surgery. If the patient reports bright red blood per rectum, monitoring of the patient's hemoglobin should also be completed.

More importantly, radiographic imaging can confirm a diagnosis. Radiopaque objects can be seen on a flat and upright abdominal plain film, which also allows evaluation of the pneumoperitoneum. Plain films can also show upstream dilated loops of bowel, which can be helpful if the object is radiolucent. More advanced imaging often is completed for the patient's chief complaint, which usually involves a CT scan to evaluate for the source of pain, bleeding, or constipation. This allows for more detailed information of the anatomy and can be helpful for radiolucent objects; however, given the cost and risk of radiation, a plain film should be the first step in diagnostic imaging for these patients. In a study of body packers, plain films had a sensitivity of 85% to 90%, and contrast-enhanced abdominal radiography had a sensitivity of 96% in one study; the operative characteristics of CT imaging are presumed to be higher and should be used if the initial screening test is negative, but large studies are lacking on this approach.[16] The 2 goals of imaging are to confirm a diagnosis and rule out perforation, both of which can be completed by a plain film.

It is important to note the limitations of imaging tests, which are often demonstrated when a radiopaque object or enhancement is encountered on a CT scan. As calcified material (ie, bones and rectal inserted toys) can be seen on CT scans, there can be calcifications from other etiologies that are not necessarily a foreign body. For instance, an 84-year-old man who arrived at our emergency department with new-onset abdominal pain underwent a CT scan that demonstrated a $1.0 \times 0.3 \times 0.9$ cm dense object in his proximal sigmoid colon (Figure 13-3A). The object was read as a possible foreign body, such as a piece of bone, that may have burrowed into the wall, and there was associated upstream bowel dilation at this calcification (Figure 13-3B). The patient denied any history of recent bone intake, but given the imaging findings, flexible sigmoidoscopy was completed. On sigmoidoscopy, colon cancer, not a foreign object, was encountered (Figure 13-3C). The patient underwent sigmoid colectomy, and the explanted tissue demonstrated no retained foreign objects.

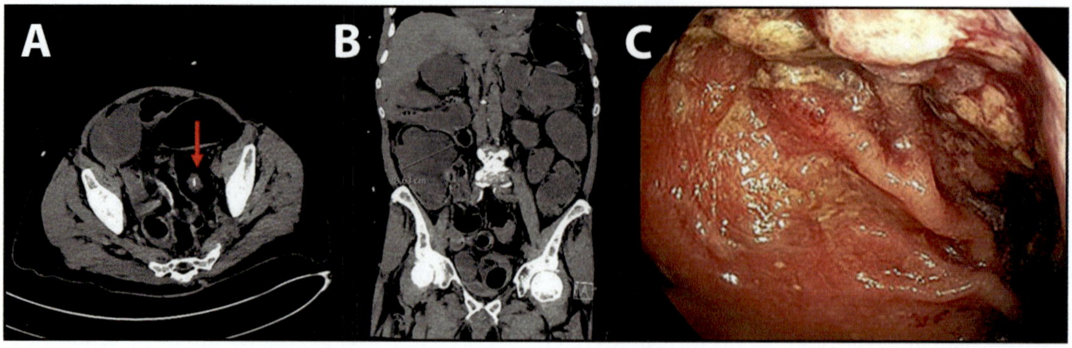

Figure 13-3. A reported retained fish bone, which on endoscopy was confirmed to be colon cancer. (A, B) CT imaging. (C) Endoscopic imaging.

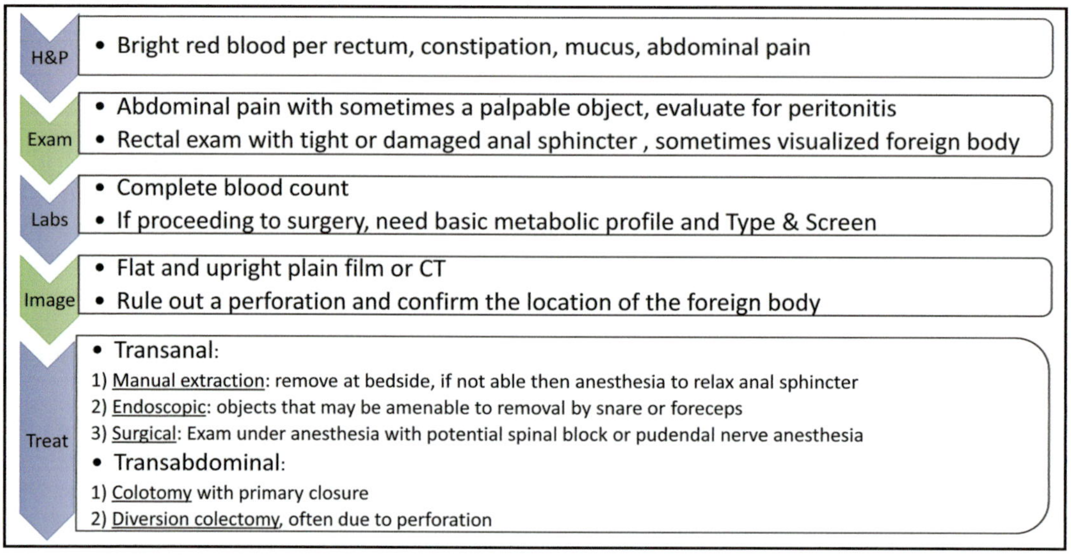

Figure 13-4. The management algorithm for a retained rectal foreign body.

Treatment and Follow-up

RULE OUT PERFORATION

The first step in the management of rectal foreign bodies is to determine if there is a perforation (Figure 13-4). Perforations can be suspected by vital signs (hypotension and tachycardia) and physical examination, supported by laboratory values, and confirmed by imaging. Free air in the abdomen is a surgical emergency and needs to be identified quickly to expedite resuscitation, antibiotics, and appropriate surgical management in the operating room. If there is no perforation and the patient is clinically stable, the foreign body can be attempted to be removed at bedside (if not a narcotic packet) or, if general anesthesia is needed, transferred to the operating room. If the object is more proximal, then a trial of nonoperative management can be attempted with close observation to see if the object will move more distally. An example of this involves a 33-year-old woman with known psychiatric issues and foreign body ingestions who swallowed multiple batteries and staples. An admission upright x-ray (Figure 13-5A) showed batteries and staples in her midabdomen with quick transit to her small bowel on repeat x-rays nonretrievable by upper endoscopy. Serial upright x-rays (Figure 13-5B-D) showed continued transit through her colon and rectal expulsion over a 6-day

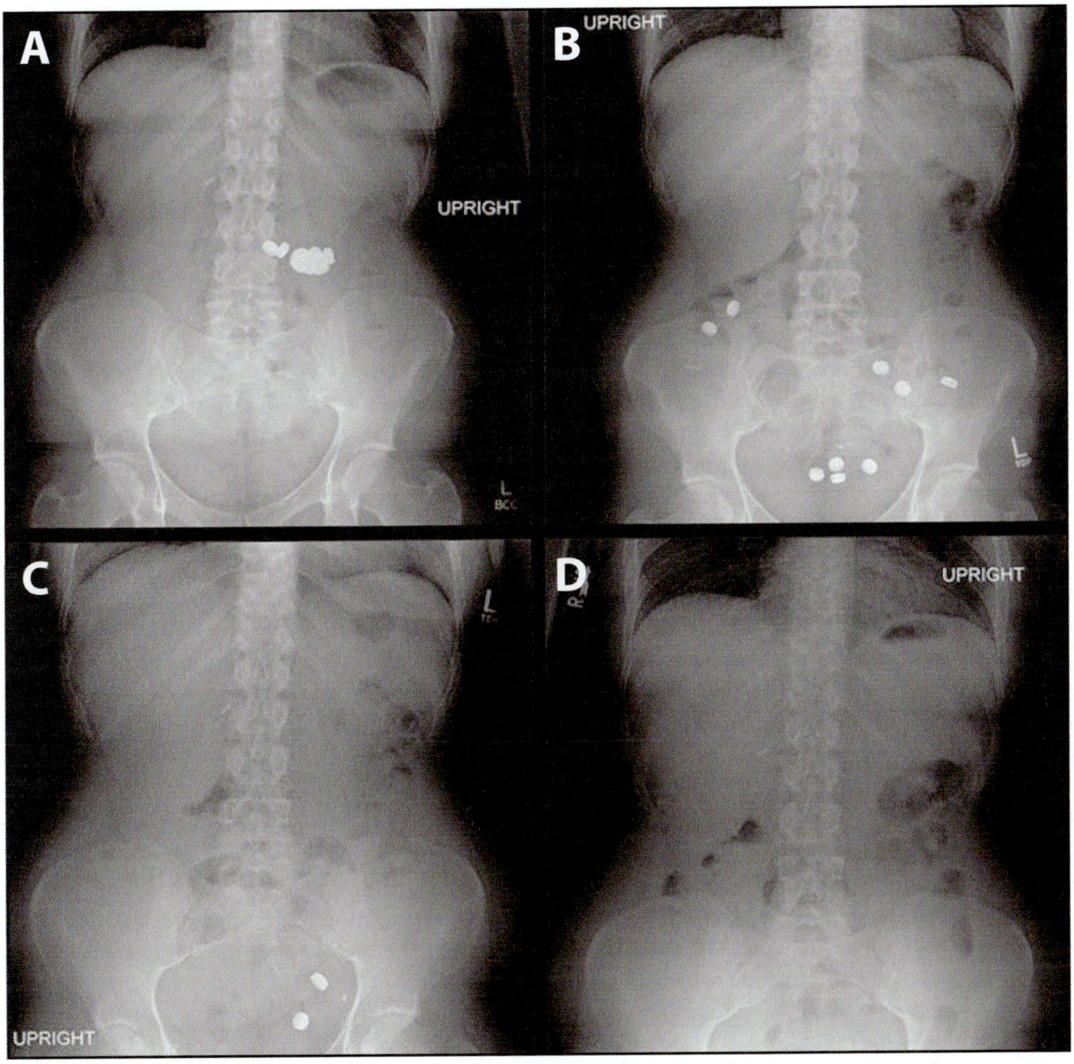

Figure 13-5. Swallowed batteries and staples managed conservatively. A through D shows transit over time.

period with the use of polyethylene glycol to facilitate colonic expulsion. Throughout the course, she remained stable with no signs of perforation. Unfortunately, many rectal foreign bodies fail to pass spontaneously and need to be removed at bedside or in the operating room. While some practitioners advocate the use of stimulants and enemas to help evacuate the foreign object, others recommend avoidance because these products can theoretically lead to more extensive rectal injury, perforation, and proximal movements of the rectal foreign object.

REMOVAL TRANSANALLY

There are 2 primary methods for the removal of rectal foreign bodies: transanal, which includes extraction at the bedside, in the operating room, or endoscopically, and transabdominal. If an object cannot be removed at bedside, the next step is often transfer to the operating room to facilitate the use of a pudendal nerve block, spinal anesthetic, and conscious or general sedation with the goal of relaxing the anal sphincter to prevent spasm and allow for improved visualization with potential extraction.[1,17-19] Once the patient has been anesthetized and sedated, he or she should be placed in the high lithotomy position in candy cane stirrups because this allows easy visualization and downward abdominal pressure to help with foreign body removal. The anal canal can be gently dilated, and, if easily visualized, the object can be removed by hand. If the object is too proximal, clamps or forceps may be used in an attempt to bring the object more distally for the surgeon to remove by hand. Some authors advocate for evaluation of the mucosa postextraction with a rigid or flexible sigmoidoscope to determine the degree of mucosal injury, evaluate for bleeding, and ensure that no additional foreign bodies are present. Less debated is the use of a postextraction x-ray to ensure there is no perforation after foreign object retrieval.

CHALLENGES FOR FOREIGN BODY REMOVAL

The variety of rectal foreign objects that can be encountered provides multiple potential challenges for removal. First, sharp objects require extra attention due to the risk of perforation to the patient and the risks of injury to the provider. When possible, removal using clamps and preventing manual extraction to prevent self-injury should be advocated. Despite the uncertain role of evaluating the mucosal wall integrity postextraction, sharp objects provide a reasonable indication for sigmoidoscopy in this setting to ensure there are no bleeding, tears, or perforation. Second, blunt objects provide a unique challenge in that they can lead to a vacuum effect that may hinder removal of the object. When the foreign object is solid and inorganic, such as jars or vibrators, creative techniques such as placing a lubricated Foley catheter alongside the object (transanal) to break the vacuum seal and help with extraction once the catheter balloon is inflated have shown to be helpful. Others have used Minnesota tubes or Sengstaken-Blakemore tubes to inflate within a retained foreign object (ie, a jar) to help aid in the extraction. Care should be made to not break the rectal foreign object, which can then cause further problems with mucosal injury and bleeding. The one case in which this can prove useful is in the extraction of fruits and vegetables because, much like an esophageal foreign object, they can be broken into smaller pieces to aid in removal given the benign nature of these natural compounds. Third, body packers provide a grave danger to the patient because certain techniques for rectal foreign body extraction can lead to immediate death of the patient if done incorrectly.

Typically, rectal foreign bodies with illegal drugs inside are wrapped (ie, in a condom). The best practice in this scenario is to serially monitor the patient and the migration of the packets, allowing them to be expelled from the patient without physical intervention because these packages can easily rupture. Unless preparing for immediate surgery or there are signs of packet rupture, whole-body irrigation with polyethylene glycol electrolyte solution is recommended at a rate of 2 L/hour.[10] Oil-based laxatives can actually reduce the tensile strength of a latex wrapping, leading to rupture of the packets, which can be life threatening and, hence, should be avoided.[20,21] If deemed necessary to extract the packets, then extreme care should be taken not to use clamps or tools because the drug released from a ruptured packet can be fatal. Conservative therapy can be completed until the packet has migrated more distally for manual digital extraction. Again, there is a risk of spontaneous packet rupture (that is increased with attempted physical extraction) and, prior to any physical extraction attempt of these objects, the health care team should have aggressive resuscitation, the antidote (ie, naloxone for heroin rupture) when available, and an operating room for exploratory laparotomy immediately available.[22]

ROLE OF ENDOSCOPY

There is limited evidence for the role of flexible sigmoidoscopy for the removal of foreign objects, mainly because the endoscope is limited in its ability to grasp foreign objects by the size of the accessory devices (ie, typically a snare or retrieval basket). The average outer diameter of these snares ranges from 13 to 27 mm, with some of the largest having an outer diameter of 33 mm. In many cases, when the object is suitable for endoscopic removal, the colonoscope can be used to insufflate and disrupt any potential vacuum that may be present. Biopsy forceps or specialty grasping forceps can also be used to remove small rectal foreign objects. Novel endoscopic attempts, including using argon plasma coagulation to incinerate an apple to facilitate removal, have also been used.[23] For larger objects that are trapped/stuck within the colon, rigid tools are preferable to flexible endoscopes.[22]

SURGICAL APPROACH

If the transanal approach is unsuccessful or if there is a confirmed perforation or rupture of a drug packet, then the next step should be surgical via a transabdominal approach.[22] This is similar to the transanal approach in the operating room, with the primary difference being that in the transabdominal approach there is a focus on advancing the rectal foreign body proximally to distally to allow for manual removal once the object is sufficiently distal. If this cannot be completed, then a colotomy would need to be performed for primary removal with subsequent primary closure. If there is clinical peritonitis, perforation with fecal contamination, or extensive damage to the mucosa, then this surgical approach should include possible diversion.

POST-REMOVAL MONITORING

Once the foreign body is removed, there is still a risk of perforation, and a repeat upright plain film (x-ray) should be completed after removal to ensure no perforation. The role of sigmoidoscopy to evaluate the mucosa has been debated; however, in the case of removal in the operating room or endoscopically, we support evaluating the mucosa to ensure there are no retained objects, to assess for mucosal damage, and to evaluate for bleeding that may be repaired endoscopically. There can also be lacerations postextraction that can lead to bleeding. Sepsis can also occur, which can lead to death. Even if simple bedside removal of the rectal foreign object is performed, close monitoring for infection, bleeding, and perforation should occur because early recognition can reduce morbidity and mortality. If a more extensive approach is required, the patient should be admitted and monitored closely for these same adverse events.

Beyond the immediate impact on trauma to the rectum, the act itself deserves attention. Whether it was voluntary or involuntary, these patients need emotional support, and often psychiatric consultation can help prevent repeat voluntary episodes. For involuntary insertions, emotional support is even more vital, and trying to ensure a safe place for disposition and checking for potential sexually transmitted infections (in the case of sexual assault and rape) are also advocated.

CONCLUSION

Rectal foreign objects are rare entities that can be initially challenging to diagnose due to the lack of forthcoming information from the patient. Detailed assessment, recognition, and potential extraction are needed to help prevent complications from the retained object (see Figure 13-4). Once diagnosed, an expeditious assessment to confirm the nature of the object, degree of harm to the patient (ie, sharp objects or body packers), and risk of perforation needs to be determined. Despite a lack of high-quality, randomized controlled trials or even prospective cohorts in multi-arm studies to determine the ideal intervention, the physiology of the retained foreign object is well understood, which involves the need to remove the retained object by relaxing the anal sphincter via anesthesia or equalizing the pressure/vacuum that may exist. Given the wide range of objects that may be retained, several novel and innovative methods have been described in the literature for foreign body retrieval. In most cases, this involves breaking any potential seal from a retained object, avoiding clamps or sharp objects in body packers, and preventing manual removal of sharp objects to prevent injury to the provider. In cases of perforation or when the object cannot be removed transanally, a surgical transabdominal approach is implemented, which can lead to a simple colotomy with primary closure or a diverting colostomy depending on the extent of damage. An evaluation of the mucosa should be completed pre- and postextraction to grade the degree of mucosal injury that would be at risk for perforation and evaluate and intervene on any potential sites of bleeding. Once the object is removed, psychiatric consultation should be completed if this was a voluntary method, which can aid in potentially mitigating future attempts. If involuntary, engagement of social work services is advised to ensure safe disposition and emotional support along with practicing the standard of care for evaluation/management of rape and assault victims.

References

1. Kurer MA, Davey C, Khan S, Chintapatla S. Colorectal foreign bodies: a systematic review. *Colorectal Dis.* 2010;12(9):851-861.
2. Lake JP, Essani R, Petrone P, Kaiser AM, Asensio J, Beart RW Jr. Management of retained colorectal foreign bodies: predictors of operative intervention. *Dis Colon Rectum.* 2004;47(10):1694-1698.
3. Cawich SO, Thomas DA, Mohammed F, Bobb NJ, Williams D, Naraynsingh V. A management algorithm for retained rectal foreign bodies. *Am J Mens Health.* 2017;11(3):684-692.
4. Ooi BS, Ho YH, Eu KW, Nyam D, Leong A, Seow-Choen F. Management of anorectal foreign bodies: a cause of obscure anal pain. *Aust N Z J Surg.* 1998;68(12):852-855.
5. Clarke DL, Buccimazza I, Anderson FA, Thomson SR. Colorectal foreign bodies. *Colorectal Dis.* 2005;7(1):98-103.
6. Bak Y, Merriam M, Neff M, Berg DA. Novel approach to rectal foreign body extraction. *JSLS.* 2013;17(2):342-345.
7. Peet TN. Removal of impacted rectal foreign body with obstetric forceps. *Br Med J.* 1976;1(6008):500-501.
8. Levin SE, Cooperman H, Freilich M, Lomas M. The use of a curved uterine vulsellum for removal of rectal foreign bodies: report of a case. *Dis Colon Rectum.* 1977;20(6):532-533.
9. Moore EE, Cogbill TH, Malangoni MA, et al. Organ injury scaling, II: pancreas, duodenum, small bowel, colon, and rectum. *J Trauma.* 1990;30(11):1427-1429.
10. Traub SJ, Hoffman RS, Nelson LS. Body packing—the internal concealment of illicit drugs. *N Engl J Med.* 2003;349(26):2519-2526.
11. Watson CJ, Thomson HJ, Johnston PS. Body-packing with amphetamines—an indication for surgery. *J R Soc Med.* 1991;84(5):311-312.
12. Krishnan A, Brown R. Plain abdominal radiography in the diagnosis of the "body packer". *J Accid Emerg Med.* 1999;16(5):381.
13. Horrocks AW. Abdominal radiography in suspected 'body packers'. *Clin Radiol.* 1992;45(5):322-325.
14. Dassel PM, Punjabi E. Ingested marihuana-filled balloons. *Gastroenterology.* 1979;76(1):166-169.
15. Goldberg JE, Steele SR. Rectal foreign bodies. *Surg Clin North Am.* 2010;90(1):173-184, Table of Contents.
16. Marc B, Baud FJ, Aelion MJ, et al. The cocaine body-packer syndrome: evaluation of a method of contrast study of the bowel. *J Forensic Sci.* 1990;35(2):345-355.
17. Koornstra JJ, Weersma RK. Management of rectal foreign bodies: description of a new technique and clinical practice guidelines. *World J Gastroenterol.* 2008;14(27):4403-4406.
18. Sharma H, Banka S, Walton R, Memon MA. A novel technique for nonoperative removal of round rectal foreign bodies. *Tech Coloproctol.* 2007;11(1):58-59.
19. Kasotakis G, Roediger L, Mittal S. Rectal foreign bodies: a case report and review of the literature. *Int J Surg Case Rep.* 2012;3(3):111-115.
20. Visser L, Stricker B, Hoogendoorn M, Vinks A. Do not give paraffin to packers. *Lancet.* 1998;352(9137):1352.
21. White N, Taylor K, Lyszkowski A, Tullett J, Morris C. Dangers of lubricants used with condoms. *Nature.* 1988;335(6185):19.
22. ASGE Standards of Practice Committee, Ikenberry SO, Jue TL, et al. Management of ingested foreign bodies and food impactions. *Gastrointest Endosc.* 2011;73(6):1085-1091.
23. Glaser J, Hack T, Rubsam M. Unusual rectal foreign body: treatment using argon-beam coagulation. *Endoscopy.* 1997;29(3):230-231.

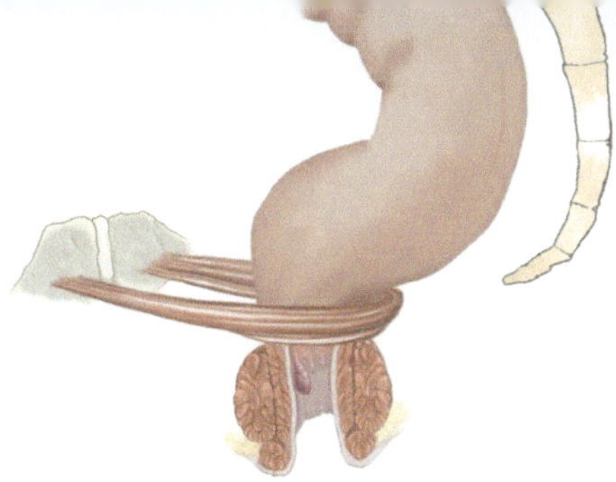

Section 4

Neoplasms

14

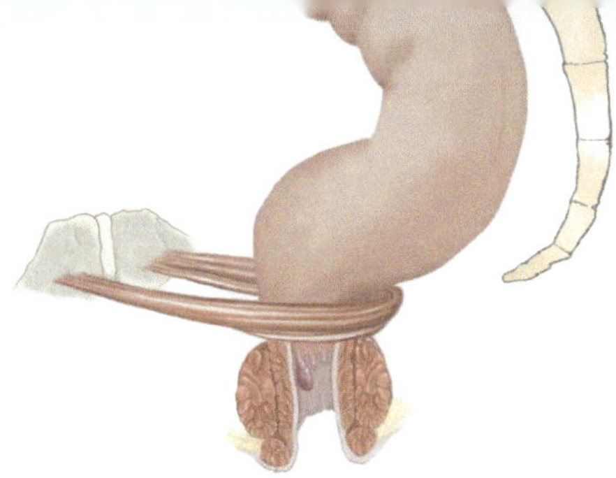

Anal Carcinoma

Zachary Yeung, MD; Tejal Mistry, MD; and Van Morris, MD

Key Points

- Anal cancer is a rare disease, with an increasing incidence in the United States and globally mediated by infection with human papillomavirus (HPV).
- Preventative vaccination against HPV is safe and effective and will decrease the global incidence of anal cancer in the decades to come.
- The majority of patients with locoregional anal cancer may be cured by treatment with concurrent chemoradiation. Abdominoperineal resection (APR) is reserved for recurrent and/or persistent disease following failure of chemoradiation.
- While cytotoxic chemotherapy has activity against metastatic anal cancer, novel immunotherapy approaches are promising and warrant further evaluation.

Anal carcinoma is a rare malignancy accounting for 2% to 3% of all gastrointestinal cancers.[1] In 2017, there were over 8000 new diagnoses of anal cancer in the United States, the majority in females, and an estimated 1000 deaths.[1] The annual incidence of anal carcinoma continues to increase, a trend noted over the past 40 years.[2-4] Anatomically, anal cancer is defined as a carcinoma arising distal to the dentate line, a specification distinguishing this disease from the more prevalent, neighboring rectal adenocarcinoma, and includes tumors of the anorectum from the anorectal ring to the anal verge.[5] Exterior anal margin cancers are treated akin to primary skin cancers. While mucosal melanomas, neuroendocrine cancers, and adenocarcinomas may arise in the anorectum, this chapter details squamous cell carcinoma of the anal canal (SCCA), the most common histologic subtype of anal cancer.

Qureshi W, ed. *Diagnosis and Management Guide for Anorectal Disease: A Clinical Reference* (pp 153-160).

Pathophysiology

By far, the strongest association for the development of anal cancer is infection with HPV,[6,7] which is responsible for greater than 90% of all SCCA cases.[8,9] Although HPV-16 is the most prevalent subtype,[10,11] other HPV subtypes, including HPV-18, -31, -33, -34, -45, -52, and -58, are also oncogenic drivers not only of SCCA, but also of head/neck, cervical, vaginal/vulvar, and penile cancers.[12] Other risk factors for the development of SCCA include a prior history of cervical cancer and/or high-grade intraepithelial neoplasia, an immunocompromised state (eg, concomitant HIV/AIDS or chronic immunosuppressant medications), prior/ongoing tobacco use, previous receptive anal intercourse, and history of a sexually transmitted disease.[13-16] Furthermore, an immunosuppressed state may predispose a patient to an impaired ability to eradicate high-risk HPV that eventually generates SCCA.[17,18]

HPV harbors a limited genome that must use replication proteins in the infected cell in order to proliferate.[19] The initial infection in the keratinized squamous epithelium occurs at sites of microtrauma whereby the virus enters into the basal layer of the skin. Here, basal cells manifest stem cell characteristics required for wound healing, and HPV successfully manipulates the proliferating nature of the basal layer for viral replication in order to amplify the episomal HPV copy number via the E1 polymerase.[20] As the HPV virions expand toward the exterior epithelium, HPV genes become activated to increase the viral copy number, produce viral capsid proteins, and shed new virus into adjacent keratinocytes for reinfection.[21] HPV oncoproteins E6 and E7 play an important role in cancer pathogenesis.[22] A major function of E6 is to bind p53 for degradation at the proteasome, essentially negating p53 activity to promote decreased apoptosis and increased cell survival of infected host cells.[23-25] Simultaneously, E7 inhibits the tumor suppressor activity of retinoblastoma and facilitates progression of the cell cycle to engender tumor cell proliferation and growth.[26] Immortalization of these tumor cells is also supported by the E6- and E7-mediated activation of the *Myc* oncogene[27] and by increased transcription of telomerase genes that maintain chromosomal length,[28] all with the ultimate result of producing a cancerous phenotype in the HPV-infected SCCA cells.

Indeed, the functional presence of these viral E6 and E7 proteins in the oncogenesis of SCCA is supported by the loss of function mutations in *TP53* and *CDKN2A* in HPV-negative anal cancers.[29] Collectively, these findings suggest that deregulation of p53 and loss of cell cycle control, whether by HPV viral oncoproteins or inactivating mutations, are essential in the cancer development of SCCA. Genomic analyses of SCCA have also revealed *PIK3CA* to be the most frequently mutated gene, occurring in about 30% of anal cancers[29,30] and promoting signaling of the phosphoinositide 3-kinase/mammalian target of rapamycin pathway, which is important in antiapoptotic tumor cell survival. Consistent with this finding, activating *PIK3CA* mutations are the most common genomic alteration in HPV-positive head/neck cancers[31] and cervical cancers,[32] suggesting an underlying commonality of pathogenic drivers among HPV-related malignancies. Indeed, anal cancers do not harbor high mutation burden; this is consistent with other HPV-associated cancers but different from non–HPV-related squamous cell lung cancers, which feature higher mutation burdens that may drive immunogenicity.[30]

Given the importance of HPV in SCCA oncogenesis, the recent development of a preventative HPV vaccine holds promise for reducing and even eradicating this disease in future decades. In 2014, a nonavalent vaccine against HPV subtypes 6, 11, 16, 18, 31, 33, 45, 52, and 58 was approved in the United States. HPV vaccination has been shown to decrease the incidence of high-grade, precancerous cervical, vaginal, and vulvar lesions in female adolescents[33] as well as high-grade anal intraepithelial neoplasia in adolescent and young men who have sex with men.[34] In 2018, the US Centers for Disease Control and Prevention recommended at least 2 doses of HPV vaccination for boys and girls as early as 9 years of age, prior to any HPV exposure; females between 13 and 26 years of age; males between 13 and 21 years of age who did not previously receive adequate vaccination; and gay, bisexual, transgender, or immunocompromised individuals 26 years of age or younger. The authors recommend referral to the Centers for Disease Control and Prevention's website for the most up-to-date recommendations regarding HPV vaccination, a likely cancer-sparing vaccine across all HPV-associated malignancies.

Signs and Symptoms

The median age of diagnosis for SCCA in the United States is 61 years.[1] Given the anatomic localization of anal cancers in the distal gastrointestinal tract, the most common symptoms at presentation for newly diagnosed SCCA are rectal bleeding and the perception of a mass in the rectal vault, often confused initially with other benign etiologies like hemorrhoids.[5] Patients may also note rectal pain, tenesmus, and changes in bowel patterns (eg, thinning of stool, sensation of incomplete evacuation, or more frequent bowel movements) at presentation. Systemic symptoms like unintentional weight loss, progressive exercise intolerance, anorexia, and bone pain warrant further consideration for distant disease.

Diagnosis/Diagnostic Evaluation

Patients presenting with such symptoms should undergo digital rectal examination to palpate for the presence of any mass. Visual inspection of the perineum should be undertaken to assess for any perianal tumor or an anal margin tumor. Given the lymph node drainage pattern for inferior rectal vessels to the external iliac and inguinal lymph nodes, examination for inguinal lymphadenopathy is a critical component of the initial visit.

Further evaluation with anoscopy or proctosigmoidoscopy is warranted for pathologic confirmation of invasive carcinoma and to identify the histologic subtype of anal cancer. Endoscopic evaluation should also report the luminal patency of the anorectum in the event that a diverting colostomy may be needed prior to treatment initiation, if pending obstruction is possible. Computed tomographic or positron emission tomographic imaging is recommended to finalize staging and to assess for the presence of distant metastases.[35,36] Alternatively, a biopsy of a palpable inguinal lymph node or distant metastatic tumor (if applicable) may confirm the presence and staging of SCCA based on the clinical impression. At our institution, we routinely check for the presence of HIV in all patients at the time of the initial evaluation given the higher risk of SCCA in HIV-infected patients. Female patients with newly diagnosed SCCA should be considered for gynecologic evaluation due to the possibility of field cancerization effects because oncogenic HPV is the predominant causative etiology for both cervical and anal cancers.

Treatment of Nonmetastatic Anal Cancer

Prior to the advent of multimodality therapy for nonmetastatic anal cancer, APR requiring a permanent colostomy was the standard treatment for patients with stage I to III anal cancer. The recurrence rates after APR were high, ranging as high as 70% in resected patients,[37] and highlighted the need for novel therapeutic approaches for the management of SCCA.

In 1974, Nigro and colleagues[38] reported a small series of 4 patients with newly diagnosed SCCA who received combined chemoradiation for their disease. Patients received a radiation dose of 30 Gy divided over 15 daily fractions and concurrent chemotherapy with 5-fluorouracil (days 1 to 5) and mitomycin C (day 1). Remarkably, all 4 patients, including one with oligometastatic disease, demonstrated complete clinical and/or pathologic responses to this treatment. Although the overall number of patients was small, this "Nigro protocol" irrevocably changed the paradigm for the treatment of SCCA by providing initial evidence that definitive chemoradiation may be curative and may spare some patients from surgery.[39,40]

To define better the roles of multimodality therapy in the management of untreated SCCA, the Anal Cancer Trial I (ACT I) investigated the added benefit of chemotherapy to radiation.[41] The trial included 577 patients with newly diagnosed, clinically (not radiographically) staged SCCA who were randomized to receive radiotherapy alone (45 Gy over 20 to 25 fractions) or radiotherapy with 5-fluorouracil and mitomycin C. Patients deemed to have a response after 6 weeks of completion of treatment were administered an additional boost of radiation. The long-term follow-up after 13 years revealed a 25% reduction in locoregional relapse for those patients treated with the combination of chemotherapy and radiation.[42] The results from this important trial emphasize that the addition of chemotherapy to radiation is beneficial for patients with newly diagnosed, untreated SCCA.

To optimize chemotherapy options, the Radiation Therapy Oncology Group 87-04/Eastern Cooperative Oncology Group 1289 Intergroup phase III trial randomized 310 patients with untreated, locoregional SCCA to chemoradiation with 5-fluorouracil alone or 5-fluorouracil in combination with mitomycin C.[43] Disease-free survival at 4 years (73% vs 51%) and the requirement of colostomy for recurrent disease (9% vs 22%) were both significantly improved for patients receiving the combination of 5-fluorouracil and mitomycin C. However, grade 4 and 5 toxicities were also higher in this group and emphasize the importance for close clinical evaluation of these patients while undergoing therapy. Ultimately, results from this trial can be applied to justify chemotherapy doublets for SCCA patients treated with chemoradiation.

The ACT II trial compared chemotherapy alternatives and assessed the use of maintenance chemotherapy following completion of chemoradiation for SCCA.[44] In this 2 × 2 study design, 940 patients with untreated, locoregional SCCA were randomized to receive chemoradiation with 5-fluorouracil plus mitomycin C or 5-fluorouracil plus cisplatin followed by a second randomization in which patients received 2 additional doses of maintenance 5-fluorouracil and cisplatin or no additional chemotherapy. The results indicated that no additional benefit in progression-free survival (but increased toxicity) was seen with maintenance chemotherapy after completion of definitive chemoradiation therapy. In addition, no differences in complete clinical response rates, rates of colostomy, or progression-free survival were seen for patients treated with 5-fluorouracil/mitomycin C relative to those treated with 5-fluorouracil/cisplatin as part of their chemoradiation, suggesting that the activities of these 2 chemotherapy doublets are similar. Importantly, the rates of grades 3 and 4 leukopenia were higher in the 5-fluorouracil/mitomycin C arm, suggesting that 5-fluorouracil/cisplatin may be the better tolerated option. Regardless, chemoradiation with 5-fluorouracil/mitomycin C with no maintenance chemotherapy remains the most commonly used regimen for locoregional SCCA at present in the United States, although 5-fluorouracil/cisplatin with radiation is equally effective and perhaps less toxic.

Post hoc analysis of the ACT II trial assessed 691 patients for response at weeks 11, 18, and 26 following the completion of treatment.[45] While 64% of patients had complete clinical responses by week 11, this rate increased to 85% by week 26 independent of any additional treatment. Given that the patients in the former group may have otherwise been referred for surgical resection after 3 months, these findings indicate that waiting a total of 6 months may render a substantial fraction of patients disease free and spare them an otherwise unnecessary surgery requiring a permanent colostomy. With APR being the recommendation for patients with persistent and/or recurrent SCCA following definitive chemoradiation, we apply these findings from the ACT II trial study to monitor for a complete clinical response up to 26 weeks after chemoradiation before referring for surgical intervention for disease failure.

Management of Metastatic Anal Cancer

Involvement by SCCA of distant organs often results in an incurable condition, necessitating the use of palliative systemic chemotherapy. As seen in Table 14-1, the reported data for the management of metastatic SCCA are sparse, with interpretation limited by small numbers of patients.[46-53]

Table 14-1

Systemic Options for Metastatic Anal Cancer

	AUTHOR	N	% RESPONSE
CISPLATIN/5-FLUOROURACIL	Ajani[46]	3	67
CISPLATIN/5-FLUOROURACIL	Faivre[47]	19	66
CARBOPLATIN/PACLITAXEL	Kim[48]	18	53
PACLITAXEL	Abbas[49]	7	57
CARBOPLATIN/PACLITAXEL/5-FLUOROURACIL	Hainsworth[50]	7	57
CISPLATIN/5-FLUOROURACIL	Eng[51]	42	53
CARBOPLATIN/PACLITAXEL	Eng[51]	24	31
NIVOLUMAB	Morris[52]	37	24
PEMBROLIZUMAB	Ott[53]	24	17

Cisplatin in combination with 5-fluorouracil remains the most commonly described regimen and has demonstrated efficacy in patients with metastatic SCCA. Carboplatin with paclitaxel also has activity in this setting and was found to have equivalent antitumor activity to cisplatin/5-fluorouracil in a phase II trial led by the International Rare Cancer Initiative in the frontline setting for patients with metastatic SCCA.[54]

A small fraction of patients with oligometastatic SCCA may be candidates for multimodality management including radiotherapy and/or surgical resection.[50] In a single-institution series of 77 patients with metastatic SCCA, 33 patients (43%) underwent multidisciplinary therapy for distant metastases, which was associated with an improved overall survival relative to patients receiving systemic chemotherapy alone (53 vs 17 months, respectively), with almost 30% of patients still alive after 6 years from the diagnosis of metastatic disease.

For patients with disease too advanced to undergo multimodality therapy, systemic options remain limited and emphasize the need for additional options in this metastatic SCCA setting. Given the role of HPV tumorigenesis in most SCCA cases, the use of immunotherapy (ie, immune checkpoint blockade agents that heighten the patient's own immune system to mediate an immune attack against the tumor[55]) warrants attention. Disruption of the programmed death-1 (PD-1):programmed death ligand-1 interaction has been associated with perpetuation of T-cell activity against tumor cells.[56] Anti–PD-1 antibodies like nivolumab and pembrolizumab augment the antitumor response by T cells and have activity in other advanced solid tumors like melanoma,[57] renal cell carcinoma,[58] non–small cell lung cancer,[59] urothelial cancer,[60] and head/neck cancers.[61] Given the immune recognition of viral antigens by T cells, it is plausible that anti–PD-1 therapy would likewise have benefit in SCCA.

Indeed, the National Cancer Institute 9673 phase II trial assessed nivolumab monotherapy in 37 patients with heavily pretreated metastatic SCCA.[51] Seven partial responses and 2 complete radiographic responses were observed for an overall response rate of 24%. The median reduction in tumor size from baseline among these responding patients was -70%. An additional 17 patients demonstrated stable disease for a disease control rate of 72%. The median progression-free survival was 4.1 months, and the median overall survival was 11 months. Correlative studies revealed that the presence of activated effector T cells with a PD-1:programmed death ligand-1 axis amenable to blockade within the tumor microenvironment prior to treatment initiation was associated with a response to treatment with nivolumab. A separate, smaller study assessing patients with metastatic anal cancer (including SCCAs and adenocarcinomas) showed similar responses with pembrolizumab.[52] Based on these results, anti–PD-1 monotherapy with nivolumab or pembrolizumab was added to the National Comprehensive Cancer Network Guidelines as a recommended therapy for refractory metastatic anal cancer.

Given the immunogenicity inherent to some HPV-associated cancers, other immunotherapy approaches have also been tested in this population. One series reported 9 patients with HPV-related unresectable cervical cancer treated with T cells reactive against HPV-specific E6 and E7 antigens.[62] Three of these patients had significant responses to this adoptive T-cell therapy, 2 of which were durable complete responses. The application of these results in larger series for all HPV-associated malignancies including SCCA is warranted. With coordinated efforts through the International Rare Cancer Initiative Consortium, novel immunotherapeutic approaches incorporating immune checkpoint blockade agents and adoptive T-cell therapy hold great promise for improving survival outcomes in the future for patients with metastatic SCCA and possibly to extend benefit to patients with locoregional anal cancer.

References

1. Siegel RL, Miller KD, Jemal A. Cancer statistics, 2017. *CA Cancer J Clin.* 2017;67(1):7-30.
2. Johnson LG, Madeleine MM, Newcomer LM, Schwartz SM, Daling JR. Anal cancer incidence and survival: the surveillance, epidemiology, and end results experience, 1973-2000. *Cancer.* 2004;101(2):281-288.
3. Nelson RA, Levine AM, Bernstein L, Smith DD, Lai LL. Changing patterns of anal canal carcinoma in the United States. *J Clin Oncol.* 2013;31(12):1569-1575.
4. Shiels MS, Kreimer AR, Coghill AE, Darragh TM, Devesa SS. Anal cancer incidence in the United States, 1977-2011: distinct patterns by histology and behavior. *Cancer Epidemiol Biomarkers Prev.* 2015;24(10):1548-1556.
5. Ryan DP, Compton CC, Mayer RJ. Carcinoma of the anal canal. *N Engl J Med.* 2000;342(11):792-800.
6. Frisch M, Glimelius B, van den Brule AJ, et al. Sexually transmitted infection as a cause of anal cancer. *N Engl J Med.* 1997;337(19):1350-1358.
7. De Vuyst H, Clifford GM, Nascimento MC, Madeleine MM, Franceschi S. Prevalence and type distribution of human papillomavirus in carcinoma and intraepithelial neoplasia of the vulva, vagina and anus: a meta-analysis. *Int J Cancer.* 2009;124(7):1626-1636.
8. Morris VK, Rashid A, Rodriguez-Bigas M, et al. Clinicopathologic features associated with human papillomavirus/p16 in patients with metastatic squamous cell carcinoma of the anal canal. *Oncologist.* 2015;20(11):1247-1252.
9. Serup-Hansen E, Linnemann D, Skovrider-Ruminski W, Hogdall E, Geertsen PF, Havsteen H. Human papillomavirus genotyping and p16 expression as prognostic factors for patients with American Joint Committee on Cancer stages I to III carcinoma of the anal canal. *J Clin Oncol.* 2014;32(17):1812-1817.
10. Steinau M, Unger ER, Hernandez BY, et al. Human papillomavirus prevalence in invasive anal cancers in the United States before vaccine introduction. *J Low Genit Tract Dis.* 2013;17(4):397-403.
11. Hoots BE, Palefsky JM, Pimenta JM, Smith JS. Human papillomavirus type distribution in anal cancer and anal intraepithelial lesions. *Int J Cancer.* 2009;124(10):2375-2383.
12. Doorbar J, Egawa N, Griffin H, Kranjec C, Murakami I. Human papillomavirus molecular biology and disease association. *Rev Med Virol.* 2015;25(suppl 1):2-23.
13. Daling JR, Madeleine MM, Johnson LG, et al. Human papillomavirus, smoking, and sexual practices in the etiology of anal cancer. *Cancer.* 2004;101(2):270-280.
14. Jimenez W, Paszat L, Kupets R, Wilton A, Tinmouth J. Presumed previous human papillomavirus (HPV) related gynecological cancer in women diagnosed with anal cancer in the province of Ontario. *Gynecol Oncol.* 2009;114(3):395-398.
15. Sunesen KG, Norgaard M, Thorlacius-Ussing O, Laurberg S. Immunosuppressive disorders and risk of anal squamous cell carcinoma: a nationwide cohort study in Denmark, 1978-2005. *Int J Cancer.* 2010;127(3):675-684.
16. Frisch M, Biggar RJ, Goedert JJ. Human papillomavirus-associated cancers in patients with human immunodeficiency virus infection and acquired immunodeficiency syndrome. *J Natl Cancer Inst.* 2000;92(18):1500-1510.
17. Patel P, Hanson DL, Sullivan PS, et al. Incidence of types of cancer among HIV-infected persons compared with the general population in the United States, 1992-2003. *Ann Intern Med.* 2008;148(10):728-736.

18. zur Hausen H. Papillomaviruses and cancer: from basic studies to clinical application. *Nat Rev Cancer.* 2002;2(5):342-350.
19. Moody CA, Laimins LA. Human papillomavirus oncoproteins: pathways to transformation. *Nat Rev Cancer.* 2010;10(8):550-560.
20. Chow LT, Broker TR, Steinberg BM. The natural history of human papillomavirus infections of the mucosal epithelia. *APMIS.* 2010;118(6-7):422-449.
21. Stanley MA. Epithelial cell responses to infection with human papillomavirus. *Clin Microbiol Rev.* 2012;25(2):215-222.
22. McLaughlin-Drubin ME, Munger K. Oncogenic activities of human papillomaviruses. *Virus Res.* 2009;143(2):195-208.
23. Huibregtse JM, Scheffner M, Howley PM. A cellular protein mediates association of p53 with the E6 oncoprotein of human papillomavirus types 16 or 18. *EMBO J.* 1991;10(13):4129-4135.
24. Scheffner M, Werness BA, Huibregtse JM, Levine AJ, Howley PM. The E6 oncoprotein encoded by human papillomavirus types 16 and 18 promotes the degradation of p53. *Cell.* 1990;63(6):1129-1136.
25. Scheffner M, Huibregtse JM, Vierstra RD, Howley PM. The HPV-16 E6 and E6-AP complex functions as a ubiquitin-protein ligase in the ubiquitination of p53. *Cell.* 1993;75(3):495-505.
26. Jones DL, Thompson DA, Munger K. Destabilization of the RB tumor suppressor protein and stabilization of p53 contribute to HPV type 16 E7-induced apoptosis. *Virology.* 1997;239(1):97-107.
27. Howie HL, Katzenellenbogen RA, Galloway DA. Papillomavirus E6 proteins. *Virology.* 2009;384(2):324-334.
28. Zhang A, Wang J, Zheng B, et al. Telomere attrition predominantly occurs in precursor lesions during in vivo carcinogenic process of the uterine cervix. *Oncogene.* 2004;23(44):7441-7447.
29. Chung JH, Sanford E, Johnson A, et al. Comprehensive genomic profiling of anal squamous cell carcinoma reveals distinct genomically defined classes. *Ann Oncol.* 2016;27(7):1336-1341.
30. Morris V, Rao X, Pickering C, et al. Comprehensive genomic profiling of metastatic squamous cell carcinoma of the anal canal. *Mol Cancer Res.* 2017;15(11):1542-1550.
31. Cancer Genome Atlas Network. Comprehensive genomic characterization of head and neck squamous cell carcinomas. *Nature.* 2015;517(7536):576-582.
32. Cancer Genome Atlas Research Network, Albert Einstein College of Medicine, Analytical Biological Services, et al. Integrated genomic and molecular characterization of cervical cancer. *Nature.* 2017;543(7645):378-384.
33. Joura EA, Giuliano AR, Iversen OE, et al. A 9-valent HPV vaccine against infection and intraepithelial neoplasia in women. *N Engl J Med.* 2015;372(8):711-723.
34. Palefsky JM, Giuliano AR, Goldstone S, et al. HPV vaccine against anal HPV infection and anal intraepithelial neoplasia. *N Engl J Med.* 2011;365(17):1576-1585.
35. Cotter SE, Grigsby PW, Siegel BA, et al. FDG-PET/CT in the evaluation of anal carcinoma. *Int J Radiat Oncol Biol Phys.* 2006;65(3):720-725.
36. Jones M, Hruby G, Solomon M, Rutherford N, Martin J. The role of FDG-PET in the initial staging and response assessment of anal cancer: a systematic review and meta-analysis. *Ann Surg Oncol.* 2015;22(11):3574-3581.
37. Boman BM, Moertel CG, O'Connell MJ, et al. Carcinoma of the anal canal. A clinical and pathologic study of 188 cases. *Cancer.* 1984;54(1):114-125.
38. Nigro ND, Vaitkevicius VK, Considine B Jr. Combined therapy for cancer of the anal canal: a preliminary report. *Dis Colon Rectum.* 1974;17(3):354-356.
39. Cummings BJ, Keane TJ, O'Sullivan B, Wong CS, Catton CN. Epidermoid anal cancer: treatment by radiation alone or by radiation and 5-fluorouracil with and without mitomycin C. *Int J Radiat Oncol Biol Phys.* 1991;21(5):1115-1125.
40. Papillon J, Chassard JL. Respective roles of radiotherapy and surgery in the management of epidermoid carcinoma of the anal margin. Series of 57 patients. *Dis Colon Rectum.* 1992;35(5):422-429.
41. Epidermoid anal cancer: results from the UKCCCR randomised trial of radiotherapy alone versus radiotherapy, 5-fluorouracil, and mitomycin. UKCCCR Anal Cancer Trial Working Party. UK Co-ordinating Committee on Cancer Research. *Lancet.* 1996;348(9034):1049-1054.
42. Northover J, Glynne-Jones R, Sebag-Montefiore D, et al. Chemoradiation for the treatment of epidermoid anal cancer: 13-year follow-up of the first randomised UKCCCR Anal Cancer Trial (ACT I). *Br J Cancer.* 2010;102(7):1123-1128.
43. Flam M, John M, Pajak TF, et al. Role of mitomycin in combination with fluorouracil and radiotherapy, and of salvage chemoradiation in the definitive nonsurgical treatment of epidermoid carcinoma of the anal canal: results of a phase III randomized intergroup study. *J Clin Oncol.* 1996;14(9):2527-2539.
44. James RD, Glynne-Jones R, Meadows HM, et al. Mitomycin or cisplatin chemoradiation with or without maintenance chemotherapy for treatment of squamous-cell carcinoma of the anus (ACT II): a randomised, phase 3, open-label, 2 × 2 factorial trial. *Lancet Oncol.* 2013;14(6):516-524.
45. Glynne-Jones R, Sebag-Montefiore D, Meadows HM, et al. Best time to assess complete clinical response after chemoradiotherapy in squamous cell carcinoma of the anus (ACT II): a post-hoc analysis of randomised controlled phase 3 trial. *Lancet Oncol.* 2017;18(3):347-356.

46. Ajani JA, Carrasco CH, Jackson DE, Wallace S. Combination of cisplatin plus fluoropyrimidine chemotherapy effective against liver metastases from carcinoma of the anal canal. *Am J Med.* 1989;87(2):221-224.
47. Faivre C, Rougier P, Ducreux M, et al. [5-fluorouracile and cisplatinum combination chemotherapy for metastatic squamous-cell anal cancer]. *Bull Cancer.* 1999;86(10):861-865.
48. Kim R, Byer J, Fulp WJ, Mahipal A, Dinwoodie W, Shibata D. Carboplatin and paclitaxel treatment is effective in advanced anal cancer. *Oncology.* 2014;87(2):125-132.
49. Abbas A, Nehme E, Fakih M. Single-agent paclitaxel in advanced anal cancer after failure of cisplatin and 5-fluorouracil chemotherapy. *Anticancer Res.* 2011;31(12):4637-4640.
50. Hainsworth JD, Burris HA 3rd, Meluch AA, Baker MN, Morrissey LH, Greco FA. Paclitaxel, carboplatin, and long-term continuous infusion of 5-fluorouracil in the treatment of advanced squamous and other selected carcinomas: results of a Phase II trial. *Cancer.* 2001;92(3):642-649.
51. Eng C, Chang GJ, You YN, et al. The role of systemic chemotherapy and multidisciplinary management in improving the overall survival of patients with metastatic squamous cell carcinoma of the anal canal. *Oncotarget.* 2014;5(22):11133-11142.
52. Morris VK, Salem ME, Nimeiri H, et al. Nivolumab for previously treated unresectable metastatic anal cancer (NCI9673): a multicentre, single-arm, phase 2 study. *Lancet Oncol.* 2017;18(4):446-453.
53. Ott PA, Piha-Paul SA, Munster P, et al. Safety and antitumor activity of the anti-PD-1 antibody pembrolizumab in patients with recurrent carcinoma of the anal canal. *Ann Oncol.* 2017;28(5):1036-1041.
54. Rao S, Sclafani F, Eng C, et al. InterAACT: A multicentre open label randomised phase II advanced anal cancer trial of cisplatin (CDDP) plus 5-fluorouracil (5-FU) vs carboplatin (C) plus weekly paclitaxel (P) in patients (pts) with inoperable locally recurrent (ILR) or metastatic treatment naïve disease: an International Rare Cancers Initiative (IRCI) trial. *Annals of Oncology.* 2018;29(suppl_8). https://doi.org/10.1093/annonc/mdy424.022
55. Ishida Y, Agata Y, Shibahara K, Honjo T. Induced expression of PD-1, a novel member of the immunoglobulin gene superfamily, upon programmed cell death. *EMBO J.* 1992;11(11):3887-3895.
56. Freeman GJ, Long AJ, Iwai Y, et al. Engagement of the PD-1 immunoinhibitory receptor by a novel B7 family member leads to negative regulation of lymphocyte activation. *J Exp Med.* 2000;192(7):1027-1034.
57. Larkin J, Chiarion-Sileni V, Gonzalez R, et al. Combined Nivolumab and Ipilimumab or Monotherapy in Untreated Melanoma. *N Engl J Med.* 2015;373(1):23-34.
58. Motzer RJ, Escudier B, McDermott DF, et al. Nivolumab versus Everolimus in Advanced Renal-Cell Carcinoma. *N Engl J Med.* 2015;373(19):1803-1813.
59. Brahmer J, Reckamp KL, Baas P, et al. Nivolumab versus docetaxel in advanced squamous-cell non-small-cell lung cancer. *N Engl J Med.* 2015;373(2):123-135.
60. Rosenberg JE, Hoffman-Censits J, Powles T, et al. Atezolizumab in patients with locally advanced and metastatic urothelial carcinoma who have progressed following treatment with platinum-based chemotherapy: a single-arm, multicentre, phase 2 trial. *Lancet.* 2016;387(10031):1909-1920.
61. Ferris RL, Blumenschein G Jr, Fayette J, et al. Nivolumab for recurrent squamous-cell carcinoma of the head and neck. *N Engl J Med.* 2016;375(19):1856-1867.
62. Stevanovic S, Draper LM, Langhan MM, et al. Complete regression of metastatic cervical cancer after treatment with human papillomavirus-targeted tumor-infiltrating T cells. *J Clin Oncol.* 2015;33(14):1543-1550.

15

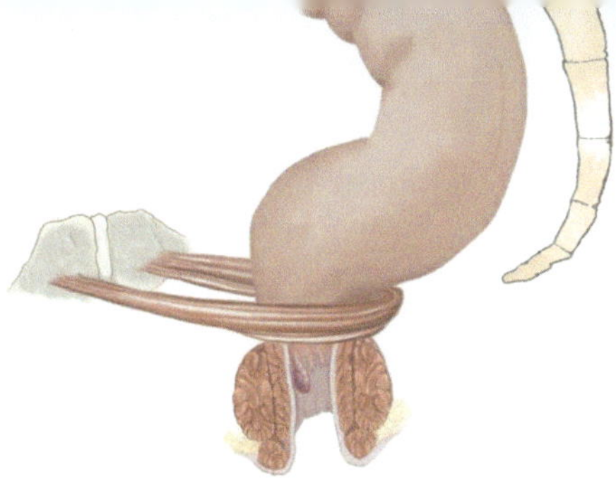

Rectal Cancer

Yasser Shaib, MD, MPH, FASGE and
Samer Doughan, MD, FRCSEd (Gen Surg)

Key Points

- Rectal cancers comprise one-third of all colorectal cancers.
- The workup should include a good rectal examination, endoscopic evaluation, and imaging as needed.
- Treatment options are highly dependent on accurate staging.
- Distant metastasis can be evaluated by computed tomographic (CT) scanning.
- Local staging is best achieved by magnetic resonance imaging (MRI) and endoscopic ultrasound (EUS) (MRI for detailed information when the disease is locally advanced and EUS for early lesions).
- Local excision should be considered for very early cancers with favorable pathologic features.
- Total mesorectal excision (TME) is the gold standard surgery. It is advocated in early cancers and following neoadjuvant treatment for locally advanced cancers.
- Organ preservation is to be considered in patients with a complete clinical response following neoadjuvant treatment.
- Close periodic follow-up is essential to detect recurrence and survey for new lesions.

Rectal cancers comprise around one-third of all colorectal cancers.[1] Unique anatomic and oncologic features greatly impact the management of rectal cancer and separate it from cancer elsewhere in the colon. This chapter focuses on the clinical features and management of rectal adenocarcinoma, which is the most common pathology of rectal cancers. Other pathologies include squamous cancers, carcinoids, lymphomas, and sarcomas.

Qureshi W, ed. *Diagnosis and Management Guide for Anorectal Disease: A Clinical Reference* (pp 161-172).

The treatment of rectal cancer has evolved markedly over the last 2 decades, and recent advances in imaging and improved surgical techniques provide clinicians with multiple options for treatment. However, rectal cancer still poses a challenging management dilemma. Optimal and successful management of rectal cancer requires careful investigation that includes accurate disease staging and patient assessment; evidence-based treatment planning that incorporates surgery, chemotherapy, and radiotherapy; and vigilant follow-up. This is best achieved using a multidisciplinary approach.

Epidemiology

Worldwide colorectal cancer is the third most common cancer in men and the second most common in women. Around 38,000 cases of rectal cancer were diagnosed in 2014, representing 28% of all colorectal cancer cases in the United States.[2] However, despite the decrease in overall incidence, some interesting trends have been reported for rectal cancer. For example, rectal cancer has been increasing in younger adults. A study examining surveillance, epidemiology, and end results data found that the age-adjusted incidence rates of rectal cancer have increased by 3.2% per year from 1974 to 2013 in adults 20 to 29 years of age. Similar trends were observed in all age groups below 55 years of age. Compared with 1989 to 1990, the proportion of rectal cancer diagnosed in adults younger than 55 years of age doubled from 14.6% to 29.2% in 2012 to 2013.[3] In addition, discrepancies in epidemiology and survival exist between different racial and ethnic groups, with African Americans having higher incidence and mortality rates when compared with others.[4] The recent application of universal screening and improving treatment outcomes are credited for increased early detection and improved survival.

Pathophysiology

While the management of rectal cancer differs markedly from cancers in the rest of the colon, they share the same risk factors, and pathogenesis appears to be the same. Most rectal cancers arise from pre-existing adenomas. Neoplastic changes involving the mucosal epithelium progress grow and eventually become invasive, invading the lymphovascular channels and adjacent lymph nodes. Rectal anatomy and blood supply allow cancers to advance locally and metastasize distantly. The anatomic restrictions (pelvic structures) and the absence of serosa confine rectal tumors and permit early local invasion.

The blood supply of the rectum provides means for distant metastasis. Low rectal cancers can metastasize to the liver through the superior hemorrhoidal vein/portal vein or the lungs through the middle hemorrhoidal vein/vena cava. Lesions located in the middle and upper rectum metastasize hematogenously to the liver through the portal circulation.

Risk factors for rectal cancer are not well defined and are usually combined with colon cancer. It is likely that a combination of environmental and genetic factors plays a role in the genesis of colorectal cancers. Several studies have examined the role of diet and lifestyle in colorectal cancer. These studies support the role of a high-fat, low-fiber diet as well as red meat consumption as strong risk factors for colorectal cancer. Alcohol, smoking, and diabetes mellitus are also associated with an increased risk of colorectal cancer.[5]

On the other hand, the use of aspirin, nonsteroidal anti-inflammatory drugs, and calcium supplements was found to be protective. Other dietary elements such as diets rich in carotene, fiber, vitamins (C, E, and D), and green vegetables might provide additional protection against colorectal cancer.[6-8] Similarly, healthy lifestyles with vigorous exercise and lean body mass provide additional protection.

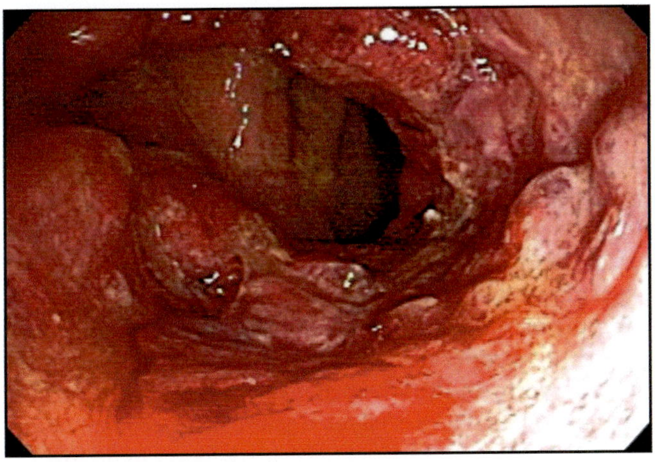

Figure 15-1. A large circumferential rectal cancer involving mid and upper rectum.

While most of these studies have examined both colon and rectal cancers together, there are data to suggest that their impact might differ between the two. For example, systematic reviews and meta-analyses of epidemiological studies suggest that, at least in Western countries, physical activity decreased the risk of colon cancer, but not of rectal cancer.[9]

In addition, some unique associations (risk and protection) for rectal cancers have been described. For example, one study found that there was no clear association between smokeless cigarette use and colorectal cancer overall. However, exclusive current smokeless cigarette users had an increased risk of rectal cancer.[10] Another study that examined coffee and tea as risk factors for colon and rectal cancers found that high coffee intake (6 cups or more) was negatively associated with the risk of colon cancer (protective) compared with low intake (1 cup or fewer). There was, however, no association with rectal cancer. For tea, the associations were the opposite; there was no association with colon cancer risk and a negative association for rectal cancer for individuals drinking 2 or more cups/day when compared with those drinking none.[11]

Signs and Symptoms

Patients with rectal cancer can present with a wide range of symptoms. These include rectal bleeding, change in bowel habits, tenesmus, and new-onset constipation. Advanced cancers can invade adjacent structures and cause pelvic and sacral pain.

Most of the early symptoms mimic those of benign conditions, such as hemorrhoids or functional bowel disorders, which might cause a delay in diagnosis. It is important that patients at risk (those with a family history or older age) be evaluated promptly. When rectal cancer is suspected, the workup should start with a thorough physical examination including rectal examination and be completed with a colonoscopy. In low-risk individuals with rectal bleeding, flexible sigmoidoscopy might be sufficient.

Diagnosis

Diagnosis is usually established via endoscopy with biopsy. On endoscopy, rectal cancers appear as large, irregular ulcerated masses, stenotic strictures, or polypoid lesions (Figure 15-1). Extensive biopsies should be taken to establish a diagnosis beyond doubt and to rule out other less likely diagnoses. The differential diagnosis includes carcinoids, stromal tumors, squamous cell carcinoma, Kaposi sarcoma (in HIV patients), lymphoma, and metastatic cancers.

Workup and Evaluation

The initial workup of rectal cancer should include a dedicated rectal examination followed by a detailed endoscopic evaluation. The rectal examination should assess the distance from the anal verge, tumor fixation, and sphincter function.

The endoscopist should make every effort to provide accurate specific information that is crucial in the management of rectal cancer patients. The endoscopist should report the exact location of the lesion from the anal verge. It is presumed that rigid sigmoidoscopy provides a better estimate than flexible sigmoidoscopy, which tends to overestimate the distance from the anal verge; however, data comparing the two are not available. Endoscopic marking with India ink tattooing is highly recommended, especially for small lesions and those in the upper rectum. This will aid in identification of the site for future reference and will aid in surgery, especially if the patient is to receive neoadjuvant therapy in which the lesion itself could disappear or if surgery is planned as the first step. Evaluation of the rest of the colon is mandatory to rule out synchronous lesions, which are found in up to 10% of cases.

When a diagnosis of rectal cancer is confirmed, carcinoembryonic antigen (CEA) levels must be obtained. These levels correlate well with the presence of advanced disease and liver metastasis and are very useful for the follow-up of patients, including those who did not have elevated CEA pretreatment.

There are several scenarios in which newly diagnosed rectal neoplasm is encountered. These include large polyps, polyps with high-grade dysplasia, unexpected cancer in a polyp, and malignancies other than adenocarcinoma such as metastatic disease or less common pathologies. Our discussion focuses on patients in whom rectal adenocarcinoma is diagnosed.

Staging

Staging of rectal cancer follows the TNM staging system and is crucial in planning therapy (Table 15-1). Disease in general is classified into 3 broad categories: early localized, locally advanced, and metastatic, with approximately 45%, 35%, and 20% of patients in each group, respectively. Staging should start with a contrast-enhanced CT scan of the abdomen and pelvis. This will help assess locoregional extension as well as distant metastasis to the liver. A chest x-ray or CT scan of the chest should be performed to evaluate for lung metastasis.

In the absence of distance metastasis, locoregional staging becomes of paramount importance because it dictates the type and sequence of treatment. Depth of invasion (T stage) and nodal involvement (N stage) are key pieces of information when planning treatment. The accuracy of CT imaging is low for these purposes and does not exceed 70%. This information can be better obtained by EUS (Figure 15-2) or MRI (Figure 15-3).

Multiple studies have evaluated the performance of EUS and MRI in this setting. The reported overall accuracy of EUS for T staging is around 90% (96% sensitivity and 90% specificity), which compared favorably with MRI (83% accuracy, 94% sensitivity, and 67% specificity).[12] More recently, the utilization of high-resolution MRI provided more accurate evaluation of depth of invasion of up to 1 mm of histopathology assessment.

The overall accuracy of EUS varies across different T stages. One report that pooled data from several studies estimates that accuracy to be 88% for T1, 78% for T2, 85% for T3, and 80% for T4.[12] EUS appears to be superior in evaluating early cancers and distinguishing T2 lesions from T1 and T3 cancers, whereas MRI provides better detailed information when adjacent organs are involved (T4) and when assessing lymphovascular invasion and/or resection margins.

Table 15-1

TNM Staging of Rectal Cancer

STAGE	T	N	M
0	Tis	N0	M0
I	T1, T2	N0	M0
IIA	T3	N0	M0
IIB	T4a	N0	M0
IIC	T4b	N0	M0
IIIA	T1-T2 T1	N1 N2a	M0
IIIB	T3-T4a T2-T3 T1-T2	N1 N2a N2b	M0
IIIC	T4a T3-T4a T4b	N2a N2b N1-N2	M0
IVA	Any T	Any N	M1a
IVB	Any T	Any N	M1b
IVC	Any T	Any N	M1c

T	T CRITERIA
TX	Primary tumor cannot be assessed
T0	No evidence of primary tumor
Tis	Carcinoma in situ, intramucosal carcinoma (involvement of lamina propria with no extension through muscularis mucosae)
T1	Tumor invades the submucosa (through the muscularis mucosa but not into the muscularis propria)
T2	Tumor invades the muscularis propria
T3	Tumor invades through the muscularis propria into perirectal tissues
T4	Tumor invades adjacent organ or structure

N	N CRITERIA
NX	Regional lymph nodes cannot be assessed
N0	No regional lymph node metastasis
N1	One to three regional lymph nodes are positive (tumor in lymph nodes measuring ≥0.2 mm), or any number of tumor deposits are present and all identifiable lymph nodes are negative
N1a	1 regional lymph node is positive
N1b	2 or 3 regional lymph nodes are positive

(continued)

Table 15-1 (continued)

TNM Staging of Rectal Cancer

N	N CRITERIA
N1c	No regional lymph nodes are positive, but there are tumor deposits in the subserosa, mesentery, or perirectal/mesorectal tissues
N2	4 or more regional nodes are positive
N2a	4 to 6 regional lymph nodes are positive
N2b	7 or more regional lymph nodes are positive
M	**M CRITERIA**
M0	No distant metastasis by imaging, etc, no evidence of tumor in distant sites or organs (this category is not assigned by pathologists)
M1	Metastasis to 1 or more distant sites or organs or peritoneal metastasis is identified
M1a	Metastasis to 1 site or organ is identified without peritoneal metastasis
M1b	Metastasis to 2 or more sites or organs is identified without peritoneal metastasis
M1c	Metastasis to the peritoneal surface is identified alone or with other site or organ metastases

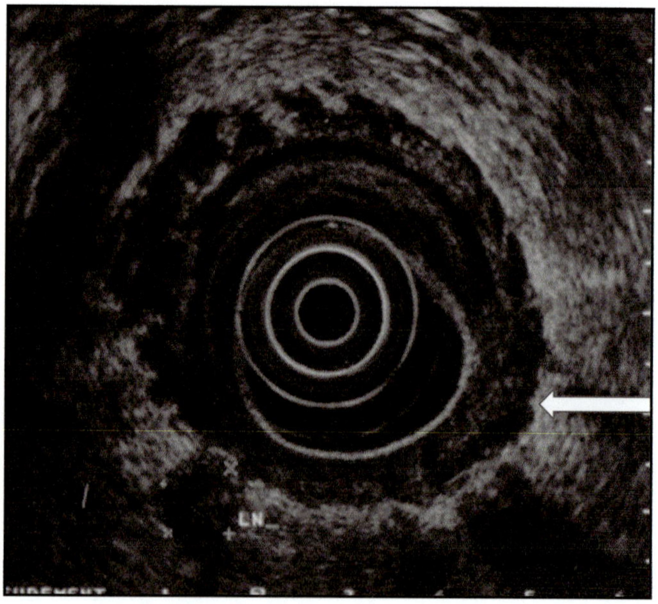

Figure 15-2. A T3 rectal tumor exhibiting the classic extensions (pseudopodia) into the perirectal fat (arrow). A round, hypoechoic perirectal lymph node (LN) is noted adjacent to the cancer.

For nodal involvement, the 2 modalities are comparable, with an overall accuracy of around 80%. EUS has an overall accuracy of around 75% with a sensitivity and specificity of 73% and 75%, respectively, according to one meta-analysis.[13] In general, it is useful in diagnosing nodal involvement rather than excluding it. However, EUS utility is limited to the perirectal area, whereas MRI can provide information about nodes in the entire mesorectum and surrounding compartments.

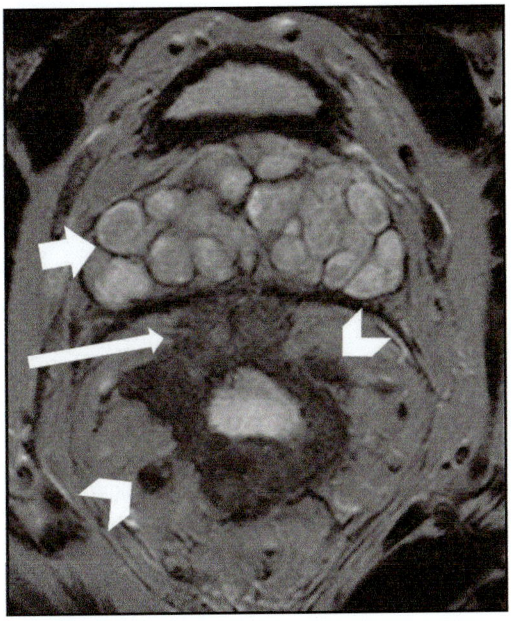

Figure 15-3. Short axis T2-weighted MRI of T4 rectal cancer. A large anterior rectal tumor (long white arrow) involves the adjacent seminal vesicles (short white arrows). There is an enlarged mesorectal lymph node and a tumor deposit (white arrowheads).

For early lesions in which surgery or local excision is considered the first step in treatment, EUS is likely to provide more useful information. It is worth noting that EUS is operator dependent, and its accuracy increases with an increased volume of cases performed.[14]

For presumably advanced lesions, it is recommended to obtain MRI of the pelvis and add EUS if additional information is needed. With diffusion-weighted imaging, MRI is also useful in assessing resectability and response to neoadjuvant therapy. For adequate quality, an MRI report is expected to provide information on the tumor height (from anal verge), size, circumference, T stage, and infiltration depth beyond the muscularis propria. Nodal disease should be described, including the number, size, borders, and distance from the tumor. In addition, extramural vascular invasion and the circumferential resection margin (CRM) should be reported.[15]

Evaluation of Response to Treatment

The evaluation of response to treatment after chemoradiation is another challenging task and is affected by peritumoral inflammation, edema, necrosis, and fibrosis that occur after therapy. These changes limit the ability of all imaging modalities to differentiate neoplastic processes from inflammation. One study that evaluated the performance of EUS staging after therapy found that EUS correctly predicted a complete response to chemoradiation in only 63% of cases, and its overall accuracy for pathologic T stage was 48%, with understaging occurring in 14% of cases and overstaging in 38%.[16] Another study that compared sensitivity and specificity of EUS and MRI in patients with locally advanced rectal cancer after therapy found that the accuracy of both EUS and MRI in patients who received neoadjuvant treatment was unsatisfactory (around 45%) in evaluating residual tumors.[17]

Treatment (Figure 15-4)

The treatment of rectal cancer has been revolutionized after the concept of TME was introduced by Bill Heald.[18] TME dissection includes 4 pillars: sharp dissection, clear radial margins, intact mesorectum, and preserved autonomic nerves. The evident improvement in local recurrence and overall

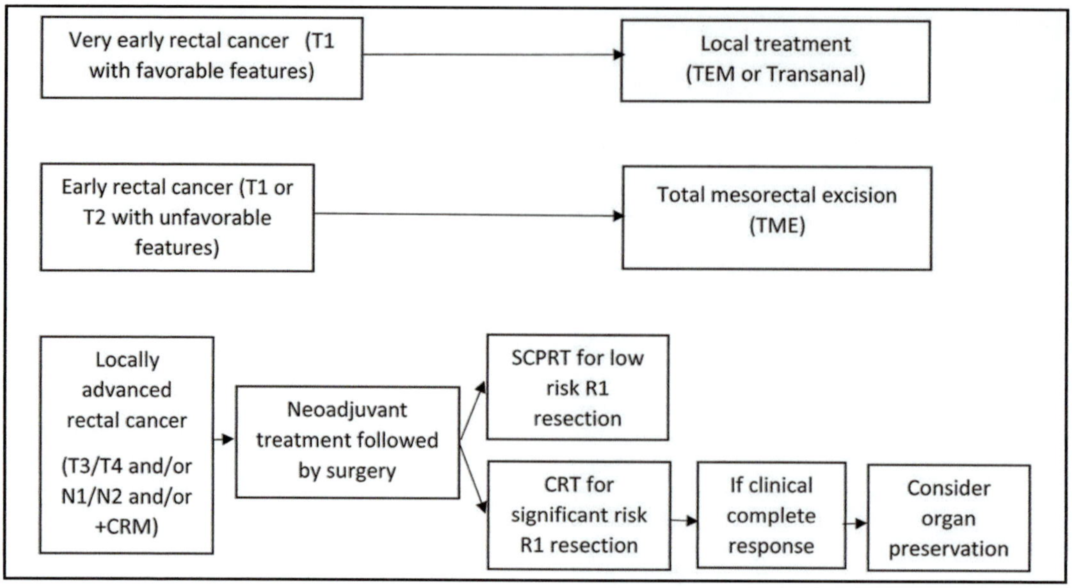

Figure 15-4. Concise schematic guideline for treatment of nonmetastatic rectal cancer.

survival[19] has led to worldwide acceptance of this technique. The data published from major colorectal centers[20-22] after the adoption of TME made it the cornerstone of rectal cancer surgery. For ultralow rectal cancers in which sphincter saving is not an option, abdominoperineal excision (APER) should be performed starting with TME and extended in a cylindrical fashion, preserving all the fascial envelopes of the rectum.

Neoadjuvant treatment following the encouraging results of the Swedish Rectal Cancer Trial[23] led to more trials in operable rectal cancer. Over the years, different modalities of neoadjuvant treatment have allowed clinicians to push the boundaries of treatment, permitting for more sphincter-saving surgeries and allowing for consideration of the option of no surgical treatment.

Optimal treatment decisions of rectal cancer should take into account the stage, size, and position of the tumor. These are best reached following extensive discussion at a multidisciplinary meeting by a team that includes surgeons, endoscopists, oncologists, radiologists, pathologists, and colorectal nurses. The consensus should be based on the extensive preoperative assessment and the ability to achieve complete resection and should take into consideration the patient's wishes and expectations.

In general, the treatment of rectal cancer can be divided into 2 large groups: the first includes those patients in whom surgery is the first line of treatment, and the other includes patients in whom neoadjuvant treatment is a must.

The treatment of patients with metastatic disease is discussed separately.

VERY EARLY RECTAL CANCER

The treatment of very early rectal cancer, defined as T1 cancer with favorable features (good cellular differentiation, absent lymphovascular invasion, and cell budding), is a simple local resection. This is usually performed either transanally or through endoscopic microsurgery.[24,25] Transanal endoscopic microsurgery (TEM) can permit accurate full-thickness local excision of the rectal tumor with outcomes very similar to standard TME without compromising anorectal function.

EARLY RECTAL CANCER

Early rectal cancer defined as T1 or T2 with less favorable features (poor cellular proliferation and/or the presence of lymphovascular invasion and/or cell budding) should be treated with formal TME resection because of the higher risk of local recurrence and the higher risk of lymph node involvement. TME can be performed either in an open or laparoscopic fashion depending on the surgeon's experience. Multiple trials (Colorectal Cancer Laparoscopic or Open Resection II, Conventional versus Laparoscopic-Assisted Surgery in Colorectal Cancer, Australasian Laparoscopic Cancer of the Rectum, etc)[26-29] have been conducted across the world and confirmed the feasibility and safety of laparoscopic surgery in rectal cancer.

For low rectal tumors, both transanal TME and robotic surgery have an important advantage of better access and exposure to the pelvis, allowing for better control of the tumor. Transanal TME still requires standardization, whereas the role of robotic surgery remains under investigation.[30] It is recommended that surgeons performing such meticulous procedures (TME or APER), whether open, laparoscopic, or robotic, be able to audit and show their outcomes in these difficult cases.

There is a potential role for TEM in T2 disease in frail or elderly patients in whom a major surgery might have an impact on their welfare. However, fit patients with T2 disease should not be offered TEM outside of an approved and well-controlled study.

LOCALLY ADVANCED RECTAL CANCER

Locally advanced rectal cancer either in size (T3-T4) or in the presence of nodal disease (N1 or N2) or threatened margins (+ CRM) should be considered candidates for neoadjuvant treatment. These will have to be divided after thorough MRI examination into tumors with nodal disease, bulky tumors with negative margins, and advanced tumors with threatened or positive margins.

Two different schedules of preoperative therapy are standards of care:

1. Short-course preoperative radiotherapy (SCPRT) with a 25-Gy total dose at 5 Gy/fraction during 1 week followed by either immediate or delayed surgery
2. Long-course chemoradiotherapy (CRT) with a recommended dose of 45 to 50 Gy in 25 to 28 fractions in addition to fluorouracil/leucovorin and oxaliplatin.

SCPRT has been proven to lower the local recurrence rate as shown in the Dutch and UK CR07 trials.[31,32] Therefore, it is advocated for those with nodal disease or bulky tumor in whom the risk of R1 resection is low. Surgery is usually performed immediately after the treatment (< 10 days from the first radiation fraction).[33] Recent data have shown that SCPRT with delayed surgery is also a useful alternative, offering similar oncologic outcomes and lower postoperative complications.[34]

CRT is advocated for tumors with threatened or positive margins because the risk of R1 resection is significant. After completing CRT, the patient is then referred for another clinical and radiologic evaluation at around 6 to 8 weeks before deciding on the type and time of surgery.[35]

In patients with both heavy nodal disease and positive margins, the addition of neoadjuvant chemotherapy before starting CRT has been used with good impact on disease control. However, in all cases in which the tumor reaches the levator, APER should be performed in a cylindrical fashion in order to prevent "waist" at the perineal body and hence avoid positive resection margins.[36]

In around 30% of patients, there is a complete clinical response of the rectal cancer following CRT or SCPRT with chemotherapy. This interesting subset of patients can be considered for the "wait and watch" protocol to allow for organ preservation, hence avoiding the morbidity of rectal resection along with the known urinary and sexual dysfunction.

Clinical Complete Response and "Wait and Watch" Approach

A clinical complete response is defined as the absence of any palpable tumor or irregularity at digital rectal examination, no visible lesion at endoscopy except a flat scar, telangiectasia, or whitening of the mucosa. These minimal criteria can be complemented by the absence of any residual tumor in the primary site and draining lymph nodes on imaging with MRI or EUS and negative biopsies from the scar. An initially raised CEA level that returns to normal (< 5 ng/mL) after CRT is associated with an increased likelihood of a clinical complete response.

Results from dedicated centers have shown encouraging oncologic and functional results for patients treated with CRT and nonoperative strategy.[37-39] However, such patients are exposed to an intensive and rigorous follow-up with MRI, endoscopic, and clinical examination for the first 2 years. This is to allow for early detection of any recurrence, and, hence, any salvage treatment can be performed in a timely and feasible fashion. More properly controlled studies are needed to validate the "wait and watch" approach.

Treatment of Patients With Metastatic Disease

The management of this particular group of patients depends on 2 critical factors: whether the primary tumor is symptomatic, and if the disease (primary and/or metastases) is amenable to resection.[40]

If the disease is resectable, chemotherapy with or without radiation should be considered before surgery. Initial chemotherapy helps by either reducing or controlling the disease and improving surgical outcomes among responders and revealing the more aggressive tumors among nonresponders. The role of radiation is less defined, but it could help surgical outcomes of the primary tumor resection.

Despite the lack of definitive studies, a reasonable approach in this group is to start with chemotherapy, assess response, and then decide (in a multidisciplinary approach) on the next step. The decision on staged resection versus synchronous resection of the metastases with the primary disease should take into account the extent of the planned resection and the overall medical condition of the patient. Resection of the primary tumor is recommended as a first step if the tumor is causing symptoms such as bleeding, obstruction, or perforation. This is followed by chemotherapy and a planned excision of the metastasis if feasible.

Among patients with unresectable metastatic disease, the management should focus on the relief of symptoms of the primary tumor if present. This includes diversion colostomy to relief obstruction and endoscopic therapies (laser and electrocoagulation) for bleeding. Endoluminal stents provide symptomatic relief; however, they are to be used with caution as they could migrate or perforate, especially if the tumor responds to treatment. Such stents are also very uncomfortable if they reach the distal rectum. In the absence of or after the control of symptoms, palliative chemotherapy is usually offered.

Detection and Treatment of Local Recurrence

Local recurrence in rectal cancer always remains a concern. Certain histopathological features have an impact on the risk of local recurrence. These features, including the pathological TNM stage, CRM status, the number/proportion of involved lymph nodes, extracapsular extension, extranodal deposits, tumor differentiation, lymphovascular invasion, extramural venous invasion, and perineural invasion should be considered when planning the follow-up.

Local recurrence after local excision might occur at the site of the tumor bed. In the presence of any unfavorable histopathological features following local excision, the value of adjuvant CRT in preventing local recurrence is unproven, and TME should remain the standard salvage option. Local radiotherapy (brachytherapy or contact) can be used as an alternative to surgery in unfit patients or in combination with CRT.[41]

Local recurrence following a good-quality TME (complete, smooth mesorectum with no defects) is not common. When encountered and if disease is localized to the pelvis, CRT should be considered if no preoperative radiation was given followed by salvage surgery by a highly specialized team. Palliative forms of treatment are to be considered for patients in whom surgery carries a substantial morbidity; these can be either in the form of CRT or local brachytherapy.[42]

Follow-up After Treatment

Patients should undergo colonoscopy at 1 year after resection. Patients who did not have a full colonoscopy due to obstructing/stricturing cancer should have a colonoscopy within 3 to 6 months. Follow-up after the first surveillance depends on the colonoscopy findings.

In addition, patients with stage 2 disease and higher are followed up with the following:

- CEA every 3 to 6 months for the first 2 years and then every 6 months for a total of 5 years
- CT abdomen/pelvis and chest scans every 6 to 12 months for a total of 5 years (consider shortening intervals for stage 4 disease)
- Proctoscopy and EUS (or MRI) every 3 to 6 months for the first 2 years and then every 6 months for a total of 5 years for patients treated with transanal excision

References

1. Bailey C, Hu C, You Y, et al. Increasing disparities in the age-related incidences of colon and rectal cancers in the United States, 1975-2010. *JAMA Surg.* 2015;150(1):17-22.
2. Joseph D, Johnson C, White A, Wu M, Coleman M. Rectal cancer survival in the United States by race and stage, 2001 to 2009: findings from the CONCORD-2 study. *Cancer.* 2017;123(suppl 24):5037-5058.
3. Siegel R, Fedewa S, Anderson W, et al. Colorectal cancer incidence patterns in the United States, 1974–2013. *J Natl Cancer Inst.* 2017;109(8).
4. Siegel R, Miller K, Fedewa S, et al. Colorectal cancer statistics, 2017. *CA Cancer J Clin.* 2017;67(3):177-193.
5. Brenner H, Kloor M, Pox CP. Colorectal cancer. *Lancet.* 2014;383(9927):1490-1502.
6. Willett W, Stampfer M, Colditz G, Rosner B, Speizer F. Relation of meat, fat, and fiber intake to the risk of colon cancer in a prospective study among women. *N Engl J Med.* 1990;323(24):1664-1672.
7. Cho E, Smith Warner SA, Spiegelman D, et al. Dairy foods, calcium, and colorectal cancer: a pooled analysis of 10 cohort studies. *J Natl Cancer Inst.* 2004;96:1015-1022.
8. Bingham SA, Day NE, Luben R, et al. Dietary fibre in food and protection against colorectal cancer in the European Prospective Investigation into Cancer and Nutrition (EPIC): an observational study. *Lancet.* 2003;361:1496-1501.
9. Pischon T, Lahmann PH, Boeing H, et al. Body size and risk of colon and rectal cancer in the European Prospective Investigation Into Cancer and Nutrition (EPIC). *J Natl Cancer Inst.* 2006;98:920-931.
10. Araghi M, Galanti MR, Lundberg M, et al. Smokeless tobacco (snus) use and colorectal cancer incidence and survival: results from nine pooled cohorts. *Scand J Public Health.* 2017;45(8):741-748.
11. Baron JA, Gerhardsson de Verdier M, Ekbom A. Coffee, tea, tobacco, and cancer of the large bowel. *Cancer Epidemiol Biomarkers Prev.* 1994;3(7):565-570.
12. Marone P, de Bellis M, Avallone A, et al. Accuracy of endoscopic ultrasound in staging and restaging patients with locally advanced rectal cancer undergoing neoadjuvant chemoradiation. *Clin Res Hepatol Gastroenterol.* 2011;35:666-670.
13. Marusch F, Ptok H, Sahm M, et al. Endorectal ultrasound in rectal carcinoma—do the literature results really correspond to the realities of routine clinical care? *Endoscopy.* 2011;43(5):425-431.
14. Lutz M, Zalcberg JR, Glynne-Jones R, et al. Second St. Gallen European Organisation for Research and Treatment of Cancer Gastrointestinal Cancer Conference: consensus recommendations on controversial issues in the primary treatment of rectal cancer. *Eur J Cancer.* 2016;63:11-24.
15. Puli SR, Reddy JB, Bechtold ML, Choudhary A, Antillon MR, Brugge WR. Accuracy of endoscopic ultrasound to diagnose nodal invasion by rectal cancers: a meta-analysis and systematic review. *Ann Surg Oncol.* 2009;16:1255-1265.
16. Vanagunas A, Lin DE, Stryker SJ. Accuracy of endoscopic ultrasound for restaging rectal cancer following neoadjuvant chemoradiation therapy. *Am J Gastroenterol.* 2004;99:109-112.
17. Mezzi G, Arcidiacono PG, Carrara S, et al. Endoscopic ultrasound and magnetic resonance imaging for re-staging rectal cancer after radiotherapy. *World J Gastroenterol.* 2009;15:5563-5567.

18. Heald RJ, Husband EM, Ryall RD. The mesorectum in rectal cancer surgery—the clue to pelvic recurrence? *Br J Surg.* 1982;69(10):613-616.
19. Heald RJ, Ryall RD. Recurrence and survival after total mesorectal excision for rectal cancer. *Lancet.* 1986;1(8496):1479-1482.
20. Kapiteijn E, Putter H, van de Velde CJ; Cooperative investigators of the Dutch ColoRectal Cancer Group. Impact of the introduction and training of total mesorectal excision on recurrence and survival in rectal cancer in The Netherlands. *Br J Surg.* 2002;89(9):1142-1149.
21. Wibe A, Møller B, Norstein J, et al. A national strategic change in treatment policy for rectal cancer—implementation of total mesorectal excision as routine treatment in Norway. A national audit. *Dis Colon Rectum.* 2002;45(7):857-866.
22. Martling A, Cedermark B, Johansson H, Rutqvist LE, Holm T. The surgeon as a prognostic factor after the introduction of total mesorectal excision in the treatment of rectal cancer. *Br J Surg.* 2002;89(8):1008-1013.
23. Cedermark B, Dahlberg M, Glimelius B, Påhlman L, Rutqvist LE, Wilking N. Improved survival with preoperative radiotherapy in resectable rectal cancer. Swedish Rectal Cancer Trial. *N Engl J Med.* 1997;336:980-987.
24. Junginger T, Goenner U, Hitzler M, et al. Long-term oncologic outcome after transanal endoscopic microsurgery for rectal carcinoma. *Dis Colon Rectum.* 2016;59:8-15.
25. Guerrieri M, Gesuita R, Ghiselli R, Lezoche G, Budassi A, Baldarelli M. Treatment of rectal cancer by transanal endoscopic microsurgery: experience with 425 patients. *World J Gastroenterol.* 2014;20(28):9556-9563.
26. Van der Pas MH, Haglind E, Cuesta MA, et al. Laparoscopic versus open surgery for rectal cancer (COLOR II): short-term outcomes of a randomised, phase 3 trial. *Lancet Oncol.* 2013;14:210-218.
27. Green BL, Marshall HC, Collinson F, et al. Long-term follow-up of the Medical Research Council CLASICC trial of conventional versus laparoscopically assisted resection in colorectal cancer. *Br J Surg.* 2013;100:75-82.
28. Stevenson AR, Solomon MJ, Lumley JW, et al. Effect of laparoscopic-assisted resection vs open resection on pathological outcomes in rectal cancer: the ALaCaRT Randomized Clinical Trial. *JAMA.* 2015;314(13):1356-1363.
29. Chen K, Cao G, Chen B, et al. Laparoscopic versus open surgery for rectal cancer: a meta-analysis of classic randomized controlled trials and high-quality nonrandomized studies in the last 5 years. *Int J Surg.* 2017;39:1-10.
30. Sun Y, Xu H, Li Z, et al. Robotic versus laparoscopic low anterior resection for rectal cancer: a meta-analysis. *World J Surg Oncol.* 2016;14:61.
31. Kapiteijn E, Kranenbarg EK, Steup WH, et al. Total mesorectal excision (TME) with or without preoperative radiotherapy in the treatment of primary rectal cancer. Prospective randomized trial with standard operative and histopathological techniques. Dutch ColoRectal Cancer Group. *Eur J Surg.* 1999;165(5):410-420.
32. Quirke P, Steele R, Monson J, et al. Effect of the plane of surgery achieved on local recurrence in patients with operable rectal cancer: a prospective study using data from the MRC CR07 and NCIC-CTG CO16 randomized clinical trial. *Lancet.* 2009;373:821-828.
33. Erlandsson J, Holm T, Pettersson D, et al. Optimal fractionation of preoperative radiotherapy and timing to surgery for rectal cancer (Stockholm III): a multicenter, randomized, non-blinded, phase 3, non-inferiority trial. *Lancet Oncol.* 2017;18(3):336-346.
34. Bujko K, Wyrwicz L, Rutkowski A, et al. Long-course oxaliplatin-based preoperative chemoradiation versus 5 × 5 Gy and consolidation chemotherapy for cT4 or fixed cT3 rectal cancer: results of a randomized phase III study. *Ann Oncol.* 2016;27:834-842.
35. Glimelius B, Tiret E, Cervantes A, et al. Rectal cancer: ESMO Clinical Practice Guidelines for diagnosis, treatment and follow-up. *Ann Oncol.* 2013;24 (suppl 6):vi81-vi88.
36. Holm T, Ljung A, Haggmark T, et al. Extended abdominoperineal resection with gluteus maximus flap reconstruction of the pelvic floor for rectal cancer. *Br J Surg.* 2007;94(2):232-238.
37. Habr-Gama A, Perez RO. Non-operative management of rectal cancer after neoadjuvant chemoradiation. *Br J Surg.* 2009;96:125-127.
38. Smith JJ, Chow OS, Gollub MJ, et al. Organ Preservation in Rectal Adenocarcinoma: a phase II randomized controlled trial evaluating 3-year disease-free survival in patients with locally advanced rectal cancer treated with chemoradiation plus induction or consolidation chemotherapy, and total mesorectal excision or nonoperative management. *BMC Cancer.* 2015;15:767.
39. Maas M, Lambregts DM, Nelemans PJ, et al. Assessment of clinical complete response after chemoradiation for rectal cancer with digital rectal examination, endoscopy, and MRI: selection for organ-saving treatment. *Ann Surg Oncol.* 2015;22(12):3873-3880.
40. Pathak S, Nunes QM, Daniels IR, Smart NJ, Poston GJ, Påhlman L. Rectal cancer with synchronous liver metastases: Do we have a clear direction? *Eur J Surg Oncol.* 2015;41:1570-1577.
41. Gérard JP, Ortholan C, Benezery K, et al. Contact X-ray therapy for rectal cancer: experience in Centre Antoine-Lacassagne, Nice, 2002–2006. *Int J Radiat Oncol Biol Phys.* 2008;72(3):665-670.
42. Bishop AJ, Gupta S, Cunningham MG, et al. Interstitial brachytherapy for the treatment of locally recurrent anorectal cancer. *Ann Surg Oncol.* 2015;22(suppl 3):S596-S602.

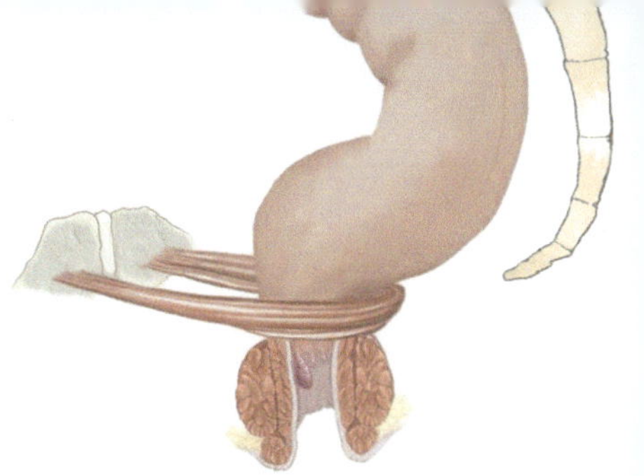

16

Miscellaneous Neoplasms

High-Resolution Anoscopy and the Role of Endoscopic Ultrasound

Stephen Landreneau, MD and Sai Sruthi Veerisetty, MD

Key Points

- Rare neoplasms of the anorectal region can present with common perianal complaints such as pruritus or bleeding.
- Careful examination of the anorectal region should include digital rectal examination and direct visualization with anoscopy, flexible sigmoidoscopy, or colonoscopy based on age/sex and risk factors.
- Endoscopic ultrasound (EUS) has utility in diagnosis and staging.
- Pelvic magnetic resonance imaging (MRI) is the recommended imaging modality to stage anorectal mass lesions.

The most common neoplasms of the anal margin, perianal skin, and rectum are adenocarcinoma and squamous cell carcinoma. The rare lesions include gastrointestinal stromal tumors (GISTs), melanoma, neuroendocrine tumors (NETs), lymphoma, Paget's disease, Kaposi sarcoma (KS), and basal cell carcinoma (BCC; Table 16-1). Diagnosing these unusual neoplasms requires a high index of suspicion because these lesions may have a benign appearance or may be discovered incidentally. Because of their rarity, our understanding and management of these lesions remain based on limited data. This chapter focuses on the miscellaneous neoplasms of the anorectal region, including their epidemiology, pathogenesis, clinical presentation, diagnosis, and surgical and nonsurgical management.

Qureshi W, ed. *Diagnosis and Management Guide for Anorectal Disease: A Clinical Reference* (pp 173-186).

Table 16-1

Miscellaneous Neoplasms of the Anorectum

NEOPLASM	PERCENTAGE DISTRIBUTION	APPEARANCE	UTILITY OF ENDOSCOPIC ULTRASOUND	MANAGEMENT
GIST	0.6% of rectal malignancies[1]	Smooth, mucosa-lined, well-circumscribed prominence of the bowel wall	Diagnosis with appearance and FNA	Resection with transanal excision, transanal endoscopic microsurgery, transanal minimally invasive surgery, or transperineal approach Imatinib
Melanoma	0.1% to 4.6% of anorectal malignancies[2]	Dark polypoid lesions	Evaluate lymph node involvement for staging	WLE or APR for invasive disease Nivolumab, ipilimumab, dabrafenib, trametinib[3]
NET	1% to 2% of rectal malignancies[3]	Yellow submucosal bulge	Evaluate tumor size, depth of invasion, and lymph node involvement to determine the ideal method of removal	Endoscopic or transanal resection or LAR/APR for invasive disease
Lymphoma	0.2% to 0.6% of colorectal malignancies[4]	Polypoid or fungating ulcerated mass or stricture	Diagnosis with FNA	Resection with systemic chemotherapy (R-CHOP or CHOP)
Paget's disease	Unknown (only 200 cases in the literature)	Erythematous, eczematous rash	None	WLE or APR for invasive disease
KS	Unknown	Dark red nodular or polypoid lesion with central umbilication or ulceration	Diagnosis with FNA	HAART, paclitaxel, interferon alpha
BCC	0.2% of all anorectal neoplasms[5]	Raised edges and central ulceration	Unknown	WLE or APR for invasive disease

APR, abdominoperineal resection; CHOP, cyclophosphamide, doxorubicin, vincristine, and prednisone; FNA, fine-needle aspiration; HAART, highly active antiretroviral therapy; LAR, low anterior resection; R-CHOP, rituximab, cyclophosphamide, doxorubicin, vincristine, and prednisone; WLE, wide local excision.

Additional Modalities for Evaluation

Anorectal complaints should initially be evaluated with visual inspection and palpation with a standard digital rectal examination and often followed with endoscopic evaluation via colonoscopy or flexible sigmoidoscopy when indicated. Additional modalities that may be used include high-resolution anoscopy, EUS, and MRI.

High-Resolution Anoscopy

High-resolution anoscopy provides detailed visual inspection of the anal canal and the transition zone from the squamous to columnar epithelium and is used primarily in the screening for anal cancer in high-risk populations, such as men who have sex with men.[7] The office-based procedure involves the use of a colposcope to examine the anal canal after the application of acetic acid or Lugol's iodine staining.[8] Although findings of squamous dysplasia have been well described, there has not been a defined role for the evaluation of miscellaneous neoplastic lesions described in this chapter.

Endoscopic Ultrasound

The role of EUS in the evaluation of anorectal disease includes sphincter evaluation in the setting of incontinence or a suspected fistula, evaluation of large or malignant-appearing polyps, staging of rectal cancer including tumor (T) and lymph node (N) status, and evaluation of subepithelial, mural, and perirectal lesions. EUS may also be used in follow-up surveillance after treatment for rectal cancer.[9] The procedure is typically performed in the outpatient setting, with or without sedation, following either preparation with enemas or, if therapeutic intervention is planned, a complete bowel preparation. EUS can provide a diagnosis in cases in which endoscopic biopsies are negative via fine-needle aspiration and fine-needle biopsy. In cases of mucosal or submucosal lesions without invasion of the muscularis propria, endoscopic mucosal resection can follow EUS, which can be diagnostic and curative for some lesions, such as small NETs. EUS findings are described for the miscellaneous neoplasms hereafter where applicable.

Magnetic Resonance Imaging

MRI has become the preferred modality for cross-sectional imaging of the pelvis for T and N staging of anorectal cancers. The strength of MRI is in its ability to delineate tissue planes, thus providing information regarding tumor invasion of adjacent structures. The National Comprehensive Cancer Network (NCCN) Guidelines recommend MRI over EUS unless there is a contraindication to MRI such as a pacemaker.[10]

Gastrointestinal Stromal Tumor

A GIST is a rare neoplasm that arises solely in the gastrointestinal tract. Over the past 3 decades, the perception, classification, and management of these tumors have changed. Previously, these tumors were noted to be smooth muscle neoplasms, such as leiomyomas, leiomyosarcomas, leiomyoblastomas, or schwannomas, based on their appearance under light microscopy.[11] Developments in immunohistochemistry and electron microscopy revealed that these tumors were derived from muscle (smooth muscle GIST), nerve (gastrointestinal autonomic nerve tumor), and/or characteristics of both (mixed GIST) or were undifferentiated (GIST not otherwise specified).[12] In 1998, with the advent of immunohistochemistry, these tumors were separated from other mesenchymal tumors with the discovery of the of c-Kit proto-oncogene.[11]

EPIDEMIOLOGY

GISTs are the most common mesenchymal tumors of the gastrointestinal tract and account for 1% to 3% of all malignant gastrointestinal tumors.[13] Less than 1% of GISTs are located in the rectum.[14] Most cases show a slight predominance in men over women and occur in the fifth and sixth decade. The annual incidence is about 5000 new cases per year in the United States.[13]

PATHOGENESIS

GISTs arise from the interstitial cells of Cajal, also known as the *intestinal pacemaker cells*. They are defined by KIT/CD117 expression, a glycoprotein that is a transmembrane receptor–type tyrosine kinase growth factor receptor detected by immunohistochemical staining. Over 95% of GISTs are positive for KIT/CD117. When this protein is phosphorylated, uncontrolled cell proliferation and differentiation result in tumor growth.

Immunohistochemistry and molecular analysis are both used to differentiate GISTs from other tumors. CD34 expression is another characteristic that can be seen in 60% to 70% of GISTs, but it can also be seen in other tumors.[11] Discovered on GIST-1 antigen expression is a specific marker also used to identify approximately 5% of GISTs that are KIT/CD117 negative.[13]

CLINICAL PRESENTATION

The signs and symptoms of clinical presentation depend on the location of the neoplasm. Usually, lesions are found incidentally on routine endoscopic procedures performed for unrelated symptoms. Most patients with rectal GISTs are asymptomatic but can have changes in bowel habits, hematochezia, or rectal pain. The size of the tumor varies and ranges from a few millimeters to greater than 30 cm.[11] Intestinal obstruction remains uncommon even with large lesions due to the exophytic growth pattern of most GISTs.[1] Patients may be asymptomatic or have vague complaints, often delaying diagnosis.

DIAGNOSIS AND MANAGEMENT

Endoscopy is the method of choice for the evaluation of GISTs. The tumor appears as a smooth, mucosa-lined, well-circumscribed protuberance of the bowel wall.[11] Occasionally, these lesions can have a central mucosal ulceration.[1] Endoscopic biopsy is usually insufficient to make a diagnosis; therefore, EUS may be useful for sampling with fine-needle aspiration or fine-needle biopsy via a core needle. Microscopic examination reveals a spindle cell lesion that requires cell block and immunohistochemistry staining to distinguish from other mural lesions, such as leiomyomas and schwannomas. The classic appearance on EUS is a well-defined hypoechoic mass arising from the fourth sonographic layer (muscularis propria) of the rectal wall.[1] An attempt at endoscopic removal with snaring the lesion can result in perforation. For nonrectal GISTs, computed tomographic (CT) imaging is the preferred method to characterize the lesion for staging and to evaluate whether metastases are present.[11] However, MRI is preferred for rectal GISTs. Prognostic factors include the size of the tumor and the mitotic index. Surgical resection remains the treatment of choice for GISTs if the tumor is localized.[13] Chemotherapy with imatinib, a selective tyrosine kinase inhibitor, is used when tumors are unresectable and as neoadjuvant therapy to decrease the size and improve the chances of successful surgery.[13] Referral should be made for surgery with options including transanal excision, transanal endoscopic microsurgery, transanal minimally invasive surgery, or the transperineal approach.[15] Adjuvant chemotherapy with imatinib for high-risk lesions has shown a survival benefit with patients initially treated for 1 year. Randomized data have shown 3 years of therapy to be superior to 1 year.[16] Three years of therapy are currently recommended, and trials are underway to determine if longer periods improve survival.[17]

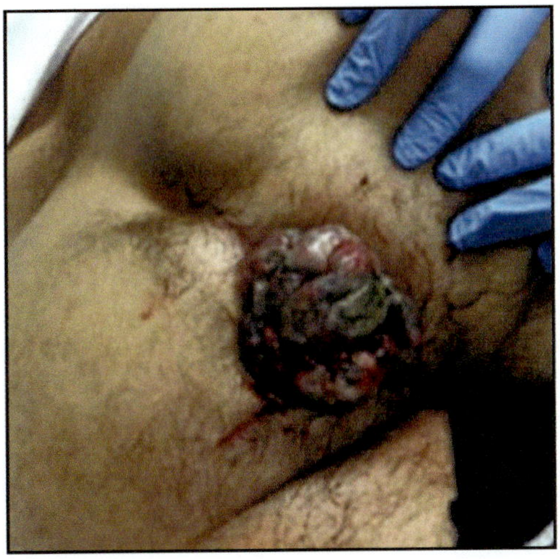

Figure 16-1. A 40-year-old individual with perianal melanoma.

Melanoma

Gastrointestinal melanomas are mucosal neoplasms that develop from melanocytes in the oropharynx, rectum, and anus. The anorectum is the most common location for primary gastrointestinal malignant melanomas.[18] After the skin and retina, the anorectum is the third most common site of origin of melanoma due to the abundance of melanocytes in the anal mucosa.[19] Anorectal melanoma is an aggressive neoplasm with a high mortality rate and high metastatic potential compared with cutaneous melanoma.[20]

Epidemiology

Anorectal melanoma has an incidence of 0.4% to 3% of all malignant melanomas and 0.1% to 4.6% of all anorectal malignancies.[19] The average age of diagnosis is in the fifth to eighth decade with a female predominance.[20] There is a higher prevalence in Whites than African Americans.[21] A family history of melanoma may be a risk factor.[20]

Pathogenesis

Melanocytes are found in the transition zone below the dentate line and increase in density distally toward the anus. There is the assumption that anorectal melanoma arises from those melanocytes and migrates to involve the rectum.[22] Multiple cell signaling pathways are involved in melanocyte migration and differentiation. Histologic features of melanoma can resemble other cancers, including lymphomas, sarcomas, and undifferentiated carcinomas. For this reason, biopsy results require immunohistochemical staining for S-100, HMB-45, melan-A, and carcinoembryonic antigen.[23]

Clinical Presentation

The most common symptom and presentation is small-volume rectal bleeding, which may be attributed to hemorrhoids. Other common complaints include changes in bowel habits, passage of mucus through the anal canal, anal pain, rectal fullness, tenesmus, pruritus, and findings of an anorectal mass or skin tag. Approximately 30% of masses are amelanotic and can resemble benign polypoid-appearing lesions resembling skin tags or hemorrhoids, leading to a delay in diagnosis.[23] Lesions are usually located in the anal canal followed by the dentate line and the rectum (Figure 16-1).[24]

DIAGNOSIS AND MANAGEMENT

Currently, there are no standardized guidelines that exist for the management of anorectal melanoma due to the rarity of the disease. Diffusion-weighted MRI is used to evaluate the anal canal and perianal region.[25] Diagnosis is made with endoscopic biopsy. EUS can be used to evaluate lymph node metastasis (LNM) for staging purposes. By the time of diagnosis, the disease is often advanced, and over half of the patients have lymph node involvement or distant metastases.[23] Positron emission tomographic–CT imaging is commonly used to evaluate inguinal and iliac LNMs that can be missed on routine contrast-enhanced CT imaging. LNMs are detected in greater than 40% of cases when the tumor has infiltrated the submucosa. LNMs are representative of lymphatic spread and can result in metastases to the lung and liver in approximately 90% of cases.[26] Multidisciplinary treatment with chemotherapy, radiation, and surgery is the mainstay of treatment. Anorectal melanoma is often resistant to radiation and shows a poor response to chemotherapy.[24] In addition, no survival benefit has been shown.[27]

The current surgical intervention is with wide local excision (WLE) or radical abdominoperineal resection (APR) and bilateral inguinal lymphadenectomy.[23] Patients with extensive disease with sphincter involvement have a poor prognosis despite the surgical approach taken. Surgical intervention is controversial because no survival benefit has been shown in studies comparing WLE or APR.[28] Achieving curative surgical margins remains challenging with WLE. APR has been reserved for lesions that are large or obstructing or infiltrate the surrounding structures.[29] Regardless of the surgical method, the prognosis is poor, with a low 5-year survival rate of 25%.[24] The median survival time is approximately 12 to 20 months.[23] Tumors with perineural invasion, infiltration of the rectal wall, or LMN have poor overall survival.[26] With the discouraging outcomes with surgical resection, medical management is a mainstay of treatment. Systemic therapy with immunotherapy agents, such as nivolumab (a programmed cell death protein 1 checkpoint inhibitor), ipilimumab (a cytotoxic T-lymphocyte–associated antigen 4 checkpoint inhibitor), dabrafenib (a BRAF gene inhibitor), and trametinib (an MEK gene inhibitor), has shown promise in increasing both progression-free survival and overall survival.[30,31]

Neuroendocrine Tumor

NETs of the gastrointestinal tract are rising due to the increase in incidental lesions found on routine endoscopy. NETs of the distal colon and rectum are considered hindgut tumors from their embryologic origin. Historically, they were considered indolent tumors.[4] Now, they are considered potentially malignant, and guidelines recommend removal.

EPIDEMIOLOGY

The incidence of NETs is approximately 1 in 100,000 and has been rising due to incidental findings on routine screening colonoscopy. Rectal NETs make up 27% of all gastrointestinal NETs and 16% of all NETs as a whole. The average age of diagnosis for rectal NETs is in the fifth decade. The incidence of rectal NETs is higher in African Americans and Asians than Whites. Rectal NETs are associated with the greatest 5-year survival rate (ie, 88%).[32]

PATHOGENESIS

NETs are derived from enterochromaffin cells located in the crypts of Lieberkühn. The tumors then progress to invade the muscularis mucosa and the submucosa, generating a submucosal appearance.[33] NETs are categorized into 3 different grades: well-differentiated (low and intermediate grade) and poorly differentiated tumors (high-grade neuroendocrine carcinomas, grade 3).

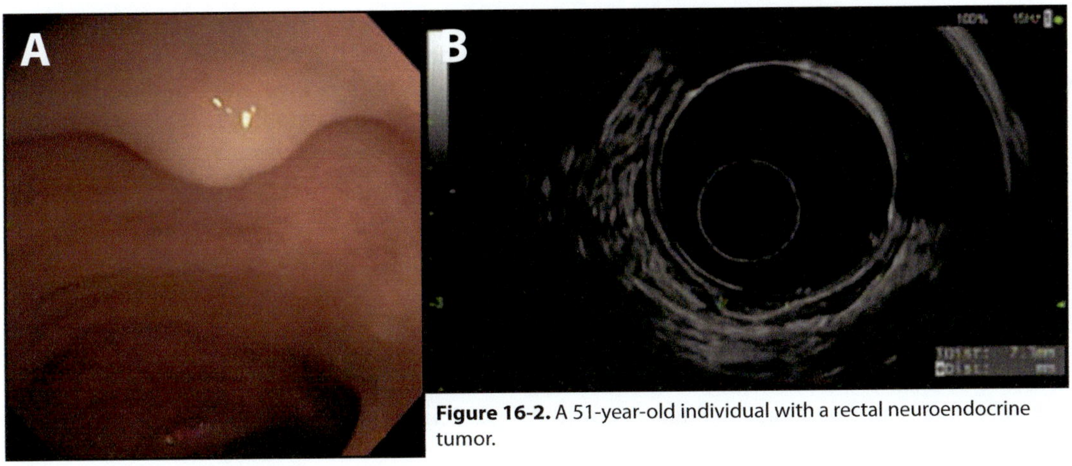

Figure 16-2. A 51-year-old individual with a rectal neuroendocrine tumor.

Well-differentiated tumors are indolent in nature, while poorly differentiated NETs are aggressive. The histologic grading system is based on mitotic counts per unit area of tumor (expressed as mitoses per 10 high-power fields) and the Ki-67 proliferation marker. If the sample size is less than 40 high-power fields, a mitotic index is not considered accurate, and Ki-67 is used to precisely measure the proliferative rate and delineate well-differentiated from poorly differentiated tumors.[32]

CLINICAL PRESENTATION

Approximately half of the patients with rectal NETs will be asymptomatic, but presenting symptoms can include changes in bowel habits, hematochezia, or rectal pain. Generally, hindgut NETs are not associated with carcinoid syndrome.[34] Most arise in the midrectum, approximately 5 to 10 cm from the anal verge. Usually, rectal NETs are small and localized at diagnosis (Figure 16-2).

DIAGNOSIS AND MANAGEMENT

The endoscopic appearance of an NET is a submucosal bulge usually located in the midrectum 5 to 10 cm above the anal verge.[32] The lesion may have a yellowish hue. EUS is able to evaluate tumor size, depth of invasion, and lymph node involvement to further evaluate the ideal approach for removal. The lesions appear isoechoic or hypoechoic and well demarcated, arising in the second sonographic layer of the rectal wall. When the lesion does not involve the muscularis propria, endoscopic mucosal resection can be performed; this can be curative as well as diagnostic if the diagnosis has not already been obtained from routine biopsy or snare polypectomy during colonoscopy. Microscopic examination shows small monotonous tumor cells, and immunohistochemistry staining confirms the diagnosis and also provides tumor grade. No significant clinical trials have been conducted regarding rectal NETs. Therefore, 2 groups of multispecialty experts with the European Neuroendocrine Tumor Society and North American Neuroendocrine Tumor Society in conjunction with the NCCN have produced consensus management guidelines.[32,35,36] The size of the tumor and depth of invasion determine malignant behavior. When the lesions are mucosal, submucosal, or < 2 cm, rectal NETs have low malignant potential and a very small risk of metastases.[32] When < 1 to 2 cm and mucosal or submucosal in nature, endoscopic or transanal resection may be the best choice for removal. If tumors are larger in size (> 2 cm) or if they invade the muscularis propria and have regional lymph node involvement, radical excision with low anterior resection or APR is the best option depending on the location. Staging radiographic imaging is not recommended for rectal NETs < 1 cm, but those with larger tumors should have EUS or MRI of the pelvis.[36] Somatostatin receptor scintigraphy (octreoscan) for staging purposes remains controversial due to the lack of evidence that it improves detection compared with standard imaging.[32] However, octreoscan is useful with metastases and can evaluate whether those tumors express somatostatin receptors.[32] Surveillance after resection depends on the size of the lesion. Stage I lesions, those ≤ 2 cm and not extending beyond the submucosa, do not require long-term surveillance because they have a low risk of metastatic spread.[32] Stage II or III lesions that invade the muscularis propria or locoregional lymph nodes require annual radiographic surveillance.[32] The North American Neuroendocrine Tumor Society guidelines do not remark on short-term surveillance with endoscopy or radiographic imaging. However, the NCCN recommends endoscopic surveillance for lesions ≥ 1 cm in size at 6 and 12 months after resection. Further surveillance should be individualized. Lesions < 1 cm in size do not require surveillance.[36]

Lymphoma

Lymphoma is a hematologic malignancy, with the gastrointestinal tract being the most common site of extranodal disease. The most common location is the stomach followed by the small intestine, colon, and rectum. Of these subtypes that present in the gastrointestinal tract, more than 90% of cases are related to diffuse large B-cell non-Hodgkin, mucosa-associated lymphoid tissue (MALT), and Burkitt lymphomas.[37] Primary gastrointestinal lymphomas are differentiated from systemic lymphomas with secondary involvement by Dawson's criteria, which was originally described in 1961. The criteria include absence of palpable superficial lymphadenopathy, absence of enlargement of the mediastinal lymph nodes on chest imaging, normal white blood cell count and differential as well as normal bone marrow biopsy, and liver and spleen without tumor.[38] In addition, only regional lymph nodes can be affected without concurrent retroperitoneal and mediastinal lymphadenopathy.[5]

Epidemiology

Colorectal lymphoma makes up only 10% to 20% of gastrointestinal lymphomas and less than 1% of all colorectal malignancies.[37] It is the third most common large bowel neoplasm after adenocarcinoma and carcinoid tumors.[39] The most common type of lymphoma that affects the gastrointestinal tract is diffuse large B-cell lymphoma, which is composed of rapidly proliferating B cells. The second most common lymphoma seen in the gastrointestinal tract is MALT lymphoma, which is a low-grade tumor of B-cell origin. Colorectal MALT lymphoma does not have an affiliation with *Helicobacter pylori* like MALT lymphoma of the stomach. Colorectal lymphoma increases in incidence with age and affects patients 50 to 70 years of age with a male predominance.[38] Immunocompromised individuals, including those with inflammatory bowel disease or HIV/AIDS and transplant recipients, are at higher risk of developing colorectal lymphoma. Only 25% of colorectal lymphomas are found in the descending colon and rectosigmoid region.[38] With primary gastrointestinal lymphoma, systemic disease with retroperitoneal or mediastinal lymphadenopathy is not necessary for diagnosis.

Pathogenesis

Non-Hodgkin lymphomas are lymphoproliferative disorders deriving from B cells, T cells, and natural killer lymphocytes.[37] The World Health Organization divides B-cell lymphomas into 5 histologic categories: extranodal marginal lymphoma (MALT), follicular lymphoma, mantle cell lymphoma, diffuse large B-cell lymphoma, and Burkitt lymphoma. Intestinal T-cell lymphomas were previously categorized into enteropathy-associated T-cell lymphoma and non–enteropathy-associated T-cell lymphoma. Now, the World Health Organization classifies them as peripheral T-cell–derived lymphomas.[39] Extranodal lymphomas are those that stem from solid organs and make up about one-third of non-Hodgkin lymphoma cases.[37]

CLINICAL PRESENTATION

Presenting symptoms include weight loss, lower gastrointestinal bleeding, and anorexia, with abdominal pain being the most common symptom. Diagnosis is made with endoscopy and findings of polypoid or fungating ulcerated mass, stricture, or multiple polypoid lesions. In rectal lymphoma, lesions can be focal or diffuse. Multiple presentations are possible, including long segment involvement, lesions that appear similar to adenocarcinoma, and aneurysmal dilatation of the wall.[37]

DIAGNOSIS AND MANAGEMENT

Diagnosis can be made with routine biopsies of the abnormal or polypoid-appearing mucosa. In cases in which biopsies are negative, EUS can be obtained with description of wall layer thickening and fine-needle aspiration. CT imaging is the radiographic imaging of choice used for diagnosis and evaluation because it can evaluate the colonic wall as well as lymph node involvement.[37]

Treatment consists of surgical resection to achieve local control with systemic chemotherapy with rituximab, cyclophosphamide, doxorubicin, vincristine, and prednisone (R-CHOP) or cyclophosphamide, doxorubicin, vincristine, and prednisone (CHOP). The recurrence rate of primary gastrointestinal lymphoma is high at approximately 33% to 75% within the first 5 years after resection.[38]

PAGET'S DISEASE

Extramammary Paget's disease (EMPD), or intraepithelial adenocarcinoma, is a rare malignancy of the perianal region. The disease is found where the apocrine glands are located and is usually noninvasive but can metastasize. EMPD is categorized as primary or secondary. Primary EMPD originates in the sweat glands of the epidermis, while secondary EMPD comes from the malignant spread of malignant cells from an underlying carcinoma.[40]

EPIDEMIOLOGY

Less than 200 cases have been reported; therefore, the incidence and prevalence of EMPD remain unknown. It represents less than 1% of all anal disease and 6.5% of all cases of Paget's disease.[41] Most documented reports are seen in small case reports. In general, older female patients are affected with a mean age of diagnosis in the sixth decade.

PATHOGENESIS

The exact etiology of Paget's disease remains unclear. The typical histologic findings are of large, rounded vacuolated cells known as *Paget's cells*.[6] Diagnosis can also be made with immunohistochemical studies for carcinoembryonic antigen and cytokeratins such as CK7, PKK1, GR53, and 35bH11.[42] Prognosis is determined by depth of invasion.[41]

CLINICAL PRESENTATION

EMPD appears as an erythematous, eczematous rash or plaque. The common presenting symptoms include intractable pruritus, rectal bleeding, and discharge.[6] Symptoms can be nonspecific and imitate benign anorectal issues like hemorrhoids and fissures or cutaneous candidiasis, which can delay diagnosis. Lesions have varying presentations with scales, crusts, oozing, or erosions.[6]

DIAGNOSIS AND MANAGEMENT

Diagnosis is made with biopsy of the lesion with histologic appearance of intraepithelial adenocarcinoma. Unlike other lesions discussed thus far, this lesion requires cutaneous biopsy rather than endoscopic biopsy, a modality typically not performed by the gastroenterologist. Referral to a provider with expertise in cutaneous biopsy, such as a surgeon or dermatologist, should be sought. Half of the patients with anal margin Paget's disease have a colorectal neoplasm and require endoscopic evaluation with colonoscopy. Treatment includes surgical management with WLE and 1-cm margins. When the lesion is locally invasive or a synchronous anorectal adenocarcinoma is present, APR is preferred.[6] There can be recurrence of disease after resection, which is why mapping biopsies or perianal biopsies in 4 quadrants taken 1 cm from the edge of the lesion to evaluate disease extent are recommended before resection.[43] The disease can reappear in a "skip"-like fashion with the spread of cells in the epidermis beyond the margin.[43]

Kaposi Sarcoma

KS is a vascular, mesenchymal tumor involving the blood vessels and lymphatics that is found in patients with altered immune systems and malignant diseases, most commonly in immunocompromised patients with HIV/AIDS.[44] The malignancy can develop at any stage of disease but tends to present in patients with advanced immunosuppression and can involve any portion of the gastrointestinal tract.[45] KS of the gastrointestinal tract has been described as both primarily occurring in the anorectum and disseminated gastrointestinal disease.[46]

EPIDEMIOLOGY

A direct correlation between KS and human herpesvirus 8 (HHV8) has been established. Approximately 8% to 12% of all KS is found in the lower gastrointestinal tract.[45] The rectum is the second most common location after the duodenum.[47] Four types of KS have been described. The classic form is described in elderly men of Mediterranean descent. The second type is associated with lymphadenopathy and affects young Bantu children in South Africa. The third type is associated with organ transplant and prolonged immunosuppressive therapy. The fourth type is AIDS-associated KS.[44] All forms of KS are affiliated with HHV8 infection.

PATHOGENESIS

KS is a spindle cell, low-grade tumor thought to derive from a proliferating vascular endothelium.[45] Histologic evaluation shows spindle cell proliferation, and immunohistochemical testing of the tumor is positive for CD34, CD31, D2-40, and the HHV8 latent nuclear antigen.[44,45]

CLINICAL PRESENTATION

Presentation is based on distribution, is variable, and is nonspecific, including asymptomatic, abdominal pain, nausea, diarrhea, gross gastrointestinal bleeding, and unexplained anemia. It may also present as an obstruction or perforation.[44] It should be suspected in a patient with known HIV/AIDs, and, if a diagnosis of HIV/AIDs is not present, it should be sought.

DIAGNOSIS AND MANAGEMENT

Diagnosis is by endoscopic appearance of a dark red nodular or polypoid lesion with central umbilication; ulceration can be seen in severe disease. Endoscopic biopsy of the lesion only results in diagnosis in 15% to 23% of cases due to the neoplasm arising in the submucosal tissue. EUS can be

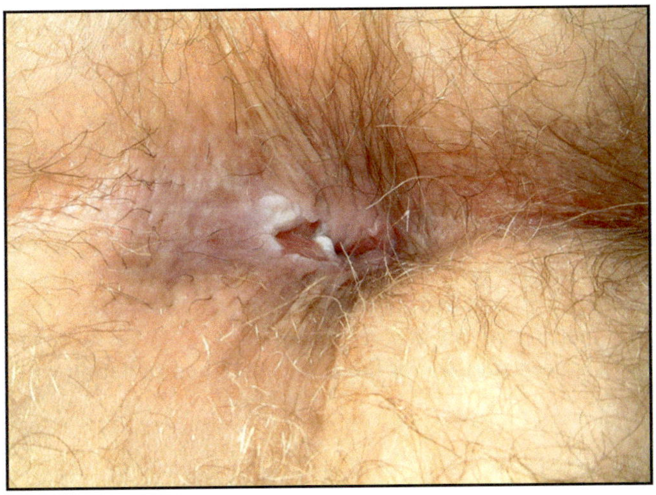

Figure 16-3. A 64-year-old individual with perianal squamous cell carcinoma.

performed with fine-needle aspiration in cases in which endoscopic biopsies are negative. The tumor is usually seen with advanced immunosuppression with HIV/AIDS; therefore, patients with extensive mucocutaneous disease and organ involvement should be treated with combined highly active antiretroviral therapy and systemic chemotherapy with doxorubicin. Currently, the malignancy is not curable. Disease relapse is about 13% per year. Other medical treatment options include paclitaxel and interferon alpha. There is currently no role for surgical resection of lesions in the absence of obstruction or perforation.[45]

Basal Cell Carcinoma

BCC is the most common nonmelanoma skin cancer, with the major risk factor being sunlight exposure. Thus, BCC of the anal margin is very rare and makes up 0.2% of all anorectal neoplasms.[6] BCCs do not have a defined precursor lesion, unlike squamous cell carcinoma (Figure 16-3). BCC must be differentiated from basaloid squamous cell carcinoma due to differences in treatment.[48]

Epidemiology

The average age of presentation is in the sixth to eighth decade with predominance in males who have a history of BCC at other skin sites, although one study showed a female preponderance.[48,49] The lesions are extremely rare, with available data only in the form of case studies and small case series.

Pathogenesis

BCC arises from the basal cell layer of the epidermis and pilosebaceous follicle units.[49] Lesions typically arise in the perianal region from the distal end of the anal canal to 5 cm from the anal verge as opposed to squamous lesions, which are commonly found in the anal canal and region of the dentate line. Lesions tend to be localized but may extend into the anal canal.[48]

Clinical Presentation

BCCs present as mass lesions in the perianal region. They are typically localized lesions but may extend into the anal canal. Symptoms can be similar to other anorectal disease benign and malignant processes. Patients may complain of bleeding, pruritus, or discharge. Visual inspection may show a perianal ulcer with central ulceration and raised edges. These findings can mimic external hemorrhoid disease or anal cysts.[48]

DIAGNOSIS AND MANAGEMENT

BCC lesions appear superficial and have a varying appearance with raised edges and central ulceration. Referral for cutaneous biopsy should be made. Care should be taken to not mislabel lesions as hemorrhoidal disease. The size of the lesion varies with an average size of approximately 1 to 2 cm, but lesions can be as large as 10 cm. BCC usually has low metastatic potential; therefore, for small lesions < 2 cm, the treatment of choice is WLE with 1-cm margins. Lesions that extend into the anal canal require more extensive resection. The recurrence rate can vary from 0% to 29% for those lesions. However, if the lesion is large or there is deep invasion of the anal canal, then radiation with possible APR is an option.[49]

CONCLUSION

Rare neoplasms of the anorectum encountered by gastroenterologists include GISTs, melanoma, NET, lymphoma, Paget's disease, KS, and BCC. These conditions can be discovered incidentally on visual inspection, palpation, or endoscopic evaluation. Although these neoplasms can be asymptomatic, they can also present with symptoms commonly attributed to benign anorectal conditions such as hemorrhoids. Any suspicious mucosal or cutaneous lesions should be sampled. EUS should be used when subepithelial lesions are suspected or mucosal biopsies fail to make a diagnosis. MRI is preferred for local staging of mass lesions. Unlike dysplastic squamous lesions, there is currently no defined role for high-resolution anoscopy in the diagnosis and management of these lesions.

REFERENCES

1. Jiang ZX, Zhang SJ, Peng WJ, Yu BH. Rectal gastrointestinal stromal tumors: imaging features with clinical and pathological correlation. *World J Gastroenterol.* 2013;19(20):3108-3116.
2. Balicevic D, Tomic K, Bekavac-Beslin M, et al. Synchronous anorectal melanoma. *World J Gastroenterol.* 2006;12(21):3453-3455.
3. National Comprehensive Cancer Network. Melanoma (version 3.2018). https://www.nccn.org/patients/guidelines/melanoma/index.html. Accessed July 21, 2018.
4. Chi Y, Du F, Zhao H, Wang JW, Cai JQ. Characteristics and long-term prognosis of patients with rectal neuroendocrine tumors. *World J Gastroenterol.* 2014;20(43):16252-16257.
5. Drolet S, Maclean AR, Stewart DA, Dixon E, Paolucci EO, Buie WD. Primary colorectal lymphoma—clinical outcomes in a population-based series. *J Gastrointest Surg.* 2011;15(10):1851-1857.
6. Leonard D, Beddy D, Dozois EJ. Neoplasms of anal canal and perianal skin. *Clin Colon Rectal Surg.* 2011;24(1):54-63.
7. Jay N, Berry JM, Miaskowski C, et al. Colposcopic characteristics and Lugol's staining differentiate anal high-grade and low-grade squamous intraepithelial lesions during high resolution anoscopy. *Papillomavirus Res.* 2015;1:101-108.
8. Alburquerque A. High-resolution anoscopy: unchartered territory for gastroenterologists? *World J Gastrointest Endosc.* 2015;7(13):1083-1087.
9. Gleeson FC. EUS in rectal cancer. *Endosonography.* Philadelphia, PA: Elsevier Saunders; 2015:260-268.
10. National Comprehensive Cancer Network. Rectal cancer (version 2.2018). https://www.nccn.org/patients/guidelines/rectal. Accessed July 21, 2018.
11. Rammohan A, Sathyanesan J, Rajendran K, et al. A gist of gastrointestinal stromal tumors: a review. *World J Gastrointest Oncol.* 2013;5(6):102-112.
12. DeMatteo RP, Lewis JJ, Leung D, Mudan SS, Woodruff JM, Brennan MF. Two hundred gastrointestinal stromal tumors: recurrence patterns and prognostic factors for survival. *Ann Surg.* 2000;231(1):51-58.
13. Lamba G, Gupta R, Lee B, Ambrale S, Liu D. Current management and prognostic features for gastrointestinal stromal tumor (GIST). *Exp Hematol Oncol.* 2012;1(1):14.

14. Liu Q, Zhong G, Zhou W, Lin G. Initial application of transanal endoscopic microsurgery for high-risk lower rectal gastrointestinal stromal tumor after imatinib mesylate neoadjuvant chemotherapy: a case report. *Medicine (Baltimore)*. 2017;96(29):e7538.
15. Fiore M, Raut CP, Gronchi A. Are we allowed to limit surgical aggressiveness with small rectal gastrointestinal stromal tumors? *Ann Surg Oncol*. 2017;24(5):1153-1156.
16. Joensuu H, Eriksson M, Hall KS, et al. One vs three years of adjuvant imatinib for operable gastrointestinal stromal tumor. *JAMA*. 2012;307(12):1265-1272.
17. National Comprehensive Cancer Network. Soft tissue sarcoma (version 2.2018). https://www.nccn.org/patients/guidelines/sarcoma. Accessed July 21, 2018.
18. Matsuda A, Miyashita M, Matsumoto S, et al. Abdominoperineal resection provides better local control but equivalent overall survival to local excision of anorectal malignant melanoma: a systematic review. *Ann Surg*. 2015;261(4):670-677.
19. Tomioka K, Ojima H, Sohda M, et al. Primary malignant melanoma of the rectum: report of two cases. *Case Rep Surg*. 2012;2012:247348.
20. Jehangir W, Schlacter N, Singh S, et al. Anorectal melanoma: a case report and an update of a rare malignancy. *World J Oncol*. 2015;6(1):308-310.
21. Khan M, Bucher N, Elhassan A, et al. Primary anorectal melanoma. *Case Rep Oncol*. 2014;7(1):164-170.
22. Carcoforo P, Raiji MT, Palini GM, et al. Primary anorectal melanoma: an update. *J Cancer*. 2012;3:449-453.
23. Limketkai BN, Chandrasekhara V, Milligan F. Primary anorectal amelanotic melanoma presenting as internal hemorrhoids. *Gastroenterol Hepatol (N Y)*. 2009;5(7):516-518.
24. Latteri S, Teodoro M, Malaguarnera M, Mannino M, Currò G, La Greca G. Abdominal perineal resection or wilde local excision in primary anorectal malignant melanoma. Case report and review. *Ann Med Surg (Lond)*. 2017;19:74-77.
25. Surabhi VR, Menias CO, Amer AM, et al. Tumors and tumorlike conditions of the anal canal and perianal region: MR imaging findings. *Radiographics*. 2016;36(5):1339-1353.
26. Falch C, Mueller S, Kirschniak A, Braun M, Koenigsrainer A, Klumpp B. Anorectal malignant melanoma: curative abdominoperineal resection: patient selection with 18F-FDG-PET/CT. *World J Surg Oncol*. 2016;14(1):185.
27. Bulut N, Dagıstanlı S, Yılmaz B, Atay OF. Surgical approach to anorectal melanoma with PET-CT staging: a case report. *Surg J (N Y)*. 2017;3(4):e177-e180.
28. Pessaux P, Pocard M, Elias D, et al. Surgical management of primary anorectal melanoma. *Br J Surg*. 2004;91(9):1183-1187.
29. Bello DM, Smyth E, Perez D, et al. Anal versus rectal melanoma: does site of origin predict outcome? *Dis Colon Rectum*. 2013;56(2):150-157.
30. Larkin J, Chiarion-Sileni V, Gonzalez R, et al. Combined nivolumab and ipilimumab or monotherapy in untreated melanoma. *N Engl J Med*. 2015;373(1):23-34.
31. Robert C, Karaszewska B, Schachter J, et al. Improved overall survival in melanoma with combined dabrafenib and trametinib. *N Engl J Med*. 2015;372:30-39.
32. Anthony LB, Strosberg JR, Klimstra DS, et al. The NANETS consensus guidelines for the diagnosis and management of gastrointestinal neuroendocrine tumors (nets): well-differentiated nets of the distal colon and rectum. *Pancreas*. 2010;39(6):767-774.
33. Rajca BP, Wagh MS. Dilemmas in endoscopic management of rectal neuroendocrine tumors: a case-based discussion. *Gastroenterol Res Pract*. 2015;2015:539861.
34. Chung TP, Hunt SR. Carcinoid and neuroendocrine tumors of the colon and rectum. *Clin Colon Rectal Surg*. 2006;19(2):45-48.
35. Ramage JK, De Herder WM, Delle Fave G, et al. ENETS consensus guidelines update for colorectal neuroendocrine neoplasms. *Neuroendocrinology*. 2016;103(2):139-143.
36. National Comprehensive Cancer Network. Neuroendocrine and adrenal tumors (version 2.2018). https://www.nccn.org/professionals/physician_gls/pdf/neuroendocrine.pdf. Accessed July 21, 2018.
37. Times M. Colorectal lymphoma. *Clin Colon Rectal Surg*. 2011;24(3):135-141.
38. Quayle FJ, Lowney JK. Colorectal lymphoma. *Clin Colon Rectal Surg*. 2006;19(2):49-53.
39. Stanojevic GZ, Nestorovic MD, Brankovic BR, Stojanovic MP, Jovanovic MM, Radojkovic MD. Primary colorectal lymphoma: an overview. *World J Gastrointest Oncol*. 2011;3(1):14-18.
40. Möller MG, Lugo-Baruqui JA, Milikowski C, Salgado CJ. Staged marginal contoured and central excision technique in the surgical management of perianal Paget's disease. *Am J Surg*. 2014;207(4):485-492.
41. Carbotta G, Sallustio P, Prestera A, Laforgia R, Lobascio P, Palasciano N. Perianal Paget's disease: a rare disorder and review of literature. *Ann Med Surg (Lond)*. 2016;9:50-52.
42. Banerjee S, Chatterjee M, Chand K. Extramammary Paget's disease. *Indian J Dermatol Venereol Leprol*. 2005;71(6):417-420.

43. Perez DR, Trakarnsanga A, Shia J, et al. Management and outcome of perianal Paget's disease: a six-decade institutional experience. *Dis Colon Rectum*. 2014;57(6):747-751.
44. Arora M, Goldberg EM. Kaposi sarcoma involving the gastrointestinal tract. *Gastroenterol Hepatol N Y*. 2010;6(7):459-462.
45. Lee AJ, Brenner L, Mourad B, et al. Gastrointestinal Kaposi's sarcoma: case report and review of the literature. *World J Gastrointest Pharmacol Ther*. 2015;6(3):89-95.
46. Lorenz HP, Wilson W, Leigh B, Schecter WP. Kaposi's sarcoma of the rectum in patients with the acquired immunodeficiency syndrome. *Am J Surg*. 1990;160(6):681-683.
47. Virmani V, Ramanathan S, Virmani VS, Ryan J, Fasih N. What is hiding in the hindgut sac? Looking beyond rectal carcinoma. *Insights Imaging*. 2014;5(4):457-471.
48. Patil DT, Goldblum JR, Billings SD. Clinicopathological analysis of basal cell carcinoma of the anal region and its distinction from basaloid squamous cell carcinoma. *Mod Pathol*. 2013;26(10):1382-1389.
49. Wietfeldt ED, Thiele J. Malignancies of the anal margin and perianal skin. *Clin Colon Rectal Surg*. 2009;22(2):127-135.

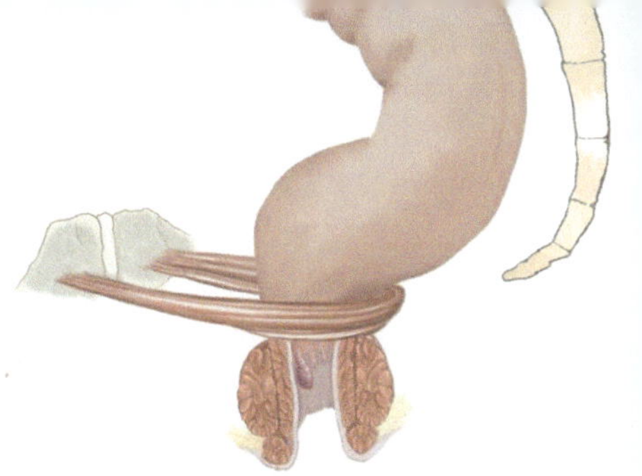

17

Anal Cytology, Anal Neoplasia, and High-Resolution Anoscopy in Patients at Risk for Anal Cancer

J. Michael Berry-Lawhorn, MD

Key Points

- The incidence of anal cancer is increasing worldwide but is uncommon in the general population.
- All persons living with HIV, other immunocompromised persons, men who have sex with men (MSM) without HIV, women with a prior history of lower genital tract precancerous lesions or cancer, and people over 35 years of age diagnosed with anal warts have an increased incidence of anal cancer.
- Anal cancer is preceded by a precancerous lesion called a *high-grade squamous intraepithelial lesion* (HSIL).
- High-resolution anoscopy (HRA) is a procedure in which the anal canal and perianus are examined using a colposcope or operating microscope after applying 5% acetic acid and is the best way to diagnose HSILs and early nonpalpable anal cancer.
- Superficially invasive squamous cell carcinoma (SISCCA) is a newly defined form of very small, early cancers with an invasive depth < 3 mm that may be treated with excision and is not palpable but can be seen during HRA.
- All patients with SISCCA should be examined with HRA whenever possible.
- Anal cancer may be preventable by treating or removing HSILs, but this has not been proven yet and is being studied in a national trial called the *Anal Cancer HSIL Outcomes Research (ANCHOR) study.*
- Gastroenterologists commonly see patients with anorectal complaints such as anal pain, bleeding, or lumps; anal cancer should be considered in the differential diagnosis.

Qureshi W, ed. *Diagnosis and Management Guide for Anorectal Disease: A Clinical Reference* (pp 187-202).

- Digital anorectal examination (DARE) is a sensitive test to detect anal cancer and differentiate it from benign conditions.
- DARE is performed by carefully palpating the walls of the entire anal canal to feel for any abnormal thickening, induration, warts, or masses.
- All patients presenting with anorectal complaints should have DARE performed.
- Gastroenterologists should have a high index of suspicion for anal cancer in patients who are known to be at increased risk.
- Most patients diagnosed with anal cancer may not be a member of a high-risk group or report a history of anal intercourse.
- Colonoscopy or flexible sigmoidoscopy provides a unique opportunity to perform DARE to screen for anal cancer and distal rectal lesions.

Background and Natural History

Anal cancer has been considered a rare cancer; more than 85% are squamous cell carcinomas related to human papillomavirus (HPV) infection, about 10% are adenocarcinomas, and the remainder are even more rare cancers such as melanoma and small cell carcinoma.[1] This chapter concentrates on squamous cell carcinomas of the anus and perianus, which will be referred to as *anal cancer*. Table 17-1 provides definitions and the significance of the relevant terminology. The incidence of anal cancer is rising worldwide at about 2% per year, with an estimated 8580 new cases in the United States in 2018 occurring in 2960 men and 5620 women.[2,3] Long-term persistent high-risk HPV (HRHPV) infection occurring over decades leads to most cases of anal cancer. HRHPV is oncogenic and responsible for squamous cell carcinomas of the cervix, vulva, anus, penis, and oropharynx. After initiating sexual activity, infection with HPV may occur in more than 80% of sexually active adults.[4,5] Vaccinating adolescents with HPV-2 or HPV-9 prior to sexual debut effectively prevents infection due to vaccine-containing types.[6,7] In the absence of an effective immune response, persistent HRHPV infection leads to the development of cancer precursors known as *HSILs*. Screening for cervical HSILs and subsequently removing these lesions have dramatically decreased the incidence and mortality of cervical cancer. Primary and secondary cervical cancer prevention programs are some of the most important advances of modern medicine.

The anus and cervix are similar tissues that are susceptible to infection with the same types of HRHPV and are therefore at risk for potentially precancerous lesions.[5] Treating cervical HSILs is an effective way of preventing cervical cancer. Standardized guidelines developed by consensus recommend specific approaches to screening and treatment. Colposcopy uses a bright light and magnification after application of 5% acetic acid to identify HSILs indicated by characteristic acetowhitening, epithelial changes, and abnormal vascular patterns. Suspected lesions are biopsied, and if they are HSILs, then a loop electrical excision of the cervical squamocolumnar junction is performed, removing the HSILs.

However, similar guidelines and standards of care do not exist for anal cancer prevention. A National Cancer Institute and Office of HIV and AIDS Malignancy–sponsored trial known as the *ANCHOR study* is currently enrolling participants. The primary objective of the ANCHOR study is to determine whether treating anal HSILs is effective in reducing the incidence of anal cancer in men and women living with HIV/AIDS. The ANCHOR study will enroll and randomize 5058 HIV-infected men and women with biopsy-proven HSILs to either active monitoring or treatment. Every 6 months, participants have an examination including anal cytology, DARE, and HRA with biopsies of any suspected HSILs annually for those in the monitoring arm and whenever seen in the treatment arm. After the last participant enrolls, follow-up continues for 5 years. The study end point is the development of anal cancer.[8]

Table 17-1

Relevant Terminology and Significance

Anal cancer	Squamous cell carcinomas of the anus and perianus
HPV	Sexually transmitted infection found in most sexually active adults (> 80%)
High-risk HPV	Oncogenic types of HPV responsible for precancerous lesions/ cancers of the entire anogenital tract and oropharynx HPV-16 and -18 cause about 70% of cancers, and the remainder are due to HPV-31, -33, -35, -39, -45, -51, -52, -56, -58, -59, and -68
Low-risk HPV	HPV-6 and -11 most common, causes anogenital warts
Low-grade squamous intraepithelial lesion	Indicative of HPV infection, not precancerous
HSIL	A high-grade squamous epithelial lesion is a potentially precancerous lesion
SISCCA	A superficially invasive squamous cell carcinoma is an early cancer excised with margins clear for cancer, but not necessarily HSIL, which invades ≤3 mm and is ≤7-mm wide
HPV-2 (Cervarix, GlaxoSmithKline)	Vaccine containing L1 capsids of HPV-16 and -18 (protects against 70% of cervical cancers; not available in the United States)
HPV-9 (Gardasil, Merck)	Vaccine containing L1 capsids of HPV-6, -11, -16, -18, -31, -33, -45, -52, and -58 (protects against 90% of genital warts and cervical/anal cancers)
DARE	Palpation of walls of the entire anal canal and perianus
HRA	Examination of the anus and perianus using a colposcope/ operating microscope after application of 5% acetic acid

Risk of Progression of Precancerous High-Grade Squamous Intraepithelial Lesions to Cancer

Although there is insufficient evidence to know whether treating anal HSILs effectively prevents anal cancer, there is strong evidence that anal HSILs are potentially precancerous. Berry et al[9] reviewed the medical records of 138 HIV-infected MSM followed at the University of California Anal Cancer Clinic, Research, and Education Center (UCSF ANCRE Clinic) who developed anal carcinoma between 1997 and 2011. Most men had been followed with regular DARE and HRA, but some were not treated despite recommendations for treatment, and some were lost to follow-up until they returned with symptomatic cancers. In 66 men, cancer was diagnosed during their first visit and considered prevalent cancer. Progression to cancer occurred while being followed in 45 men, but a direct relationship of the cancer to biopsy-proven HSILs could not be established.

By reviewing medical records and pathology reports and comparing HRA pictures of the preceding HSILs and subsequent cancer, it was demonstrated conclusively in 27 men that their anal cancer developed in exactly the same location as a previously biopsied HSIL. In this group of 27 MSM, cancers were detected by DARE in 85%, underscoring the importance of DARE as an anal cancer screening tool. This is particularly relevant because only 53% had symptoms that might have prompted medical attention. An additional 4 cancers were identified solely by a biopsy of changes detected during HRA. Anal HSILs have clear potential to progress to anal cancer in HIV-infected MSM.[9]

Additional observations substantiating that an HSIL is precancerous include the following. In new patients referred to the UCSF ANCRE Clinic, prevalent anal cancer is diagnosed primarily in patients who have either never been screened or, more to the point, were lost to follow-up after being diagnosed with an HSIL and never treated.[10] It is less common to find cancers in patients treated for HSILs and followed regularly. HSILs adjacent to cancers are usually seen in both types of patients. In addition, SISCCA can be seen to arise or "bud off" directly from HSILs. In cohort studies, untreated patients have a higher rate of progression compared with treated patients.[11-13] Therefore, many providers choose to treat HSILs based on the limited evidence available while awaiting the outcome of the ANCHOR study. This lack of conclusive evidence of the effectiveness of HSIL treatment in anal cancer prevention, however, should be discussed as part of the consent process prior to treatment.

Anal SISCCAs are minimally invasive squamous cell carcinomas that have been completely excised with clear margins and are no more than 7 mm in horizontal extent and invade no more than 3 mm in depth. SISCCA is a newly defined pathologic entity that originated from the Lower Anogenital Squamous Terminology Standardization consensus conference in 2012.[14] The definition is based on microinvasive cervical carcinoma, which can be treated conservatively with cone excision with good results. Although the optimal management of SISCCA has yet to be determined, there is a suggestion both historically and in currently published reports that excision may be a viable option that may spare some patients the need for radiation and chemotherapy. Although chemotherapy is highly curative and allows preservation of anal function, it causes lifelong morbidity in some patients, including anal urgency, relative anal stenosis, and sexual dysfunction. When patients are managed conservatively, any concomitant HSIL must be ablated and patients followed every 3 to 4 months for the first 2 years after excision. If SISCCA is found during office-based HRA, patients can be referred for excision if it appears that the lesion can be completely excised with at least a 1-mm margin. This approach is currently being evaluated in patients living with HIV/AIDS in a National Cancer Institute and AIDS Malignancy Consortium–sponsored trial.[8]

Epidemiology of Anal Human Papillomavirus, Anal High-Grade Squamous Intraepithelial Lesions, and Anal Cancer

Anal cancer affects more women than men worldwide; however, the highest incidence of anal cancer occurs in MSM living with HIV/AIDS[15-19] (Table 17-2). Immunosuppressed men or women due to HIV, organ transplantation, or other chronic immunosuppressive therapy and women who have a history of lower genital tract neoplasia such as a cervical HSIL/cancer and a vulvar HSIL/cancer have a higher incidence of anal cancer than men and women without these risk factors.[20] The true prevalence of anal neoplasia in the general population of women is uncertain because there have been no large natural history studies of women specifically looking at anal neoplasia in which women were examined with well-performed HRA.[21] Anal receptive intercourse is a risk factor but is not required to acquire anal HPV infection or develop anal cancer.

Although anal HPV infection in women may be common, it is often transient. A consensus paper on anal cancer screening in women states that screening may be considered in women at high risk for anal cancer.[20] Experts in anal neoplasia state that routine screening of normal women is not recommended based on the likely low prevalence of HSILs combined with the observed low incidence of anal cancer in the overall population.[20] In a recently published study from Homerton Anal Neoplasia Service in London, women with a prior history of anogenital neoplasia had HSILs/cancer demonstrated in 33% (105/323) of HRA-directed biopsies.[22] The goal of the study was to evaluate the performance characteristics of anal cytology when compared with results from HRA-guided biopsies; it is not a true prevalence rate but substantiates that women with prior lower genital tract neoplasia

Table 17-2

Epidemiology of Anal Cancer, Anal HPV Infection, and Anal High-Grade Squamous Intraepithelial Lesions[5,15-19,25,26,29]

	ANAL CANCER INCIDENCE PER 100,000	ANAL HPV INFECTION PREVALENCE	ANAL HSIL PREVALENCE
HIV-positive MSM	77.8 to 131	80% to 95%	29.1% to 52%
HIV-negative MSM	5.1 to 36.9	60%	21.5% to 24.7%
HIV-positive women	9.4 to 30	66% to 80%	9% to 27%
Women	1.5 to 2.1	32% to 42%	4% to 9%
Men	1.0	18%	Not available

require closer attention and are at higher risk. In another study based on surveillance, epidemiology, and end results data, women with a prior history of either in situ or invasive gynecologic neoplasm were significantly more likely to develop anal cancer compared with the general population. Women with in situ or invasive vulvar lesions were at highest risk, with a standardized incidence ratio of 22.2 (95% confidence interval [CI], 16.7-28.4) and 17.4 (95% CI, 11.5-24.4), respectively. The mean time to the development of anal cancer was shorter for vulvar in situ than cervical in situ disease at 8.9 and 15.7 years, respectively, and also for vulvar cancer and cervical cancer, which was 7.1 and 11.4 years, respectively.[23] These data are consistent with the proximity of the anus to the vulva and are not surprising; they highlight a group of women at particular risk.

It is also true that many women who develop anal cancer do not have obvious risk factors. In a population-based, case-control study from Toronto, women who developed anal cancer were significantly more likely to have had a prior history of lower genital tract cancer than women who did not develop anal cancer (odds ratio = 10.5; 95% CI, 3.6-30.3).[24] However, less than 2% of the women who developed anal cancer had such a history, emphasizing that, at least in this study, 98% of women did not have a prior history of lower genital tract cancer. Women who present with anal symptoms should be evaluated carefully; consider early referral for HRA or to someone experienced in managing anal neoplasia.

MSM living with AIDS or HIV have the highest incidence of anal cancer (131/100,000); HSILs are found in 50% or more of MSM when examined by HRA by experienced providers.[25,26] Much of the published natural history data on anal HPV and neoplasia are from these groups. Preliminary results presented at the 31st International Papillomavirus Conference in Cape Town, South Africa (February 28-March 4, 2017) from a study evaluating screening methods in HIV-positive women found a prevalence of anal HSILs of 27%.[27] What is notable in this report is that none of the women had ever previously been screened, and all were examined with HRA; this is the highest prevalence of HSILs reported to date and is consistent with observations from the UCSF ANCRE Clinic. All men and women living with HIV/AIDS are at increased risk for anal cancer and may benefit from anal cancer screening. However, MSM not infected with HIV are also considered to be a high-risk group, with an estimated incidence rate as high as 36.9 per 100,000 of anal cancer and a prevalence of HSILs of 25% or more.[15,28,29] Because the incidence of anal cancer is uncommon below 35 years of age, many experts recommend screening MSM beginning at 35 or 40 years of age.

The impact of immunosuppression on the prevalence of HRHPV and resulting precancerous lesions and cancers cannot be understated. An increased risk of HPV-related anogenital cancers occurring at a young age is associated with congenital dedicator of cytokinesis 8 deficiency.[30] More commonly, providers will encounter patients who have had solid organ transplants, bone marrow transplants, and iatrogenic immunosuppression for autoimmune disease including inflammatory bowel disease (IBD). The increased rates of HPV-related anogenital cancers have been well documented in solid organ transplant recipients. Standardized incidence ratios comparing observed cancers with expected cancers in the general population were highest for in situ compared with invasive cancer and for anal cancer at 11.6 (95% CI, 8.7-15.2) and 5.4 (95% CI, 4.4-6.6), respectively. The risk of cancer was increased with the length of time since transplantation consistent with the effect of prolonged immunosuppression. The rates were lowest for cervical neoplasia, which was attributed to the effectiveness of regular screening programs.[31] Experts have recommended screening for anal cancer precursors in this group, but the uptake even for cervical cancer screening has been lower than expected.[32]

Anal Neoplasia and Patients With Inflammatory Bowel Diseases

Published data are limited in scope and conflicting about whether anal cancer or HSILs are significantly increased in patients with IBD. In a systematic review of anal cancer in IBD, the authors concluded that anal cancer is rare, particularly in patients with ulcerative colitis, based on the small number of cases reported in the literature.[33] In a population-based cohort study from Denmark, chronic immunosuppression used to treat autoimmune diseases in 242,114 patients moderately increased the rate of anal cancer compared with controls. This varied according to diseases; for the 40,535 IBD patients, the standardized incidence ratio was highest for Crohn's disease at 3.1 (95% CI, 1.2-6.4) but was not increased for ulcerative colitis.[34]

Conflicting data were reported in 2 recent studies that examined anal HPV infection and anal neoplasia in IBD patients. In a pilot study of 46 patients with IBD, 41 (89.1%) had anal HPV infection, including 65.2% who had HPV-16, and 19 of 21 women had vaginal HPV. Moreover, 21 of 46 (45.7%) had abnormal anal cytology, and 33 were examined with HRA. Anal lesions were diagnosed in 28 of 46 (60.9%) women, including an HSIL in 4 (8.7%) and a low-grade squamous intraepithelial lesion (LSIL) in 24 (43.5%).[35] This contrasts to a larger study of 194 subjects with IBD and 76 age-matched healthy controls without a history of IBD in which 5 of 270 (1.86%) had HRHPV.[36] Cytologic abnormalities were only minor, with 17 of 194 (8.8%) IBD patients and 2 of 76 (2.6%) healthy controls having atypical squamous cells of undetermined significance (ASCUS), but this higher trend was not statistically significant ($P = .10$). Of the total cohort, 20 of 290 (6.9%) were excluded because the cytology samples had insufficient cellularity. Condylomata were seen in 2 of 6 patients who had HRA, but HSILs were not found. The prevalence of HRHPV was higher in those with ASCUS, and cytologic abnormalities were statistically more significant in patients with Crohn's disease.

These disparate results may be partially explained by the different methods of HPV testing used in the 2 studies (ie, polymerase chain reaction vs hybrid capture). Also, the results presented by Cranston et al[35] are from an experienced in-office HRA provider. They may be a more accurate reflection of the impact of immunosuppression in this group of patients. The low rates of HPV infection and abnormal cytology reported by Shah et al[36] may reflect inadequate sampling of the anal canal even though study staff were reportedly trained in the proper collection technique. It is well established that differences in the collection technique can contribute to an increased insufficiency rate.[37] Further research is required to clarify the true prevalence of HPV and HSILs in this population and the possible role of screening.

Recently, a case report of HPV-related HSILs extending up to 10 to 25 cm above the anal verge in 3 patients with longstanding refractory ulcerative colitis was published.[38] During HRA, lesions were

Table 17-3

Patients With an Increased Incidence of Anal Cancer in Whom Anal Cytology Screening Should Be Recommended if High-Resolution Anoscopy Is Available

CAVEATS	• Screening using anal cytology should only be performed if you have a resource to refer patients for HRA. • Screening should be performed in patients who have a reasonable life expectancy. • Begin screening at 25 years of age if immunosuppressed. • Begin screening at 35 to 40 years of age if immunocompetent.
WHO SHOULD BE SCREENED?	• All men and women living with HIV/AIDS, particularly MSM • Immunocompetent MSM • Women with a prior history of lower genital tract HPV-related precancerous lesions or cancer • Older patients (> 35 years) with condyloma • Solid organ transplant recipients and other severely immunocompromised patients

seen in the anus that extended beyond the anoscope into the distal rectum, requiring colonoscopy to define the proximal extent. We have recently seen 2 similar patients in the UCSF ANCRE Clinic, and an HSIL was documented by biopsy up to the second rectal valve in one. We have used a transanal minimally invasive GelPort (Applied Medical Resources) adapted from laparoscopy to access and treat these lesions using electrocautery in the operating room. Based on the paucity of data available, it is difficult to recommend screening in this group, but it is likely that there is some increase in HPV infection related to immunosuppressive medication, inflammation from IBD itself, and some as-yet-unexplained additional intrinsic immunosuppression that has been speculated to exist in patients with Crohn's disease. Although anal cancer is uncommon, it is reasonable for providers caring for patients with IBD to have an increased awareness of the possibility of HPV-related anorectal lesions based on the widespread rates of anal HPV in sexually active adults and to have a low threshold for biopsy of any unusual-appearing lesions in the anorectum. It is particularly important that patients who present with new anal symptoms or a change in chronic symptoms with irritation, pain, bleeding, or palpable lumps be evaluated promptly and properly with consideration of referral for HRA.

Diagnosis of Anal Lesions

Diagnostic methods to evaluate anal neoplasia include anal cytology, anal HPV testing, DARE, and HRA with biopsy. Anal cytology and HPV testing are screening tests used to identify patients who require further testing to determine if an HSIL is present. Groups recommended for screening are listed in Table 17-3. When these tests are negative, an HSIL is less likely. HRA is the next step when anyone is diagnosed with abnormal anal cytology of any level; it is the best way to identify and histologically confirm an HSIL and also rule out anal cancer. DARE is a screening test specifically for anal cancer. If simple anoscopy or perianal inspection reveals lesions such as anal warts or condyloma, friable plaquelike lesions, thickened leukoplakic lesions, erythematous raised lesions, or perianal ulcerations, then patients should be referred for HRA. Although simple anoscopy may reveal macroscopic, gross anal lesions, including anal cancer, the sensitivity for diagnosing anal HSIL is limited. Because HSIL is likely to be missed with simple anoscopy, patients may be falsely reassured that they are not at risk for anal cancer if they are only examined with simple anoscopy. Recently, 1417 anal cytology results were reported from a single urban academic institution following a high-risk population. HSIL cytology was found in 106 (7.5%), a high prevalence for HSIL cytology. Only 376 were examined with simple anoscopy, revealing a prevalence of histologic HSILs of 80 out of 1417 or 5.6% and indicating that a relatively large proportion of likely true HSILs in the population were missed using simple anoscopy as opposed to HRA.[39]

Likewise, colonoscopy and flexible sigmoidoscopy are not very sensitive methods for diagnosing anal HSILs, although narrow band imaging has been advocated as a way to enhance sensitivity. The primary role of colonoscopy is in the detection and removal of adenomas to prevent colorectal cancer; however, it provides a unique opportunity to examine the anus. Quality indicators for colonoscopy were reviewed in "Standardized Colonoscopy Reporting and Data System: Report of the Quality Assurance Task Group of the National Colorectal Cancer Roundtable."[40] Two issues stand out in these very comprehensive recommendations. Although DARE, or at least digital rectal examination, is commonly performed prior to inserting the colonoscope, it was not listed as required or even mentioned. Retroflexion and visualization of the anorectum during colonoscopy are controversial in terms of how much they add to adenoma detection. In this report, it was stated that retroflexion of the rectum simply be indicated as done or not done but not required as a measure of quality.[40] Others have suggested that retroflexion may play an important adjunctive role in detecting rectal polyps.[41]

In the UCSF ANCRE Clinic, we commonly see patients referred to us after colonoscopy when anal lesions were seen. More commonly, patients referred for routine anal cancer screening have reported a recent normal colonoscopy. Subsequent HRA may frequently find extensive HSILs, particularly in high-risk patients. Even patients who are not considered at high risk but are found to have condyloma during colonoscopy have a high likelihood of having HSILs when examined using HRA. Although anal cancer is uncommon in the general population, it is recommended that if abnormalities are noted during colonoscopy they be biopsied. DARE and retroflexion should be a standardized part of the examination for patients reporting bleeding or pain with bowel movements with consideration for referral for HRA if available. Given the low incidence of anal cancer in the general population, specific assessment of anal neoplasia cannot be recommended in the absence of symptoms during colonoscopy unless an abnormality in the anorectum is incidentally noticed. Thorough DARE if performed during colonoscopy, however, provides an opportunity to potentially identify patients who may otherwise go undetected.

Anal cytology is commonly used as a screening test to determine whether someone should be referred for HRA by identifying whether abnormal cells indicative of anal neoplasia are present. When anal cytology is performed simultaneously prior to HRA, it functions as an objective quality assessment; if HSIL cytology is present, histologic HISL should be found greater than 90% of the time within 3 months.[42] Currently, most anal cytology is processed using ThinPrep (Hologic, Inc.) or SurePath (Becton, Dickinson and Company) liquid–based medium, as opposed to spreading a swab on a glass slide. The liquid-based medium is then centrifuged, and cells are placed and stained on a slide, yielding a more interpretable specimen. The residual liquid can be used for HPV testing. Specimens with adequate cellularity have 2000 to 3000 nucleated squamous cells with 1 to 2 nucleated cells per high-power field; anything less is considered insufficient. Cytology results include no evidence of intraepithelial lesions or malignancy; ASCUS; LSIL; atypical squamous cells, cannot exclude high-grade squamous intraepithelial lesion (ASC-H); HSIL; or squamous cell carcinoma.

The test characteristics and positive or negative predictive value of anal cytology are dependent on the prevalence of the disease in the population being studied. Most of the preliminary work in developing anal cytology has been in persons at high risk for disease. This means that anal cytology performed in persons with HIV infection will have a higher sensitivity compared with anal cytology in MSM not living with HIV or in the general population.[43] Serially repeated testing over time is one approach to increase sensitivity as opposed to a single testing episode. Cytology often underestimates the severity of disease; in a group of MSM living with and without HIV with simultaneous cytology and HRA, histologic HSIL was found in about 15% of patients with normal cytology, 40% with ASCUS, 57% with ASC-H, 38% with LSIL, and 88% with HSIL.[29] It is recommended that all persons with ASCUS or greater cytology be referred for HRA in order to determine whether HSIL is present. Using a threshold of ASCUS for referral, the sensitivity of anal cytology is comparable to cervical cytology. A sensitivity of anal cytology ranging from 69% to 93% and a specificity ranging from 32% to 59% have been reported.[44]

ANAL CYTOLOGY COLLECTION

A polyester-tipped, nonscored swab is moistened with tap water and inserted into the anal canal prior to placing lubricant to perform DARE. In the left lateral position, the verge is separated, and the tip of the swab is inserted through the verge into the anal canal until it bypasses the internal sphincter or anorectal ring and abuts the distal rectal wall. Slightly rotating the swab as it is inserted or asking the patient to retract the right buttocks as the examiner gently opens the verge by pushing down on the right side can facilitate insertion. Since the depth of the anal canal varies, it is recommended that the swab be fully inserted in order to adequately sample the anal transformation zone. Pressure is applied to the swab so that it is bowed as it is rotated and slowly withdrawn over 15 to 20 seconds. The swab is immediately placed in liquid cytology medium and vigorously agitated for 30 seconds and then discarded. The top of the vial should be secured tightly to avoid leakage and is then is sent to the cytology laboratory for processing. The specimen should be marked as anal or nongynecologic to distinguish it from a cervical Pap. It is also recommended to alert the laboratory specifically and discuss their experience with anal cytology. In the absence of significant prior experience, it is best to have the sample interpreted by a cytopathologist with experience interpreting cervical specimens as opposed to a gastrointestinal specialist.

It is logical based on the role of persistent HRHPV infection in causing cervical anal HSIL and cancer that HPV testing may play a role in screening for HSIL. Primary HPV testing is becoming the preferred method for cervical cancer screening as opposed to cervical cytology. and new guidelines are in the process of being developed because of its very high sensitivity and negative predictive value. Currently, HPV testing is not recommended as a primary screening tool for anal cancer screening because of the high prevalence of anal HRHPV in the highest-risk populations. Many experts recommend using HRHPV testing for its high negative predictive value, meaning that anal HSIL is less likely in persons with a negative HRHPV test and suggesting that it may play a role in screening lower-risk groups.[43,45] If HRHPV is found, then further genotyping can be done specifically to look for HPV-16 or -18 in order to identify patients at highest risk of HSIL who may benefit from immediate cervical colposcopy or HRA.[45]

DARE is a screening test for anal cancer not for HSIL. DARE was coined as an alternative to digital rectal examination to emphasize the importance of assessing the entire anal canal. DARE is a low-cost resource that can be applied to all persons at risk and when performed properly is relatively sensitive at detecting anal cancer. There is often a significant delay between the onset of symptoms and the actual diagnosis of anal cancer; many patients report that they never were examined with DARE. Symptoms are often attributed to benign anorectal conditions such as hemorrhoids, fissures, and fistulas, all of which are highly common but can be distinguished by DARE if performed. The shift away from recommending routine digital rectal examination as part of the annual physical or gynecologic examination means that primary care providers and even specialists may be less likely to perform this simple examination or be familiar with how to distinguish between normal and abnormal findings. It is a procedure not routinely included in the medical curricula, and many providers, including gastroenterologists and some colorectal surgeons, may not have been specifically trained.[43]

Published guidelines for performing DARE are lacking, but the International Anal Neoplasia Society (IANS) is working on a set of guidelines.

In the series of cancers that progressed from previous biopsy-proven HSIL published by Berry et al,[8] findings were palpable in 23 of 27 MSM with cancer and 4 cancers were detected only during HRA. In 2014, a systematic review of guidelines recommending DARE for anal cancer screening in MSM living with HIV was published.[46] Only 2 guidelines, the European AIDS Clinical Society guidelines and the US guidelines for prevention and treatment of opportunistic infections in HIV-infected adults and adolescents, mentioned DARE, but neither was based on strong evidence just expert opinion. The recommendation was "DARE should be performed every 1 to 3 years" and "may be useful to detect masses."[46] In 2015, the "German-Austrian Guidelines on Anal Dysplasia and Anal Cancer in HIV-Positive Individuals: Prevention, Diagnosis, and Treatment" were published and included a complex algorithm recommending annual assessment of risk including prior and current history of anal lesions, inspection, palpation, cytology, and HRA when indicated.[47] In a systematic review of screening for anal cancer in women, DARE is recommended as a screening tool for women at high risk, including women living with HIV, women following organ transplantation, women with systemic lupus erythematosus and Crohn's disease, and women with either vulvar or cervical neoplasia, but is not specifically recommended in women in the general population unless they specifically report symptoms.[20]

The following approach is recommended for performing DARE, which should be performed after anal cytology is collected (if planned) in order to get an optimal specimen. Explain to the patient why the examination is being performed and obtain consent; in the left lateral decubitus position, using a gloved finger apply lubrication with or without 2% to 5% lidocaine jelly or anorectal cream, place gentle pressure on the verge and, as the sphincter muscle relaxes, insert the lubrication into the anal canal. Once lubrication has been placed and the sphincter relaxed, insert the index finger fully and rotate the hand so the pad of the finger is able to palpate the walls of the anorectal canal beginning at the anorectal ring and continuing outward to the verge, moving from the right lateral position in a counterclockwise direction to systematically examine each octant until you return to the right lateral position. Then, palpate the anorectal ring and distal rectum by sweeping with a curved finger from anterior to posterior, palpating the posterior space, and then palpating anteriorly on either side of the prostate in men ending with the prostate or the rectovaginal septum in women. After examining the anal canal, palpate the entire perianal surface from the verge 5 cm outward. The examiner is feeling for focal thickening, nodularity, textural changes such as granularity or cragginess, scarring, defects, induration, masses, anal papillae, or anal warts. Internal hemorrhoids are usually not palpable unless thrombosed, and patients who present with anal symptoms suspected of hemorrhoids but in whom DARE reveals palpable findings or in whom simple anoscopy reveals anything other than simple hemorrhoids such as heaped-up friable epithelial tissue should be referred for HRA.

HIGH-RESOLUTION ANOSCOPY

HRA is defined as examination of the anal canal and perianus after application of 5% acetic acid (AA) using high-power magnification and bright light provided by either a colposcope or operating microscope in order to identify epithelial and vascular changes that can be targeted for biopsy. Histology may reveal normal findings such as normal or reactive squamous metaplasia, LSIL, HSIL, SISCCA, or invasive squamous cell carcinoma. Most HSILs are invisible until after the application of AA, with the exception of thicker lesions that may appear as plaquelike friable areas and some larger raised perianal lesions that may be visible during simple anoscopy or even to the naked eye. Lugol's iodine is used judiciously after the application of AA within the anal canal to help identify HSILs by characteristic yellow staining due to the absence of glycogen. These epithelial and vascular characteristics have been validated for the anus, and guidelines for performing HRA were recently published by the IANS.[42,48,49] HRA is considered the gold standard for determining HSILs. In many places, HRA has replaced the earlier procedure known as operative mapping, in which 20 or more

Table 17-4

Patients Who Should Be Referred for High-Resolution Anoscopy

- All patients with abnormal cytology, including ASCUS or greater
- Anal canal or perianal condyloma (particularly if found during colonoscopy)
- Women who have vulvar HSIL/cancers that extend to the perineum
- Serendipitous SISCCA or HSIL in hemorrhoidectomy or colonoscopy specimens
- Symptomatic patients with extensive perianal lesions (likely to be HSIL or SISCCA)
- Suspected diagnosis of SISCCA (preferably to guide excision)
- Prior to excision of perianal or anal margin HSIL/SISCCA (coexistent HSIL within anal canal found in > 70%)

biopsies were obtained from predetermined locations from the anal canal and perianus. Table 17-4 lists who should be considered for referral for HRA.

HRA is commonly performed in the office; AA causes abnormal areas to turn acetowhite, and abnormal vascular patterns become prominent. Visible lesions are biopsied. Recognition of specific vascular patterns distinguishes LSILs from HSILs and highlights areas suspicious for cancer. Most SISCCAs are not palpable and, unless serendipitously removed while excising benign lesions such as hemorrhoids, tags, or what appears to be "warts," are only recognizable during HRA. Directly visualizing these lesions facilitates treatment and recognizing early cancers. Although this procedure was adapted from colposcopy in the early 1990s, it is technically more challenging to examine the anus because of mucosal folds, hemorrhoids, and the pressure of the sphincter muscle on the anoscope. Because of these anatomic challenges, the learning curve is quite steep to develop the proficiency to readily recognize these vascular changes that identify HSIL or SISCCA.

A brief history of HRA will help to provide a perspective on why there are a limited number of providers performing HRA. Using a colposcope to examine the anus was first mentioned in the literature in 1977.[50] Later in the 1990s, groups in San Francisco, London, and New York began to develop the procedure in response to the alarming number of anal cancers seen in people living with AIDS. Natural history studies were performed, which allowed providers to become more experienced and optimize HRA. Office-based treatment was developed in 2001. The first educational course to teach HRA was held in 2005 in San Francisco organized by Dr. Joel Palefsky and colleagues from UCSF in conjunction with the American Society of Colposcopy and Cervical Pathology. This is not a procedure that is taught as part of any medical school, residency, or fellowship curricula. The IANS was created as the first professional society dedicated to the pathogenesis, diagnosis, treatment, and prevention of anal neoplasia. IANS held its Inaugural Scientific Meeting in San Francisco in November 2013. HRA education continues to evolve, and members of IANS are leading the effort to train enough providers worldwide to meet this fast growing need.

No formal certification process currently exists to document that a provider has been trained and is proficient in performing HRA. HRA providers who participate in the ANCHOR study must complete specific training requirements. Suggestions for training provided in the IANS guidelines for practice standards in the detection of anal cancer precursors include attending a basic HRA didactic course; acquiring knowledge about anal cancer epidemiology, pathophysiology, anatomy, and principles of management of anal neoplasia; visiting an established site to observe HRA performed by an experienced provider; mentorship by an experienced HRA provider to receive individual feedback on performance of HRA; documenting cytology and histology in a log of 50 cases with an adequate percentage of HSILs and minimal discordance between HSIL cytology and histology; and, ideally, observation of a series of HRA examinations in new patients by a more senior skilled provider.[42] HRA is currently performed by a wide variety of providers with different skill sets. Surprisingly, a survey of colon and rectal surgeons found that less than half who state they perform HRA had ever been formally trained. Most did not use the basic techniques for performing HRA established by recognized experts in the field.[51] As the nascent field of HRA has grown, it has been established that novice HRA providers require a sustained level of experience seeing patients at high risk for HSIL in order to become proficient. For novice providers, the ability to find HSIL is directly related to the number of HRA procedures performed.[52,53] When examinations are not preformed adequately, areas of HSIL can be missed, which means that early cancers may also be missed. Similarly, a lack of recognition of all HSILs has an impact on the outcome of treatment of HSILs. These statements are based on the author's 25 years of experience performing HRA, particularly patients referred to the UCSF ANCRE Clinic who had been managed by other providers.

A discussion of how to specifically perform HRA and the characteristics of specific types of lesions is beyond the scope of this chapter.[49,54] However, some discussion of the limitations of HRA may be useful. After completing HRA, the provider should have an impression as to whether HSIL or cancer is present. In all cases, this impression should be verified with histology. When someone is skilled at performing HRA, progressively abnormal vascular changes can be seen by reviewing pictures of earlier examinations, which may indicate an area of potential progression to cancer. Examples of these vascular changes include coarse punctation, coarse mosaic pattern, and atypical vessels that are very bizarrely shaped. Other characteristics that help to indicate possible cancer include more dilated caliber vessels, a more disorganized pattern of punctation or mosaic pattern as opposed to a regular one, nonbranching vessels, and friability.[8]

The ultimate goals of HRA are to determine if HSIL, changes consistent with SISCCA, or if invasive cancer is present or conversely to confirm that the examination is completely normal and not clinically worrisome. This clinical impression coupled with the cytology and histology results can be used to design a specific management plan for each patient detailing when he or she should return for ongoing follow-up based on his or her potential risk of developing cancer. If only HSIL is present with no suspicion of cancer, then many experts would treat these lesions using a variety of ablation techniques such as infrared coagulation, electrocautery, laser ablation, or argon plasma coagulation. If cancer is suspected, a large enough representative sample of the lesion must be excised for histology. Often this is one of the indications in our clinic for referring patients for HRA-guided surgery. The significance of finding SISCCA is that radiation and chemotherapy may be able to be avoided. Based on our initial clinical experience managing patients with SISCCA, it is highly recommended that patients be referred for HRA and HRA-guided excision whenever SISCCA is suspected. Two cases will be presented to emphasize the critical role that HRA plays in managing patients with anal neoplasia.

Case Discussion

Patient 1 is a 47-year-old man living with HIV who was diagnosed 7 years earlier. He immediately began antiretroviral therapy with subsequent excellent control of HIV and no opportunistic infections, and he never had a low CD4 lymphocyte nadir. He self-referred for ongoing anal cancer screening after his surgeon retired. He had a prior history of anal warts treated by a local surgeon several times in the office with electrocautery beginning shortly after his HIV diagnosis. He was never diagnosed with HSIL and never had HRA, although he was examined periodically with simple anoscopy by a very experienced provider. The initial cytology 7 years earlier was ASCUS but positive for HRHPV. When seen at the UCSF ANCRE Clinic for further care, he reported no specific anal symptoms, except for occasional bleeding during receptive anal sex. A colonoscopy was performed 1 month prior and was normal, except for hemorrhoids. Anal cytology was HSIL. DARE was normal,

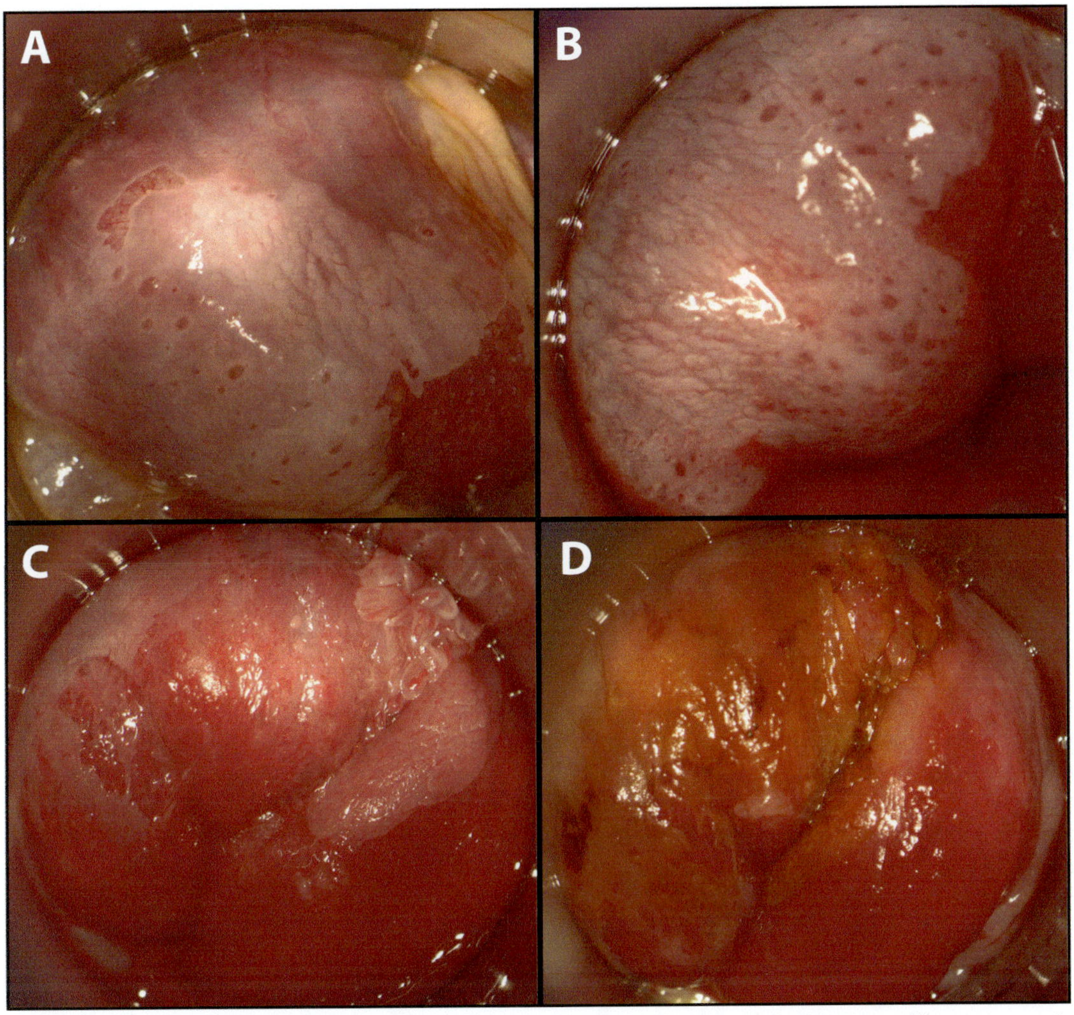

Figure 17-1. Case 1. (A) A histologic HSIL in the right lateral canal identified by acetowhitening and a coarse mosaic pattern. At the top of the figure is the normal epithelium. (B) A histologic HSIL in the right posterior canal with a coarse mosaic pattern most clearly seen on the left side of the picture. (C) A histologic HSIL in the right anterior canal in atypical-appearing condyloma. (D) Lugol's negative staining of the condyloma shown in C.

and HRA revealed diffuse lesions consistent with HSIL including a friable, atypical condyloma using Lugol's negative staining. Five representative areas were biopsied. Histology was HSIL in all biopsies, including the presumed condyloma, now confirmed to be papillary HSIL. Treatment options are being discussed (Figure 17-1).

Patient 2 is a 47-year-old man living with AIDS who had been diagnosed and treated using HRA-guided surgery for anal canal HSIL and condyloma and perianal HSIL 13 years earlier. He moved and never returned for follow-up but was examined several years prior to returning to the UCSF ANCRE Clinic and had a reportedly normal examination. Three months prior to being seen, he developed anal pain, presumably due to an anal abscess, but ultimately was diagnosed with chlamydia proctitis and treated with a 21-day course of doxycycline with significant improvement. He returned to the clinic noting anal leakage of mucous, a sense that his anus was scarred in some way, and recurring external irritation with physical activity. Anal cytology was HSIL. DARE was abnormal with palpable fullness in the right lateral anal canal and thickening and scarring posteriorly. A large, erythematous ulcerated right perianal lesion was noted consistent with HSIL but was highly suspicious for occult invasion. HRA revealed mucosal bulging on the right and an area of unusual-appearing

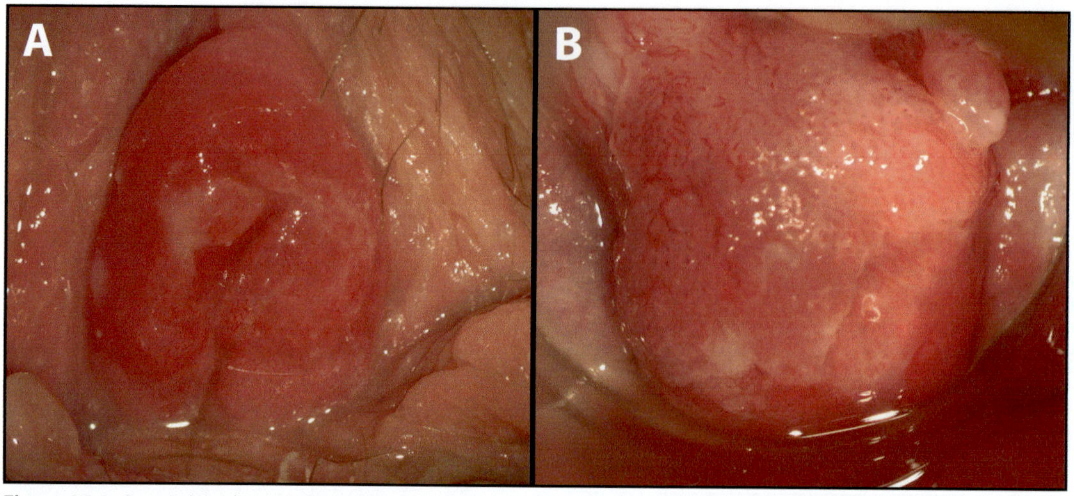

Figure 17-2. Case 2. (A) A large, velvety red ulcerated lesion in the right lateral perianus suspicious for cancer. The lesion was excised in the operating room, and it was discovered that it was only HSIL. (B) An area of atypical vessels in the right posterior anal canal that was targeted for excision in the operating room. Histology of the right posterior anal canal lesion show an atypical squamous submucosal nodule with central keratinous debris. The nodule is surrounded by desmoplastic stroma and small tongues of invasive squamous cell carcinoma. The overlying mucosa is the colonic epithelium, and the nodule does not obviously connect with the surface.

vessels adjacent in the right posterior anal canal. The examination was quite uncomfortable, and he was referred for HRA-guided surgery. The right lateral mass shown in Figure 17-2A was only HSIL with no invasion, but an excisional biopsy of the area of abnormal vessels in the right posterior anal canal revealed invasive cancer, which was unsuspected by palpation (Figure 17-2B). Careful HRA and recognition and biopsy of atypical vessels yielded a diagnosis of cancer. He was referred for radiation and chemotherapy.

Conclusion and a Pragmatic Approach to Patients With Anorectal Complaints

The objective of this chapter is to provide a better understanding of who is at risk for anal HSIL or cancer, how they may present, some of the pros and cons of various tests to diagnose anal neoplasia, and the important role of HRA and DARE in patients suspected of having anal neoplasia. Recommendations for best practices for approaching a patient with anorectal complaints who needs further evaluation to rule out possible neoplasia have been made. Although the vast majority of such patients will have benign disease, a small number will not. Sexually transmitted infections such as chlamydia, gonorrhea, syphilis, and herpes should be excluded and treated. If symptoms persist, then the anal canal can be easily sampled for anal cytology or HPV infection and DARE performed. If cytologic abnormalities are identified, then patients should be referred for HRA. If HRA is not available, then performing a thorough DARE is recommended. If the patient has a palpable abnormality and HRA is not available, then they should be referred to a colorectal surgeon or a surgeon experienced in managing anal diseases. Although it is possible to identify patients with an increased risk of having either HSIL or possibly cancer, there are a substantial number of patients who present with anorectal complaints who will not appear to belong to one of these groups. Having an increased awareness of possible anal HSIL or cancer that may occur even in the absence of receptive anal sexual activity or having any obvious risk factors for anal cancer will allow providers to examine patients thoroughly and appropriately refer them if a diagnosis cannot be made or if they have persistent symptoms.

References

1. Nelson VM, Benson AB 3rd. Epidemiology of anal canal cancer. *Surg Oncol Clin N Am*. 2017;26(1):9-15.
2. American Cancer Society. *Cancer Facts & Figures 2018*. Atlanta, GA: American Cancer Society; 2018.
3. Wang CJ, Sparano J, Palefsky JM. Human immunodeficiency virus/AIDS, human papillomavirus, and anal cancer. *Surg Oncol Clin N Am*. 2017;26(1):17-31.
4. Schiffman M, Doorbar J, Wentzensen N, et al. Carcinogenic human papillomavirus infection. *Nat Rev Dis Primers*. 2016;2:16086.
5. Stier EA, Sebring MC, Mendez AE, Ba FS, Trimble DD, Chiao EY. Prevalence of anal human papillomavirus infection and anal HPV-related disorders in women: a systematic review. *Am J Obstet Gynecol*. 2015;213(3):278-309.
6. Arbyn M, Xu L, Simoens C, Martin-Hirsch PP. Prophylactic vaccination against human papillomaviruses to prevent cervical cancer and its precursors. *Cochrane Database Syst Rev*. 2018;5:CD009069.
7. Schiffman M, Wentzensen N. Human papillomavirus infection and the multistage carcinogenesis of cervical cancer. *Cancer Epidemiol Biomarkers Prev*. 2013;22(4):553-560.
8. Berry-Lawhorn JM, Palefsky JM. Progression of anal high-grade squamous intraepithelial lesions to anal squamous cell carcinoma and clinical management of anal superficially invasive squamous cell carcinoma. *Semin Colon Rectal Surg*. 2017;28(2):91-96.
9. Berry JM, Jan N, Cranston RD, et al. Progression of anal high-grade squamous intraepithelial lesions to invasive anal cancer among HIV-infected men who have sex with men. *Int J Cancer*. 2014;134(5):1147-1155.
10. Pineda CE, Berry JM, Jay N, Palefsky JM, Welton ML. High-resolution anoscopy targeted surgical destruction of anal high-grade squamous intraepithelial lesions: a ten-year experience. *Dis Colon Rectum*. 2008;51(6):829-835; discussion 835-837.
11. Kreuter A, Potthoff A, Brockmeyer NH, et al. Anal carcinoma in human immunodeficiency virus-positive men: results of a prospective study from Germany. *Br J Dermatol*. 2010;162(6):1269-1277.
12. Weis SE, Vecino I, Pogoda JM, Susa JS. Treatment of high-grade anal intraepithelial neoplasia with infrared coagulation in a primary care population of HIV-infected men and women. *Dis Colon Rectum*. 2012;55(12):1236-1243.
13. Swedish KA, Lee EQ, Goldstone SE. The changing picture of high-grade anal intraepithelial neoplasia in men who have sex with men: the effects of 10 years of experience performing high-resolution anoscopy. *Dis Colon Rectum*. 2011;54(8):1003-1007.
14. Darragh TM, Colgan TJ, Cox JT, et al. The Lower Anogenital Squamous Terminology Standardization Project for HPV-Associated Lesions: background and consensus recommendations from the College of American Pathologists and the American Society for Colposcopy and Cervical Pathology. *Arch Pathol Lab Med*. 2012;136(10):1266-1297.
15. Machalek DA, Poynten M, Jin F, et al. Anal human papillomavirus infection and associated neoplastic lesions in men who have sex with men: a systematic review and meta-analysis. *Lancet Oncol*. 2012;13(5):487-500.
16. Chin-Hong PV, Vittinghoff E, Cranston RD, et al. Age-specific prevalence of anal human papillomavirus infection in HIV-negative sexually active men who have sex with men: the EXPLORE study. *J Infect Dis*. 2004;190(12):2070-2076.
17. Castro FA, Quint W, Gonzalez P, et al. Prevalence of and risk factors for anal human papillomavirus infection among young healthy women in Costa Rica. *J Infect Dis*. 2012;206(7):1103-1110.
18. Eleuterio J Jr, Benício GC, Giraldo PC, et al. Liquid-based cytology and HPV DNA testing using intra-anal specimens from HIV-negative women with and without genital HPV-induced lesions. *Diagn Cytopathol*. 2015;43(5):360-365.
19. Sudenga SL, Nyitray AG, Torres BN, et al. Comparison of anal HPV natural history among men by country of residence: Brazil, Mexico, and the United States. *J Infect*. 2017;75(1):35-47.
20. Moscicki AB, Darragh TM, Berry-Lawhorn JM, et al. Screening for anal cancer in women. *J Low Genit Tract Dis*. 2015;19(suppl 1):S27-S42.
21. Stier EA, Chiao EY. Anal cancer and anal cancer precursors in women with a history of HPV-related dysplasia and cancer. *Semin Colon Rectal Surg*. 2017;28(2):97-101.
22. Albuquerque A, Sheaff M, Stirrup O, et al. Performance of anal cytology compared with high-resolution anoscopy and histology in women with lower anogenital tract neoplasia. *Clin Infect Dis*. 2018;67(8):1262-1268.
23. Saleem AM, Paulus JK, Shapter AP, Baxter NN, Roberts RL, Ricciardi R. Risk of anal cancer in a cohort with human papillomavirus-related gynecologic neoplasm. *Obstet Gynecol*. 2011;117(3):643-649.
24. Jimenez W, Paszat L, Kupets R, Wilton A, Tinmouth J. Presumed previous human papillomavirus (HPV) related gynecological cancer in women diagnosed with anal cancer in the province of Ontario. *Gynecol Oncol*. 2009;114(3):395-398.
25. Silverberg MJ, Lau B, Justice AC, et al. Risk of anal cancer in HIV-infected and HIV-uninfected individuals in North America. *Clin Infect Dis*. 2012;54(7):1026-1034.
26. Palefsky JM, Holly EA, Efirdc JT, et al. Anal intraepithelial neoplasia in the highly active antiretroviral therapy era among HIV-positive men who have sex with men. *AIDS*. 2005;19(13):1407-1414.

27. Chiao E, Wiley D, Lee J, et al. Multiple-test anal HSIL screening strategies improves anal HSIL detection in HIV-positive women. Paper presented at: 31st International Papillomavirus Conference Clinical Research: Anal Cancer and Its Precursors; March 2, 2017; Cape Town, South Africa.
28. Daling JR, Weiss NS, Klopfenstein LL, Cochran LE, Chow WH, Daifuku R. Correlates of homosexual behavior and the incidence of anal cancer. *JAMA*. 1982;247(14):1988-1990.
29. Berry JM, Palefsky JM, Jay N, Cheng SC, Darragh TM, Chin-Hong PV. Performance characteristics of anal cytology and human papillomavirus testing in patients with high-resolution anoscopy-guided biopsy of high-grade anal intraepithelial neoplasia. *Dis Colon Rectum*. 2009;52(2):239-247.
30. Chu EY, Freeman AF, Jing H, et al. Cutaneous manifestations of DOCK8 deficiency syndrome. *Arch Dermatol*. 2012;148(1):79-84.
31. Madeleine MM, Finch JL, Lynch CF, Goodman MT, Engels EA. HPV-related cancers after solid organ transplantation in the United States. *Am J Transplant*. 2013;13(12):3202-3209.
32. Chin-Hong PV. Human papillomavirus in kidney transplant recipients. *Semin Nephrol*. 2016;36(5):397-404.
33. Slesser AA, Bhangu A, Bower M, Goldin R, Tekkis PP. A systematic review of anal squamous cell carcinoma in inflammatory bowel disease. *Surg Oncol*. 2013;22(4):230-237.
34. Sunesen KG, Nørgaard M, Thorlacius-Ussing O, Laurberg S. Immunosuppressive disorders and risk of anal squamous cell carcinoma: a nationwide cohort study in Denmark, 1978-2005. *Int J Cancer*. 2010;127(3):675-684.
35. Cranston RD, Regueiro M, Hashash J, et al. A pilot study of the prevalence of anal human papillomavirus and dysplasia in a cohort of patients with IBD. *Dis Colon Rectum*. 2017;60(12):1307-1313.
36. Shah SB, Pickham D, Araya H, et al. Prevalence of anal dysplasia in patients with inflammatory bowel disease. *Clin Gastroenterol Hepatol*. 2015;13(11):1955-1961.e1.
37. Wiley DJ, Hsu H, Bolan R, et al. Comparison of 2 anal cytology protocols to predict high-grade anal intraepithelial neoplasia. *J Low Genit Tract Dis*. 2013;17(4):414-424.
38. Connolly JG, Goldstone SE. Squamous cell dysplasia in the proximal rectum of three patients treated for ulcerative colitis on immunomodulators. *Int J Colorectal Dis*. 2017;32(5):753-756.
39. Morency EG, Harbert T, Fatima N, Samolcyzk J, Maniar KP, Nayar R. Anal cytology: institutional statistics, correlation with histology, and development of multidisciplinary screening program with review of the current literature. *Arch Pathol Lab Med*. 2019;143(1):23-29.
40. Lieberman D, Nadel M, Smith RA, et al. Standardized colonoscopy reporting and data system: report of the Quality Assurance Task Group of the National Colorectal Cancer Roundtable. *Gastrointest Endosc*. 2007;65(6):757-766.
41. Ruiz-Rebollo ML. Should rectal retroflexion be included as a quality indicator for colonoscopy? *Gastrointest Endosc*. 2015;82(2):421.
42. Hillman RJ, Cuming T, Darragh T, et al. 2016 IANS international guidelines for practice standards in the detection of anal cancer precursors. *J Low Genit Tract Dis*. 2016;20(4):283-291.
43. Cuming TNM. Anal cancer screening: techniques and guidelines. *Semin Colon Rectal Surg*. 2017;28(2):69-74.
44. Darragh TM, Palefsky JM. Anal cytology. In: Nayar R, Wilbur DC, eds. *The Bethesda System for Reporting Cervical Cytology Definitions, Criteria, and Explanatory Notes*. New York, NY: Springer International Publishing; 2015:263-286.
45. Jeronimo J, Castle PE, Temin S, et al. Secondary prevention of cervical cancer: ASCO resource-stratified clinical practice guideline. *J Glob Oncol*. 2017;3(5):635-657.
46. Ong JJ, Chen M, Grulich AE, Fairley CK. Regional and national guideline recommendations for digital ano-rectal examination as a means for anal cancer screening in HIV positive men who have sex with men: a systematic review. *BMC Cancer*. 2014;14:557.
47. Esser S, Kreuter A, Oette M, et al. German-Austrian guidelines on anal dysplasia and anal cancer in HIV-positive individuals: prevention, diagnosis, and treatment. *J Dtsch Dermatol Ges*. 2015;13(12):1302-1319.
48. Jay N, Berry JM, Hogeboom CJ, Holly EA, Darragh TM, Palefsky JM. Colposcopic appearance of anal squamous intraepithelial lesions: relationship to histopathology. *Dis Colon Rectum*. 1997;40(8):919-928.
49. Jay N, Berry JM, Miaskowski C, et al. Colposcopic characteristics and Lugol's staining differentiate anal high-grade and low-grade squamous intraepithelial lesions during high resolution anoscopy. *Papillomavirus Res*. 2015;1:101-108.
50. O'Connor JJ. The study of anorectal disease by colposcopy. *Dis Colon Rectum*. 1977;20(7):570-572.
51. Factor SH, Pereira GA, Goldstone SE. Are colon and rectal surgeons ready to screen for anal dysplasia? Results of a survey on attitudes and practic. *Sex Transm Dis*. 2014;41(4):246-253.
52. Hillman RJ, Gunathilake MP, Jin F, Tong W, Field A, Carr A. Ability to detect high-grade squamous anal intraepithelial lesions at high resolution anoscopy improves over time. *Sex Health*. 2016;13(2):177-181.
53. Richel O, Prins JM, de Vries HJ. Screening for anal cancer precursors: what is the learning curve for high-resolution anoscopy? *AIDS*. 2014;28(9):1376-1377.
54. Jay N. High-resolution anoscopy: procedure and findings. *Semin Colon Rectal Surg*. 2017;28:75-80.

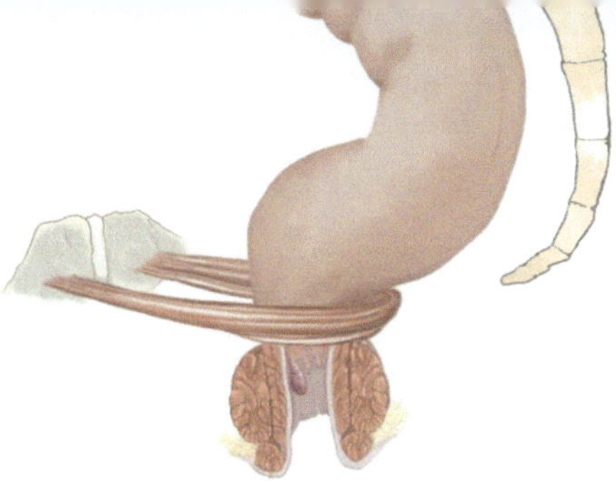

Financial Disclosures

Dr. Ihsan Al-Bayati has no financial or proprietary interest in the materials presented herein.

Dr. Sarah Al-Obaidi has no financial or proprietary interest in the materials presented herein.

Dr. Avo Artinyan has no financial or proprietary interest in the materials presented herein.

Dr. Noemi Baffy has no financial or proprietary interest in the materials presented herein.

Dr. J. Michael Berry-Lawhorn received a one-time honoraria from Antiva Bioscienes.

Dr. Lisa S. Brubaker has no financial or proprietary interest in the materials presented herein.

Dr. Bidhan Das has no financial or proprietary interest in the materials presented herein.

Dr. Samer Doughan has no financial or proprietary interest in the materials presented herein.

Dr. Gulchin A. Ergun is on the speaker's bureau for Medtronic.

Dr. Yezaz A. Ghouri has no financial or proprietary interest in the materials presented herein.

Dr. Vineet S. Gudsoorkar has no financial or proprietary interest in the materials presented herein.

Dr. Mitchel Guttenplan is Medical Director of CRH Medical Corp.

Dr. Lisa M. Haubert has no financial or proprietary interest in the materials presented herein.

Dr. Stephen Landreneau has no financial or proprietary interest in the materials presented herein.

Dr. Richard McCallum has no financial or proprietary interest in the materials presented herein.

Dr. Tejal Mistry has no financial or proprietary interest in the materials presented herein.

Dr. Van Morris is a consultant for Array Biopharma, and he receives research support from Array Biopharma, Bristol-Myers Squibb, and EMD Serono.

Dr. Rishi D. Naik has no financial or proprietary interest in the materials presented herein.

Dr. Leila Neshatian has no financial or proprietary interest in the materials presented herein.

Dr. Keith L. Obstein has no financial or proprietary interest in the materials presented herein.

Dr. Waqar Qureshi has no financial or proprietary interest in the materials presented herein.

Dr. Roman Sargsyan has no financial or proprietary interest in the materials presented herein.

Dr. Mehnaz A. Shafi has no financial or proprietary interest in the materials presented herein.

Dr. Yasser Shaib has no financial or proprietary interest in the materials presented herein.

Dr. Bo Shen is a consultant for Janssen and a consultant and speaker for Abbvie and Takeda.

Dr. Andy Tau has no financial or proprietary interest in the materials presented herein.

Dr. Sarah B. Umar has no financial or proprietary interest in the materials presented herein.

Dr. Sai Sruthi Veerisetty has no financial or proprietary interest in the materials presented herein.

Dr. Zachary Yeung has no financial or proprietary interest in the materials presented herein.

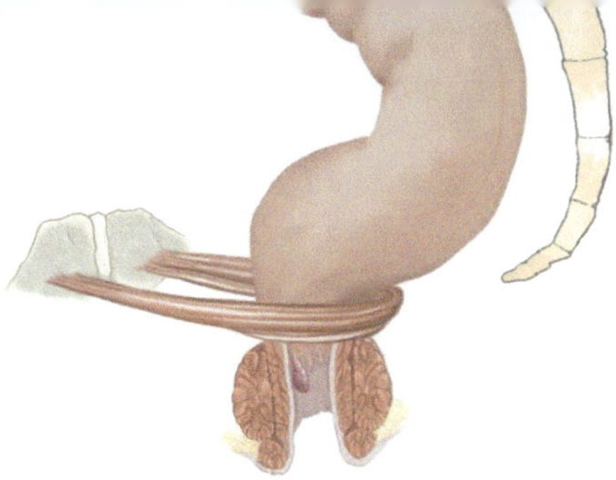

Index